SMALL MOLECULE THERAPY FOR GENETIC DISEASE

This book summarizes the substantial work that has been accomplished with simple molecules in the treatment of inborn errors of metabolism. These agents are discrete, often of natural origin, and provide predictable therapeutic responses. As such, they avoid many of the practical difficulties associated with gene and protein therapies.

This book will enable interested clinician/scientists and others to rapidly survey the field, thus ascertaining what has been done as well as future directions for therapeutic research. Its important introductory chapters discuss the infrastructure of the field. These chapters focus on an introduction to pharmacokinetics and pharmacodynamics, a description of the FDA Office of Orphan Products, and a summary of the operation of the National Institutes of Health Office of Rare Diseases Research. The remainder of the book is devoted to a review of small molecule therapy for genetic diseases. The book closely analyzes the cofactors used to augment the function of defective enzymes and the compounds that are able to use an alternative pathway to avoid the consequences of the metabolic block present in the patient. Among other therapies, the authors discuss the use of zinc and tetrathiomolybdate to treat Wilson disease and the use of cysteamine to treat nephropathic cystinosis.

Dr. Jess G. Thoene is currently Director of the Biochemical Genetics Laboratory in the Division of Pediatric Genetics at the University of Michigan in Ann Arbor and an Active Emeritus Professor of Pediatrics. He has held positions in numerous organizations, including Director of the Hayward Center for Human Genetics at Tulane University Health Sciences Center; Fellow and Medical Director of the Joseph P. Kennedy Jr. Foundation; member of the Board of Directors of Copley Pharmaceuticals; and Chairman of the Board of Directors of the National Organization for Rare Disorders. He has authored numerous articles on inborn errors of metabolism, holds three U.S. patents, and is certified in pediatrics and clinical biochemical genetics.

Small Molecule Therapy for Genetic Disease

Edited by

Jess G. Thoene

University of Michigan

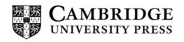

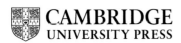

Shaftesbury Road, Cambridge CB2 8EA, United Kingdom

One Liberty Plaza, 20th Floor, New York, NY 10006, USA

477 Williamstown Road, Port Melbourne, VIC 3207, Australia

314–321, 3rd Floor, Plot 3, Splendor Forum, Jasola District Centre, New Delhi - 110025, India

103 Penang Road, #05-06/07, Visioncrest Commercial, Singapore 238467

Cambridge University Press is part of Cambridge University Press & Assessment,
a department of the University of Cambridge.

We share the University's mission to contribute to society through the pursuit of
education, learning and research at the highest international levels of excellence.

www.cambridge.org
Information on this title: www.cambridge.org/9780521517812

© Cambridge University Press & Assessment 2010

First published 2010

A catalogue record for this publication is available from the British Library

Library of Congress Cataloging-in-Publication data
Small molecule therapy for genetic disease / edited by Jess G. Thoene.
    p. ; cm.
Includes bibliographical references and index.
ISBN 978-0-521-51781-2 (hardback)
1. Metabolism, Inborn errors of - Chemotherapy - Handbooks, manuals, etc.   2. Metabolism,
Inborn errors of - Gene therapy - Handbooks, manuals, etc.   3. Genetic disorders -
Chemotherapy - Handbooks, manuals, etc.   I. Thoene, Jess G.   II. Title.
[DNLM: 1. Genetic Diseases, Inborn - drug therapy.   2. Orphan Drug Production.   3. Rare
Diseases - drug therapy.   4. Small Molecule Libraries - therapeutic use. QZ 50 S635 2010]
RC627.8.S55   2010
616.3′9042–dc22   2010002899

ISBN   978-0-521-51781-2   Hardback

....

Every effort has been made in preparing this book to provide accurate and up-to-date
information which is in accord with accepted standards and practice at the time of
publication. Although case histories are drawn from actual cases, every effort has been
made to disguise the identities of the individuals involved. Nevertheless, the authors,
editors and publishers can make no warranties that the information contained herein
is totally free from error, not least because clinical standards are constantly changing
through research and regulation. The authors, editors and publishers therefore
disclaim all liability for direct or consequential damages resulting from the use of
material contained in this book. Readers are strongly advised to pay careful attention
to information provided by the manufacturer of any drugs or equipment that they plan
to use.

Contents

Color plates follow page 130.

Contributors

Hans C. Andersson, MD, FACMG
Director, Hayward Genetics
  Center
Karen Gore Professor of Human
  Genetics
Tulane University Medical Center
New Orleans, LA

George J. Brewer, MD
Morton S. and Henrietta K. Sellner
  Emeritus Professor of Human
  Genetics
Emeritus Professor of Internal
  Medicine
Departments of Human Genetics and
  Internal Medicine
University of Michigan School of
  Medicine
Ann Arbor, MI

Neil R. M. Buist, MB, ChB, FRCPE
Professor Emeritus
Departments of Pediatrics and Medical
  Genetics
Oregon Health & Science University
Portland, OR

Barbara K. Burton, MD
Professor of Pediatrics
Northwestern University Feinberg
  School of Medicine
Division of Genetics, Birth Defects,
  and Metabolism

Children's Memorial Hospital
Chicago, IL

Gregory M. Enns, MB, ChB
Associate Professor of Pediatrics
Director, Biochemical Genetics
  Program
Division of Medical Genetics
Stanford University
Stanford, CA

William A. Gahl, MD, PhD
Clinical Director, National Human
  Genome Research Institute
National Institutes of Health
Bethesda, MD

Stephen C. Groft, PharmD
Director, Office of Rare Diseases
  Research
Department of Health and Human
  Services
National Institutes of Health
Bethesda, MD

Marlene E. Haffner, MD, MPH
Haffner Associates LLC
Rockville, MD
Former Director, Office of Orphan
  Products Development
U.S. Food and Drug Administration
Adjunct Professor, Departments of
  Medicine and Preventive Medicine
  and Biometrics

F. Edward Hébert School of Medicine
and Biometrics
Uniformed Services University of the
Health Sciences
Bethesda, MD

Wendy J. Introne, MD
Staff Clinician, Office of the Clinical
Director
National Human Genome Research
Institute
National Institutes of Health
Bethesda, MD

Stephen G. Kaler, MD
Head, Unit on Human Copper
Metabolism; Program in Molecular
Medicine
Eunice Kennedy Shriver National
Institute of Child Health and
Human Development
National Institutes of Health
Bethesda, MD

Amy Lawson-Yuen, MD, PhD
Physician in Clinical Genetics and
Pediatrics
Woodcreek Healthcare
Puyallup, WA

Juan J. L. Lertora, MD, PhD
Director, Clinical Pharmacology
Program
NIH Clinical Center
National Institutes of Health
Bethesda, MD

Harvey L. Levy, MD
Senior Physician in Medicine
Children's Hospital Boston
Professor of Pediatrics
Harvard Medical School
Boston, MA

Tan T. Nguyen, MD, PhD
Associate Professor of Pathology
Department of Pathology

F. Edward Hébert School of Medicine
and Biometrics
Uniformed Services University of the
Health Sciences
Bethesda, MD

Kevin J. O'Brien, RN, MS-CRNP
Staff Clinician, Office of the Clinical
Director
National Human Genome Research
Institute
National Institutes of Health
Bethesda, MD

Kirit Pindolia, PhD
Department of Medical Genetics
Henry Ford Hospital
Center for Molecular Medicine and
Genetics
Wayne State University School of
Medicine
Detroit, MI

Brian Schreiber, MD
Assistant Professor, Department of
Medicine, Division of Nephrology
Medical College of Wisconsin
Milwaukee, WI
Vice President, Medical Affairs
Sigma Tau Pharmaceuticals
Gaithersburg, MD

James A. Shayman, MD
Professor of Internal Medicine and
Pharmacology
Associate Vice President for Research,
Health Sciences
University of Michigan School of
Medicine
Ann Arbor, MI

Jess G. Thoene, MD
Director, Biochemical Genetics
Laboratory
Active Professor Emeritus of Pediatrics
University of Michigan School of
Medicine
Ann Arbor, MI

Konstantina M. Vanevski, MD
Special Volunteer Fellow
Clinical Pharmacology Program
NIH Clinical Center
National Institutes of Health
Bethesda, MD

Susan C. Winter, MD
Clinical Professor of Pediatrics
University of California, San
  Francisco
Medical Director, Medical Genetics

Children's Hospital Central California
Madera, CA

Barry Wolf, MD, PhD
Chair, Department of Medical
  Genetics
Henry Ford Hospital
Professor, Center for Molecular
  Medicine and Genetics
Wayne State University School of
  Medicine
Detroit, MI

Preface

The problem of recognition and treatment of rare diseases has been a topic of interest since Representative Henry Waxman held hearings on this issue in 1980. Led by Representative Waxman, clinician/scientists, legislators, patient interest groups, and drug companies all participated in the formation and passage of the Orphan Drug Act of 1983 (PL 97–414). In that legislation, an orphan disease was defined as a condition that affects fewer than 200,000 Americans. In testimony during hearings while the bill was being drafted, it was learned that treatments for more than 100 rare diseases existed but were not being developed because of lack of interest by pharmaceutical companies because of the small market and thus, lack of potential profitability. The Act provided tax incentives for clinical trials of these agents, grants to assist investigators in performing the trials, and a structure at the U.S. Food and Drug Administration (FDA; The Office of Orphan Products; see Chapter 2) to help shepherd applications through the agency. The Act has been an unqualified success. In fact, President Reagan, who initially threatened to veto the legislation, later described it as " . . . one of the most significant and successful pieces of health care legislation during my presidency . . . "[1,2]

The topics addressed in this book are all rare diseases within the meaning of the Orphan Drug Act. The success of these therapies is recognition of the hard work expended by clinical investigators (many of whom are authors of chapters in this book) to bring successful treatment for these serious and often life-threatening conditions to new drug approval.

This book is published with several goals in mind. One is to provide a convenient repository for the substantial work that has been accomplished by individual investigators treating rare genetic disorders with simple molecules. In the current era in which macromolecular therapy is looked to as the ultimate treatment for diseases as disparate as cancer, coronary artery disease, and genetic disease, it is somewhat reassuring to realize the broad scope that small molecules have in treating many serious, life-threatening disorders across the age span. These agents are discrete, often of natural origin, and provide predictable therapeutic responses. As such, they avoid many of the practical difficulties associated with gene and protein therapies.

Another goal is to provide a handbook that will enable potential clinician/scientists and others to rapidly survey the field, thus ascertaining what has been done and what can yet be done. Assisting implementation of these aspects of the book are three very important chapters in **Section I, Infrastructure**. This section includes an introduction to pharmacokinetics and pharmacodynamics, which, although covered in the usual medical school curriculum, are often not retained in the depth needed to plan and execute a Phase I or Phase II drug trial. Readers will find definitions of terms to assist in reading the pharmacologic literature, important examples of parameters required to prepare a viable FDA New Drug Application, and substantial references to assist in further reading.

Chapter 1, on the FDA Office of Orphan Products, written by the second director of that office, Dr. Marlene Haffner, and Dr. Tan Nguyen, provides an outstanding review of the functions of that office. It behooves everyone considering undertaking a therapeutic trial for an orphan disease to read this chapter. Grants for clinical trials in rare diseases are funded by this office, and protocol assistance is provided to help otherwise naïve investigators wend their way through the new drug approval process at the FDA.

Those who wish to embark on a clinical trial of a small molecule to treat a rare disease will benefit by reading Chapter 2 on the National Institutes of Health (NIH) Office of Rare Diseases Research, written by its director, Stephen Groft, PharmD. This chapter contains substantial and varied information that will assist investigators in accessing many resources at NIH, including finding funding for clinical trials and access to specialized analytical facilities that will be useful in many of these endeavors.

The remainder of the book is devoted to a review of small molecule therapy for genetic diseases. **Section II** is a review of cofactors used to augment the function of defective enzymes by increasing production of more active holoenzyme through treating the patient with that enzyme's specific cofactor. When successful, the results are startling, as described in Chapter 4, by Dr. Kirit Pindolia and Dr. Barry Wolf, on treatment of biotin-responsive disorders.

Section III is devoted to compounds that are able to use an alternative pathway to avoid the adverse consequences of the metabolic block present in the patient. A number of ingenious molecules have been devised and approved by the FDA to treat diseases in this category.

The final section, **Section IV**, covers the use of metal ions to treat severe disorders including Wilson disease, which has the distinction of being one of the first approved orphan products, and Menkes disease and other acquired and inherited copper deficiency syndromes.

From the perspective of rare disease patients, a book like this can serve many purposes, including assisting them in educating their health care providers. It was well documented by the National Commission on Orphan Diseases that patients and their families must first become experts in their rare disorder and then educate their health care professional. According to a survey commissioned by the National Commission on Orphan Diseases, one-third of rare disease patients wait between one and five years to receive a correct diagnosis, and one in seven such patients waits six years or more.[3] We hope this book will assist in reducing that interval. Additionally, by drawing attention to rare disorders, it is hoped that this book may encourage practitioners treating such patients to consult the growing number of Web-based registries that facilitate locating an appropriate clinical trial.

To the extent that this book succeeds in meeting any of these goals, the effort expended will have been justified.

ACKNOWLEDGMENTS

An editor's job is greatly facilitated by cooperative authors who meet deadlines and submit quality writing on the first draft. Such was the case in the current volume and I thank this group for meeting those criteria and making it a pleasure to complete this work. The same goes for Barbara Walthall at Aptara, who made the nuts and bolts of copyediting painless and efficient.

It is also critical to acknowledge the contributions of the many patients and their families whose courage to volunteer for clinical trials enables all such studies and new drug approvals. On behalf of all the authors, I salute our patients and hope that clinical trials of orphan drugs continue to improve their health and quality of life. Lastly, I thank my wife, Dr. Marijim Thoene, DMA , whose constant support inspires my efforts.

REFERENCES

1. Ronald Reagan. Letter to Jess Thoene, February 23, 1993
2. Thoene J. Orphan drugs and orphan tests in the USA. *Community Genet.* 2004;7:169–172
3. Report of the National Commission on Orphan Diseases. U.S. Department of Health and Human Services, Public Health Service, February 1989

SECTION I
INFRASTRUCTURE

1 The U.S. Food and Drug Administration and the regulation of small molecules for orphan diseases

Marlene E. Haffner and Tan T. Nguyen

THE ORPHAN DRUG ACT

Responding to heightened public appeal by a coalition of patient representatives, Representative Henry Waxman introduced into the United States Congress, in 1981, legislation to address the lack of interest in the pharmaceutical sector to develop drugs for rare but often serious or fatal diseases.[1] These "orphan" diseases do not present sufficiently viable markets for drug makers to recover the drug-development costs, much less to expect profitability. In December 1982, Congress passed the Orphan Drug Act ("the Act") amending the Federal Food, Drug, and Cosmetic Act (FDCA) to establish incentives for the development of promising drugs for rare diseases or conditions in the United States. On January 4, 1983, President Ronald Reagan signed the Act into law.[2] To implement the provisions

3

of the Act, the United States Food and Drug Administration (FDA) issued the Orphan Drug Regulations Final Rule in 1992.[3]

WHAT ARE THE ORPHAN DRUG INCENTIVES?

The Act initially defined an orphan drug on the basis of unprofitability: one intended for the diagnosis, treatment, or prevention of a rare disease or condition in the United States, such that there was no reasonable expectation that the costs of developing the drug would be recovered from its sales in the United States. This definition was amended in 1984 to provide, in addition, a prevalence threshold of 200,000 persons affected by the disease or condition of interest in the United States as a surrogate for the lack of profitability. The Act, as amended, provided financial and regulatory incentives to encourage the development of potentially promising orphan drugs as discussed below.

Orphan drug marketing exclusivity

This is the most important incentive of the Act. After the FDA has approved the orphan drug for marketing, the drug sponsor receives a seven-year exclusivity period for the rights to market the drug for the approved orphan indication.[4] That is, during this period, the FDA may not approve another same drug for the same indication (see the section "How Does the FDA Protect the Marketing Exclusivity of the Pioneer Drug?" for further discussion on the protection of marketing exclusivity). Exclusivity may be withdrawn by the FDA only if the sponsor fails to assure an adequate supply of the drug to meet the needs of patients. In this instance, which has never occurred, the marketing approval status of the drug would not be affected.

Orphan products grants

The Orphan Products Grants Program is administered by the FDA Office of Orphan Products Development (OOPD).[5] Its objective is to provide seed money for clinical investigations on the safety and effectiveness of drugs, medical devices, and medical foods for the diagnosis, treatment, and prevention of rare diseases or conditions in the United States. Grants are awarded on a competitive basis to foreign or domestic, private or public, for-profit or not-for-profit, state or local units of government, and federal agencies (not part of the Department of Health and Human Services). In fiscal year 2009, a Phase I clinical study is eligible for grant support of up to $200,000 per year for a period of three years, and Phase 2, 3, and 4 clinical investigations (see the section "How Has the FDA Approved Nonbiological Orphan Drugs for Genetic Disorders?" for explanations on phases of drug development) may be eligible for support of $400,000 per year for up to four years.[6] Except for medical foods, clinical investigation on a drug or a medical device supported by orphan product grants must be conducted under an approved Investigational New Drug (IND) application or an Investigational Device Exemption (IDE) application, respectively.

Written recommendations for investigation of an orphan drug

The FDA, upon request, will issue written recommendations to the sponsor of an orphan drug for the nonclinical (in vitro and in vivo laboratory animal testing) and clinical drug research and development programs necessary for the drug's approval. This regulatory incentive – initially intended for orphan drugs – has been replaced by the FDA-wide informal consultation process known as the pre-IND program.[7]

Open protocols for investigation of orphan drugs

The sponsor of an orphan drug under clinical investigation is encouraged to expand the *treatment use* of the drug to patients who are not eligible to be in the clinical trials and who cannot be satisfactorily treated by available alternative drugs. Such expanded use is governed by the regulations on treatment use protocol of an IND.[8] To initiate such an open protocol, the sponsor must demonstrate to the FDA that (1) the disease or condition is serious or immediately life-threatening, (2) the drug is under active clinical investigation with sufficient evidence of safety and effectiveness, and (3) there is no comparable or satisfactory alternative therapy.

Tax credit

The sponsor of the orphan drug can claim an orphan drug tax credit against federal taxes equal to 50% of the clinical testing expenses incurred between the date the drug is designated as an orphan drug by the FDA and the date of its marketing approval.[9,10] To be eligible, the clinical testing must be conducted under an approved IND. The tax credit may apply to foreign clinical investigation expenses if there is an insufficient testing population in the United States. As currently allowed, the unused tax credit can be carried back one year and then forward 20 years.

Waiver of user fees

In 1992, Congress passed the Prescription Drug User Fee Act authorizing the FDA to collect user fees from drug sponsors to support the costs of drug reviews in exchange for FDA agreement to meet drug-review performance goals in a timely fashion.[11] These fees include the application fee levied on the sponsor's New Drug Application (NDAs) for marketing approval of the drug, the annual establishment fee, and the product fee. Subsequently, the Food and Drug Administration Modernization Act of 1997 exempted sponsors of designated orphan drugs from the application fee. The Food and Drug Administration Amendments Act (FDAAA) of 2007 further allowed exemption of the establishment fee and product fee, if the sponsor's gross worldwide revenue is less than $50 million in the preceding year.[12,13] These exemptions represent substantial financial incentives. For example, the application fee, establishment fee, and product fee in 2009 each amount to $1,247,200, $425,600, and $71,520, respectively. These fees continue to increase annually.

HOW DOES A SPONSOR SEEK AND OBTAIN ORPHAN DRUG DESIGNATION?

To be eligible for the aforementioned incentives, a sponsor must submit to the OOPD a request for orphan drug designation of a drug previously unapproved for the rare disease or condition of interest.[14] The OOPD, an office located in the FDA's Office of the Commissioner, administers the Act. The request can now be submitted electronically.[15] As of May 2008, sponsors of orphan drugs may also use a common application form to submit their designation requests to the FDA and the European Medicines Agency (EMEA).[16] The request to the FDA must contain the following information:

- the sponsor's contact information (or the authorized United States resident agent if the sponsor is not a United States–based entity);
- the generic and trade name (if available) of the drug;[17]
- the formulation, chemical and physical properties, proposed dosage form, and route of administration;
- the contact information of the drug's manufacturer;[18]
- the proposed orphan designation;
- a description of the rare disease or condition in question;
- the reasons why the drug is needed;
- the scientific basis for the use of the drug;[19]
- for a treatment drug, documentation showing that the rare disease or condition affects fewer than 200,000 persons in the United States at the time the request is submitted;[20,21]
- for a diagnostic drug, preventive drug, or a vaccine, documentation showing that the number of persons to whom the drug may be administered annually is less than 200,000;
- if the prevalence *exceeds* the statutory threshold of 200,000 persons, documentation to support the lack of reasonable expectation on cost recovery, even if the drug is solely marketed in the United States for seven years;
- a summary of the regulatory history and development status of the drug; and
- a statement attesting that the sponsor is the real party of interest in the development, production, and sales of the orphan drug.

The designation request may be submitted to the FDA at any time during the drug-development process, preferably before the commencement of clinical investigation to maximize the tax credit benefit. It must, however, be filed before the sponsor submits its own marketing application of the drug.[22] Until such orphan drug is approved, another sponsor may file a separate designation request for the same drug for the same use.

An orphan designation, after being granted, may be revoked only if the FDA later finds material facts that the drug was ineligible for orphan designation at the time the sponsor submitted the request.[23] To protect the sponsor from unpredictable investment risks, the designation status cannot be revoked even if the prevalence of the disease or condition (e.g., because of an outbreak or advancement in diagnosis) subsequently surpasses the threshold of 200,000.[24] At any time before the drug is approved, the sponsor may request an amendment to the designation on the basis of unexpected findings, if such amendment does not render the drug ineligible for orphan designation.[25]

WHAT IS A MEDICALLY PLAUSIBLE SUBSET?

In general, an orphan designation is granted to a drug intended for use by all patients with a rare disease or condition. Nevertheless, the Orphan Drug Regulations also stipulate that a drug may be designated for use in a defined subset of patients with a *common* disease or condition, provided that the sponsor can plausibly demonstrate that the drug will be developed for use solely in that subset – in other words, the remaining patients are not appropriate candidates for the drug.[26] The subset is often referred to, in regulatory parlance, as a *medically plausible subset*.[27]

Medically plausible subsets have been legitimately defined by the drug's toxicity profile (e.g., a toxic drug to be used in only patients refractory to all lesser toxic treatments); mechanism of action (e.g., a receptor-specific drug for use in receptor-positive patients); unique biopharmaceutical property (e.g., a prodrug requiring metabolic conversion in responders to be effective); route of administration (e.g., an inhalation drug to treat lung-transplant rejection); or previous clinical experiences (e.g., clinical trials showing the drug to be safe and effective in only adult patients). It is reasonable to expect also that a drug targeting a rare genotype-encoded mutation of a common disease phenotype may qualify for orphan designation for the subset of individuals affected by the mutation. In recognizing pediatric patients as "therapeutic orphans," the OOPD has, for years, granted orphan designation to drugs without approved pediatric indication to spur the development of drugs for use in this population.[28]

HOW DOES THE FDA PROTECT THE MARKETING EXCLUSIVITY OF THE PIONEER DRUG?

Under the Orphan Drug Regulations, two drugs are considered the same if they contain the same active substance (i.e., the *active moiety* of a small-molecule drug, or the *principal molecular structural feature* of a large-molecule drug.[29] These regulatory stipulations are solely intended to maximize exclusivity protection to the first approved orphan drug. For example, a second sponsor can neither produce a new salt or an ester form of the same active moiety nor introduce a different glycosylation pattern of a protein drug – a relatively insignificant undertaking in either case – to circumvent the first sponsor's orphan drug exclusivity.

Nevertheless, the Orphan Drug Regulations allow orphan designation of a newly developed drug containing the same active substance as a previously approved drug for the same rare disease or condition, if the sponsor of the newly developed drug can present a *plausible hypothesis* that the former is *clinically superior* to the latter.[30] This provision was put forth to encourage the development of better orphan drugs and to advance public health. Clinical superiority may be based on greater safety, greater effectiveness, or, when neither can be shown, the drug making a major contribution to patient care.[31] The marketing approval of such a drug, however, is conditioned upon definitive evidence of clinical superiority. If this superiority is proven, the sponsor will receive the seven-year marketing exclusivity for this drug.

It is notable that an orphan drug sponsor, despite marketing exclusivity for the orphan indication, may still be vulnerable to marketing competition. This situation may occur when one or more comparable generic versions of the protected drug already exist on the market for other, nonorphan indications. Although the FDA will not permit generic drugs to be labeled for the exclusive orphan indication, the existence of the generic version of the product may not prevent off-label use of the possibly less-expensive versions of the protected drug for the same indication.

OVERVIEW OF NONBIOLOGICAL ORPHAN DRUGS APPROVED FOR GENETIC DISORDERS

As of March 2009, the FDA has approved 24 nonbiological orphan drugs for 21 indications related to genetic disorders (Table 1–1). Sixteen (67%) drugs were considered to be *new molecular entities* – innovator drugs that had not been previously approved by the FDA for any other uses (Table 1–2). The prevalence of the diseases or conditions of interest at the time the sponsor made the orphan-designation request ranged from several hundred to 127,000 persons (median ~15,000). The rate of FDA marketing approval was, on average, one drug per year (Figure 1–1). The FDA also granted priority review of marketing application to the majority (80%) of these drugs.[32]

Of the 21 indications, 17 (81%) are for treatment or management of the disease or condition, three (14%) for preventive use, and one (5%) for diagnostic purposes. One drug was concurrently approved for dual indications: desmopressin for treatment of hemophilia A and for von Willebrand disease type I.

Of the 24 approved drugs, Ucephan (sodium benzoate and sodium phenylacetate) and synthetic porcine secretin are no longer available on the market. The

Table 1-1. Nonbiological orphan drugs approved by the FDA for genetic disorders

Generic name	Trade name	Source*	Indication	Prevalence at designation
Ambrisentan	LETAIRIS®	Gilead Sciences	Treatment of pulmonary arterial hypertension	127,000
Apomorphine	APOKYN®	Vernalis Pharmaceuticals	Treatment of off episodes in Parkinson disease	112,500
Benzoate/phenylacetate	UCEPHAN®	Kendall McGaw Pharmaceuticals	Treatment/prevention of hyperammonemia in UCD	100
Benzoate/phenylacetate	AMMONUL®	Ucyclyd Pharma	Treatment of acute hyperammonemia/encephalopathy in UCD	1,000
Betaine	CYSTADANE®	Jazz Pharmaceuticals	Treatment of homocystinuria	1,000
Bosentan	TRACLEER®	Actelion Pharmaceuticals	Treatment of pulmonary arterial hypertension	69,000
Cysteamine	CYSTAGON®	Mylan Pharmaceuticals	Treatment of nephropathic cystinosis	800
Desmopressin	DDAVP®	Sanofi Aventis	Treatment of hemophilia A/von Willebrand disease (type I)	22,000
Epoprostenol	FLOLAN®	GlaxoSmithKline	Treatment of pulmonary arterial hypertension	60,400
Iloprost	VENTAVIS®	Actelion Pharmaceuticals	Treatment of pulmonary arterial hypertension	127,800
Levocarnitine	CARNITOR®	Sigma-Tau Pharmaceuticals	Treatment of primary carnitine deficiency	100
Miglustat	ZAVESCA®	Actelion Pharmaceuticals	Treatment of type 1 Gaucher disease	11,000
Nitisinone	ORFADIN®	Rare Disease Therapeutics	Treatment of hereditary tyrosinemia type 1	2,500
Riluzole	RILUTEK®	Sanofi Aventis	Treatment of amyotrophic lateral sclerosis	30,000
Sapropterin	KUVAN®	BioMarin Pharmaceutical	Treatment of hyperphenylalaninemia	19,500
Selegiline	ELDEPRYL®	Somerset Pharmaceuticals	Adjunct treatment of Parkinson disease	30,000
Synthetic porcine secretin		ChiRhoClin	Diagnosis of gastrinoma	25,000
Phenylbutyrate	BUPHENYL®	Medicis	Chronic adjunctive treatment of hyperammonemia in UCD	1,000
Tiopronin	THIOLA®	Mission Pharmacal	Prevention of cystine stone in homozygous cystinuria	1,000
Tobramycin	TOBI®	Novartis Pharmaceuticals	Management of CF patients with *Pseudomonas aeruginosa*	30,000
Tranexamic acid	CYKLOKAPRON®	Pfizer	Prevention of tooth-extraction hemorrhage in hemophilia	20,000
Treprostinil	REMODULIN®	United Therapeutics	Treatment of pulmonary arterial hypertension	5,500
Trientine	SYPRINE®	Aton Pharma	Treatment of penicillamine-intolerant Wilson disease	700
Zinc acetate	GALZIN®	Gate Pharmaceuticals	Maintenance treatment of Wilson disease	5,000

* Last known source (as of March 2009). UCD: urea cycle disorders; AIP: acute intermittent porphyria; CF: cystic fibrosis.

Table 1–2. Timeline of orphan drug designation and marketing approval

Drug	Date of orphan designation	Date of marketing approval	Marketing application review*	Exclusivity status as of March 2009	Generic(s) by another manufacturer	Time from designation to approval[†]
Ambrisentan	7/16/2004	6/15/2007	P	Yes	No	2 Y 11 M
Apomorphine	4/22/1993	4/20/2004	P	Yes	No	11 Y
Benzoate/phenylacetate[‡]	1/21/1986	12/23/1987	P	No	No	1 Y 11 M
Benzoate/phenylacetate	11/22/1993	2/17/2005	P	Yes	No	11 Y 3 M
Betaine	5/16/1994	10/25/1996	P	No	No	2 Y 5 M
Bosentan	10/6/2000	11/20/2001	S	No	No	1 Y 1 M
Cysteamine	1/25/1991	8/15/1994	P	No	No	3 Y 7 M
Desmopressin	1/22/1991	3/7/1994	P	No	Yes	3 Y 1 M
Desmopressin	1/22/1991	3/7/1994	P	No	Yes	3 Y 1 M
Epoprostenol	9/25/1985	9/20/1995	P	No	Yes	10 Y
Iloprost	8/17/2004	12/29/2004	P	Yes	No	4 M
Levocarnitine	2/28/1984	4/10/1986	P	No	Yes	2 Y 1 M
Miglustat	5/29/1998	7/31/2003	S	Yes	No	15 Y 2 M
Nitisinone	5/16/1995	1/18/2002	P	No	No	6 Y 8 M
Riluzole	3/16/1993	12/12/1995	P	No	Yes	2 Y 9 M
Sapropterin	1/29/2004	12/13/2007	P	Yes	No	3 Y 10 M
Selegiline	11/7/1984	6/5/1989	S	No	Yes	4 Y 7 M
Synthetic porcine secretin[‡]	6/18/1999	4/4/2002	P	Yes	No	2 Y 10 M
Phenylbutyrate	1/22/1993	4/30/1996	P	No	No	3 Y 3 M
Tiopronin	1/17/1986	8/11/1988	P	No	No	2 Y 7 M
Tobramycin	10/13/1994	12/22/1997	P	No	No	3 Y 2 M
Tranexamic acid	10/29/1985	12/30/1986	S	No	No	1 Y 2 M
Treprostinil	6/4/1997	5/21/2002	P	Yes	No	5 Y
Trientine	12/24/1984	11/8/1985	P	No	No	11 M
Zinc acetate	11/6/1985	1/28/1997	S	No	No	11 Y 3 M

* P: priority review; S: standard review (see text for explanation).
[†] Time rounded to the nearest month/year.
[‡] No longer available on the market.

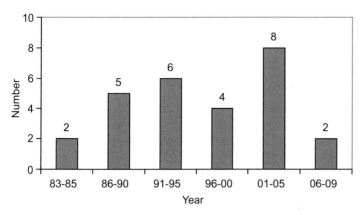

Figure 1–1: Number of biological orphan drugs approved by the FDA for genetic disorders over time.

remaining 22 orphan drugs are currently made available by 19 sponsors – six (27%) of which (Actelion Pharmaceuticals, Allschwil/Basel, Switzerland; Gilead Sciences, Foster City, CA: GlaxoSmithKline, Brentford, Middlesex, United Kingdom; Novartis Pharmaceuticals, Basel, Switzerland; Pfizer, New York, NY; and Sanofi Aventis, Bridgewater, NJ) are among the top 20 pharmaceutical or biotechnology companies ranked by sales in 2008.[33]

At the time this chapter was written, seven (32%) orphan drugs still retained orphan drug marketing exclusivity for the orphan indication (Table 1–2). Of the remaining 15 (68%) drugs with expired exclusivity, 9 (60%) currently have no competitive sources. Among the six drugs with generic counterparts, it is notable that three are relatively costly (epoprostenol – approximately $100,000/year; riluzole – approximately $9,600/year; and desmopressin – approximately $600/dose), two have other approved uses (desmopressin and levocarnitine), and one shares a growing target population (selegiline).[34,35,36] The seeming lack of interest by pharmaceutical manufacturers to offer generic versions of relatively unprofitable orphan drugs following the expiration of their exclusivity underlines the need for incentives not only for development, but also for assurance of their long-term marketing availability.

The time from orphan designation to marketing approval of the orphan drugs of interest varied greatly, from as short as 4 months 13 days for iloprost to as long as 15 years 2 months for miglustat (Table 1–2). The median time was approximately three years one month. This length of time may closely approximate how long it took for clinical testing of these drugs , because, for the most part, orphan designation occurred early in the clinical development phase. The actual overall time for a drug-development program (nonclinical and clinical testing) would be substantially longer. As stated earlier, the request for designation must be received by the OOPD prior to the receipt of the NDA by the FDA Review Division of the marketing application of the drug.

Several of these drugs were approved for the treatment of manifestations common to both genetic and nongenetic forms of the disease: ambrisentan, bosentan, epoprostenol, iloprost, and treprostinil for pulmonary hypertension; selegiline and apomorphine for Parkinson disease. The latter two drugs were approved for use in medically plausible subsets of a relatively common disease: apomorphine for treatment of off episodes in the subset of patients with advanced Parkinson disease, and selegiline for adjunctive treatment in the subset of Parkinson patients who experience deteriorating response to dopamine agonists.

A recent search in the registry of ongoing clinical trials maintained by the National Library of Medicine revealed that at least 20 (91%) of these drugs are undergoing safety and efficacy clinical trials for new, unrelated orphan or nonorphan indications.[37] This "fringe benefit" is seen in a number of drugs initially developed with orphan drug incentives for legitimate orphan diseases or conditions, and subsequently has been found to have broader and, occasionally, more profitable uses.[38] Hence, one may argue that orphan drug incentives benefit more than just patients with certain rare diseases or conditions.

HOW HAS THE FDA APPROVED NONBIOLOGICAL ORPHAN DRUGS FOR GENETIC DISORDERS?

Nonbiological drugs are approved pursuant to section 505 of the FDCA (21 U.S.C. § 355). In seeking FDA approval of a *new drug*,[39] the applicant must provide evidence in the marketing application, or NDA, that the drug is safe and effective through nonclinical studies and adequate and well-controlled clinical investigation. The latter must be conducted through an IND application process.[40] Upon receipt of an IND, the FDA has 30 days to approve it. After approval, the proposed clinical investigation may proceed. Alternatively, the FDA may place an IND on *clinical hold* to delay a proposed clinical investigation, typically because there is insufficient nonclinical information for assessing the potential risks to subjects of the proposed clinical investigation.[41]

In general, the clinical investigation of many drugs proceeds through four phases.[42] Phase I usually involves a small number of healthy volunteers or patients to primarily delineate the drug's pharmacological, pharmacokinetic, and, in applicable cases, pharmacodynamic characteristics. In Phase 2, the drug is typically evaluated in controlled studies with a relatively limited number of patients to determine its preliminary efficacy, safety, and optimal dosages. Phase 3 studies may be controlled or uncontrolled in design, and involve a substantially larger number of patients with more heterogenic disease status to gather additional information on the drug's safety and effectiveness to establish its risk–benefit relationship. During Phase 3, a sponsor may also obtain the FDA's approval to open a *treatment use* IND to allow additional patients who are otherwise ineligible for clinical trials to receive the promising investigational drug.[43] Concurrent with marketing approval, the FDA may enter an agreement with the sponsor to conduct additional postmarketing (Phase 4) studies to delineate the drug's optimal use – for example, in additional patient populations, other stages of the disease, or longer-term use of the drug.[44]

The FDA will approve a new drug if the applicant can demonstrate that there is sufficient information that the drug is safe, and that there is "…substantial evidence that the drug will have the effect it purports or is represented to have under the conditions of use prescribed, recommended, or suggested in the proposed labeling thereof…"[45] *Substantial evidence* of the drug's effectiveness is defined as data from adequate and well-controlled investigations. The regulatory term *adequate and well-controlled investigations* implies not only the quality of the required data, but also the quantity of requisite evidence. As defined in 21 CFR § 314.126, an adequate and well-controlled clinical study is one with (1) clear objectives; (2) a design that permits a valid comparison with a control (e.g., placebo, dose comparison, no treatment, active treatment, historical data) to provide a quantitative assessment of drug effect; (3) adequate measures to minimize bias; and (4) well-defined and reliable analysis to assess treatment response. Uncontrolled or partially controlled studies are not acceptable as the *sole* basis for approving the claims of effectiveness.

Traditionally, substantial evidence is established by data from at least two persuasive, adequate and well-controlled studies. As pointed out in FDA's Guidance for Industry entitled *Providing Clinical Evidence of Effectiveness for Human Drug and Biological Products*, in most cases of drug development the needs to (1) determine an optimal dose, (2) study patients of varied disease severity, (3) compare the drug to other therapy, and (4) study an adequate number of patients for safety purposes often require more than one adequate and well-controlled study to base an effectiveness determination. Nevertheless, evidence of effectiveness may also be established on a single adequate and well-controlled study. For example, if the first study has provided highly reliable and statistically robust evidence of a clinically meaningful effect – such as survival, irreversible morbidity, or prevention of a disease with a potentially serious outcome – a second confirmatory study may be impractical or ethically impossible.[46]

The FDA has made it clear in the Orphan Drug Regulations that the approval standards for orphan drugs would not be different from those for nonorphan drugs.[47] Nevertheless, recognizing that orphan drugs are developed for serious, life-threatening, or severely debilitating diseases without satisfactory alternative interventions, the FDA appears to have applied broad flexibility in applying the statutory standards to expedite their approvals.[48] The majority of nonbiological orphan drugs for genetic disorders were approved through clinical investigations involving a relatively small number of patients, and clinical studies understandably flexible, but no less robust, in their designs compared with conventional drug for nonorphan diseases (Table 1–3).[49] Figure 1–2 summarizes the types of clinical studies pivotal to their approvals. The majority (89%) were in the form of controlled studies spanning the FDA's stipulations for adequate and well-controlled study (i.e., placebo-controlled, dose-comparison control, active-treatment control, no-treatment control, and historical control). Placebo-controlled (39%) and dose-comparison control (31%) designs were the prevailing types. The use of uncontrolled studies for two drugs – miglustat and sapropterin – was complemented with either an active-treatment control or a placebo-controlled study,

Table 1–3. Clinical development of selected orphan drugs for genetic disorders

Drug	Year of approval	Number of studies	Study design	Pivotal clinical studies* — Study endpoints	Number of patients	Pediatric information
Ambrisentan	2007	2	R, DB, PC†, DC	Six-minute walk, time to clinical worsening	393	No
Sapropterin	2007	3	OL, U	Blood phenylalanine levels	659	Yes
		1	R, DB, PC	Blood phenylalanine levels	88	N/A
Apomorphine	2004	3	R, DB, PC, DC	UPDRS motor scores	108	No
Iloprost	2004	1	R, DB, PC†, DC	Composite clinical response (six-minute walk test, NYHA class, death, clinical deterioration)	203	No
Miglustat	2003	2	OL, U, DC	Liver/spleen volume, hemoglobin levels, platelet counts	46	Yes
		1	R, OL, AC	Liver/spleen volume, hemoglobin levels, platelet counts	36	No
Nitisinone	2002	1	OL, HC	Survival, death/transplant for liver failure, incidence of liver cancer, porphyric crisis	207	No
Treprostinil	2002	2	R, DB, PC†, DC	Six-minute walk test, Borg dyspnea index	470	No
Bosentan	2001	2	R, DB, PC†, DC	Six-minute walk test, hemodynamic parameters	245	Yes
Tobramycin	1997	2	R, DB, PC	Pulmonary function, *Pseudomonas aeruginosa* CFUs, hospitalization, parenteral antibiotic treatment	258	Yes
Zinc acetate	1997	1	DC, NC	Copper balance	60	No
		2	Obsv	Neuropsychiatric function, liver function tests, clinical signs/symptoms, plasma copper, copper balance	190	
Epoprostenol	1994	3	R, OL, AC	Survival, six-minute walk test, Borg dyspnea index, dyspnea-fatigue index, NYHA class, hemodynamic parameters	162	No
Riluzole	1994	2	R, PC, DC	Survival, muscle strength, neurological function	1,114	No
Cysteamine	1994	?	HC, DC	Serum creatinine levels, creatinine clearance, growth	~240	Yes
Trientine	1985	2	OL, DC	Clinical response	41	Yes
		1	OL, NC	Survival, clinical response (neurological status, Kayser–Fleicher rings, serum copper, liver function tests)	13	

* Based on available labeling information.

† Added to concurrent conventional therapy.

AC: active-treatment control; DB: double-blind; DC: dose-comparison control; HC: historical control; NC: no-treatment control; OL: open-label; Obsv: observational; PC: placebo-controlled; R: randomized; U: uncontrolled; N/A: not applicable; NYHA: New York Heart Association functional classification of heart failure; UPDRS: Unified Parkinson's Disease Rating Scale; CFU: colony-forming unit.

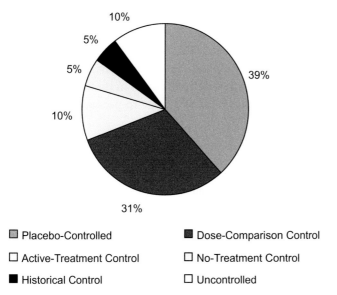

Placebo-Controlled   Dose-Comparison Control

Active-Treatment Control   No-Treatment Control

Historical Control   Uncontrolled

Figure 1–2: Types of pivotal clinical studies of nonbiological drugs for genetic disorders. In some of these studies, the investigational drug or placebo was added to the concurrent therapy.

respectively. The number of studies ranged from one (nitisinone) to three. Where possible, the studies were randomized and blinded in nature. Whereas most drugs for genetic disorders were approved on the basis of demonstrable effects on clinical endpoints (i.e., survival or irreversible morbidity), three were approved essentially on surrogate endpoints that are predictive of clinical benefit (cysteamine – serum creatinine levels, creatinine clearance, growth, leukocyte cystine depletion; miglustat – liver/spleen volume, hemoglobin levels, platelet counts; and sapropterin – blood phenylalanine levels).

CONCLUSIONS

Since their inception in 1983, orphan drug incentives have spurred the development and marketing approval of more than 300 drugs benefiting up to 12 million Americans affected by nearly 180 rare diseases.[50] Of these, 24 nonbiological drugs – the majority of which were new molecular entities – were approved for the diagnosis, prevention, and treatment of manifestations related to at least 16 serious or debilitating genetic disorders. The FDA appears to have exercised its flexibility in approving these drugs, balancing delicately between the statutory demands for safety and effectiveness and the real-world impracticality for "perfect" data.

Collectively, these drugs benefit approximately 450,000 patients in the United States and many more in the rest of the world. Some of these disorders are "ultra-rare" – affecting at most a few hundred patients. Hence, without orphan drug incentives, it is unlikely that drugs for these disorders would ever be developed, given the substantial costs and unpredictable financial returns associated with such an endeavor. As pointed out earlier, 60% of orphan drugs with expired exclusivity remain "orphans," in that their manufacturers remain the sole suppliers. Nonetheless, it is heartening to note that these drugs, following their initial approval, find their potential uses in other diseases or conditions affecting many-fold more patients. In the end, the taxpayers' investments in these orphan drugs are a win–win opportunity that brings relief and hope to persons in desperate need of a cure.

NOTES

1. The word "drug" herein refers to both small-molecule chemical drugs and large-molecule biological products.
2. Pub. L. No. 97–414; codified as amended at 21 U.S.C. §§ 360aa-360ee (1988). The Orphan Drug Act added four sections to the FDCA: section 525 (21 U.S.C. § 360aa) directs the FDA to provide written recommendations for nonclinical and clinical investigations of orphan drugs; section 526 (21 U.S.C. § 360bb) contains provisions on orphan drug designation; section 527 (21 U.S.C. § 360cc) contains provisions on orphan drug marketing exclusivity; and section 528 (21 U.S.C. § 360dd) concerns the open protocol (treatment use) provision of orphan drugs.
3. See Orphan Drug Regulations Final Rule (21 CFR Part 316) at http://www.fda.gov/orphan/odreg.htm. (accessed March 2009). Title 21 of the Code of Federal Regulations is reserved for FDA rules and can be electronically accessed at http://www.accessdata.fda.gov/scripts/cdrh/cfdocs/cfcfr/CFRSearch.cfm.
4. This exclusivity does not extend to the nonorphan indications for use of the drug if the drug can be used for other diseases.
5. http://www.fda.gov/orphan/ (accessed March 2009).
6. http://www.fda.gov/orphan/grants/index.htm (accessed March 2009).
7. http://www.fda.gov/cder/about/smallbiz/pre_IND_qa.htm (accessed March 2009).
8. *Treatment use*, or more well known as *compassionate use*, is a regulatory term defined in 21 CFR § 312.34. Note: Title 21 of the Code of Federal Regulations is reserved for FDA rules and can be accessed electronically at http://www.accessdata.fda.gov/scripts/cdrh/cfdocs/cfcfr/CFRSearch.cfm.
9. The tax credit is regulated by the Internal Revenue Service (26 U.S.C. § 45C and 326 CFR § 1.28–1).
10. The tax credit is not applicable to expenses funded by a grant, contract, or by a government entity.
11. Pub. L. No. 102–571.
12. See section 736 (a)(1)(F) of the FDCA.
13. See section 736(k) of the FDAAA.
14. http://www.fda.gov/orphan/ (accessed March 2009).
15. http://www.fda.gov/orphan/esub/esub.htm (accessed March 2009).
16. The *Common EMEA/FDA Application for Orphan Medicinal Product Designation* (FDA Form 3617) can be found at http://www.fda.gov/opacom/morechoices/fdaforms/FDA-3671.pdf (accessed March 2009).
17. If the drug has no generic or trade names, the sponsor should identify the drug by its scientific name, chemical name, amino acid sequence, or nucleotide sequence.
18. The name and address of the manufacturer(s) of the drug's active substance and finished drug product, if the sponsor does not manufacture them.
19. Such information should include all available nonclinical and clinical data, if any, and even preliminary, published or unpublished, and positive, negative, or nonconclusive.
20. The prevalence of a rare disease or condition is typically established by epidemiologic data from authoritative textbooks, peer-reviewed journals, or databases maintained by government agencies (e.g., the Surveillance, Epidemiology and End Results [SEER]

program database for cancer prevalence by the National Cancer Institute) or proprietary sources. In the absence of any prevalence data on a particular disease, testimonies by experts in the field may be submitted.

21. For diseases of short duration (i.e., less than one year), the annual incidence of the disease has been accepted by FDA as surrogate for prevalence. This does not apply to those with a chronic relapsing and remitting course.

22. Prior to May 6, 1986, the FDA allowed retroactive orphan drug designation of certain drugs after they had been approved for marketing (51 Fed. Reg. 4505 [1986]).

23. 21 CFR § 316.29(a).

24. 21 CFR § 316.29(c).

25. 21 CFR § 316.26.

26. 21 CFR § 316.20(b)(6). *See* also section II.B, paragraph 6, of notice of proposed rulemaking entitled "Orphan Drug Regulations" (56 Fed. Reg. 3338 [1991]) for the preamble discussion on this *medically plausible subset* concept. The subset must meet the statutory prevalence threshold or unprofitability eligibility for orphan drug designation.

27. The regulatory concept of medically plausible subset is occasionally misinterpreted by unsuspecting sponsors as a medically distinct or recognizable subset. More often, sponsors artificially define subsets ("salami slicing") of a common disease or condition simply to meet this well-intended but ill-defined provision because of the lack of cogent regulatory definitions for a *disease* or *condition*. For example, epoetin alfa initially received orphan designation in 1986 for anemia associated with end-stage renal disease. In 1991, it was designated for anemia associated with human immunodeficiency virus (HIV) infection. These types of anemia were, at the time, considered to be distinct *diseases*. Eventually the drug was found to be useful for the treatment of all chemotherapy-related and surgery-induced anemias – conditions affecting significantly larger patient populations. Had the latter developments been anticipated, it is unlikely that the drug would have received the initial orphan designations, because anemia, and not subsets thereof, would have been considered to be the drug's target disease. Notwithstanding, without early orphan drug incentives, the development of this drug could have been delayed. The confusion surrounding the medically plausible subset issue is further compounded by the opacity in regulatory decisions by the FDA. For example, the FDA has for years refused to designate any drug targeting a B-cell receptor for use solely in follicular B-cell lymphoma, contending that it is a subset of B-cell lymphoma (prevalence of approximately 400,000 persons) and that the drug could potentially be used in other subtypes of B-cell lymphoma. Recently, the FDA appeared to have reversed this policy without any notice.

28. http://www.fda.gov/orphan/designat/pediatric.html (accessed March 2009).

29. 21 CFR § 316.3(b)(3),(13).

30. 21 CFR § 316.20(b)(5).

31. There is no regulatory definition of a *major contribution* to patient care. Such determination is made on a case-by-case basis and is based on a significant improvement in the drug's formulation or route of administration that is truly beneficial (not just providing minor conveniences) to the patients. Recently, a case for a major contribution to patient care was made for reintroducing a previously approved drug that is no longer available on the market without any discernible evidence for clinical superiority.

32. Upon receipt of the drug's marketing application, the FDA may designate it for *priority review* if the drug potentially provides a safe and effective diagnosis, treatment, or prevention of a disease or condition without satisfactory alternative intervention or if it represents a significant improvement over available drugs. A priority review sets the target date for FDA action on the application at six months, as opposed to ten months for a *standard review*. *See* http://www.fda.gov/cder/mapp/6020.3R.pdf (accessed March 2009).

33. See http://www.contractpharma.com/articles/2008/07/2008-top-20-pharmaceutical-companies-report (accessed March 2009).

34. http://www.phassociation.org/Learn/treatment/epo.asp (accessed March 2009).

35. http://www.alsa.org/files/cms/Resources/FYI_07_Presumptive%20Disability.pdf (accessed March 2009).
36. http://www.nytimes.com/1990/08/19/business/wall-street-did-the-short-sellers-stumble.html?sec=&spon= (accessed March 2009).
37. http://clinicaltrials.gov/ct2/home (accessed March 2009).
38. See Note 27.
39. The term *new drug* does not connote whether a drug is new or old. It is statutorily defined under 21 CFR 201(p)(1) as a drug that has not been "...generally recognized, among experts qualified by scientific training and experience to evaluate the safety and effectiveness of drugs, as safe and effective for use under the conditions prescribed, recommended, or suggested in the labeling thereof...."
40. See 21 CFR Part 312 for regulations and requirements related to an IND application.
41. See 21 CFR § 312.42 for stipulations concerning *clinical hold* and procedures to address it. The FDA may also suspend an ongoing clinical investigation if there is reason to believe that the investigational drug is unsafe or ineffective.
42. 21 CFR § 312.21.
43. See "Open protocols for investigation of orphan drugs" section.
44. 21 CFR § 312.85.
45. See section 505(d) of the FDCA.
46. In section 115(a) of the FDAMA of 1997, Congress amended section 505(d) of the Act to allow the FDA to consider "data from one adequate and well-controlled clinical investigation and confirmatory evidence" to constitute *substantial evidence* if FDA determines that such data and evidence are sufficient to establish effectiveness.
47. See the FDA's response to comment 74 in the Supplementary information of Orphan Drug Regulations, final rule (57 Fed. Reg. 62,076 [1992]). See also Haffner M. Adopting orphan drugs – two dozen years of treating rare diseases. *N Engl J Med.* 2006;354(5):455–457.
48. The FDA's established procedures designed to expedite the development, evaluation, and marketing of new therapies intended to treat persons with life-threatening and severely debilitating illnesses, especially where no satisfactory alternative therapy exists, are stipulated under 21 CFR Part 312, Subpart E, *Drugs Intended to Treat Life-threatening and Severely-debilitating Illnesses. See* also 21 CFR Part 314, Subpart H, *Accelerated Approval of New Drugs for Serious or Life-Threatening Illnesses* for FDA's regulations on drug approval based on a surrogate endpoint or on an effect on a clinical endpoint other than survival or irreversible morbidity.
49. Information obtained from the available drug labels.
50. Nguyen T. The development of orphan drugs. In: Pisano DJ, Mantus D, eds. *FDA Regulatory Affairs: A Guide for Prescription Drugs.* Boca Raton, FL, CRC Press, 2008.

2 The Office of Rare Diseases Research: Serving a coordinating function at the National Institutes of Health

Stephen C. Groft

INTRODUCTION

The National Institutes of Health (NIH) presents numerous grant and contract mechanisms to the research community, as well as sources of information to patients, the public, health professionals, and the research community, to provide a focus on rare diseases. Most of the research activities and programs have traditionally been the responsibility of 27 research institutes and centers (ICs). The Office of Rare Diseases at the NIH was established in 1993 within the Office of

The statements and opinions presented in this chapter are those of the author and do not represent the position of the NIH or the Department of Health and Human Services.

the NIH Director. In 2002, Public Law 107–280 provided a legislative mandate for the office. Since that time, the office has been renamed the Office of Rare Diseases Research (ORDR), with a primary goal of providing a focus on research-related activities.[1] The ORDR serves in a coordinating role for the NIH and develops programs that will bring research emphasis to the more than 6,500 rare diseases and conditions. The disorders and conditions in the rare diseases category are defined by the prevalence figure of fewer than 200,000 people in the United States with the specific disease. An estimated 25 million to 30 million people in the United States have a rare disease or condition. There are no treatments proven to be effective for most of these individuals.

This chapter will focus on many of the activities of the ORDR and include other significant activities related to rare diseases research and orphan products development. It is important to note that the NIH ICs have many other areas of research interest in rare diseases that cannot be covered in this discussion. The ORDR interacts with individual investigators and program directors in both the Intramural and Extramural Research Programs at the NIH and those individuals responsible for the development and dissemination of information. One major change in the research of rare diseases is the recognition of the need for a multidisciplinary approach. The scope and breadth of activities reflected in the programs supported by the NIH affirm the need for an all-inclusive approach to rare diseases. The NIH provides this emphasis by encouraging interdisciplinary and multidisciplinary research teams and programs by providing resources to effect the required collaborations. The ORDR uses the Trans-NIH Working Group on Rare Diseases Research to provide guidance on research strategies to increase the understanding of rare diseases.

The goals of the ORDR are (1) to increase research of rare diseases by fostering collaboration and cooperative research partnerships, (2) to improve the development and dissemination of information on rare diseases, and (3) to reduce time to diagnosis and treatment, with improved access to investigational and approved interventions. All of the research activities note the substantial contributions of patient advocacy groups (PAGs) as research partners and major links to the public and the rare diseases community.

The following are examples of ongoing ORDR- and NIH-sponsored programs to achieve these overarching goals.

COORDINATED EFFORTS FOR SUCCESSFUL RARE DISEASES RESEARCH AND ORPHAN PRODUCTS DEVELOPMENT

Despite the program emphasis and financial commitments by the pharmaceutical and biotechnology industries to orphan-product development, there remains insufficient interest in the development of products for most rare diseases and conditions. This apparent lack of emphasis has motivated ORDR efforts to facilitate the research and development of potential products for rare diseases using the strengths and resources from multiple partners. Organizations such as the Cystic

Fibrosis Foundation, the Muscular Dystrophy Association, Alpha-1 Foundation, Friedreich Ataxia Research Association, and Parent Project for Duchenne Muscular Dystrophy, the Progeria Research Foundation, and others have expanded their traditional roles to move rare diseases research into the area of emphasis on orphan-products development. Their new role requires the expertise usually possessed by the pharmaceutical, biotechnology, and medical device industries and contract research organizations.

A systematic, coordinated approach to research and product development is needed and requires numerous partners from around the world, including industry collaborators. Required partners include the following:

- Academic research communities reflecting the needs of a multidisciplinary approach required for rare disease research;
- PAGs, foundations, and other philanthropic organizations, including global partners;
- Health care providers and medical specialty societies with clinical expertise in specific rare diseases; and
- Federal government departments and agencies, including:
  - Regulatory organizations (Food and Drug Administration [FDA]);
  - Research-supporting institutions (NIH, Department of Veterans' Affairs [VA], Agency for Healthcare Research and Quality [AHRQ], Department of Defense [DoD]);
  - Disease monitoring and prevention (Centers for Disease Control and Prevention [CDC] and the NIH);
  - Health care services and newborn-screening programs (Health Resources and Services Administration [HRSA]); and
  - Reimbursement:
    - Social Security Administration,
    - Centers for Medicare and Medicaid Services, and
    - Other insurers.

This novel model provides a focused approach to an individual rare disease or related disorders and to development of specific compounds and devices that may be effective. To implement this approach, collaboration is a major requirement in establishing a research and product-development agenda.

SCIENTIFIC CONFERENCES, WORKSHOPS, AND MEETINGS

The NIH and ORDR recognize the value of the coordination, exchange, and dissemination of information on the investigation of the basic and clinical research aspects of rare diseases. The ORDR cosponsors a broad array of scientific meetings with NIH ICs and other federal agencies, including the FDA, CDC, and HRSA. Support for scientific meetings is always dependent on the scientific interests of the research ICs and the availability of funds. Frequent cosponsors for these meetings also include academic investigators, PAGs, foundations, industry, and scientists. The collaborative efforts are a prime example of the usefulness of public–private partnerships. These conferences have been shown to be successful in producing outcomes such as (1) identification of research opportunities; (2) establishment of research priorities; (3) program announcements to solicit research applications; (4) agreement on diagnostic or monitoring criteria; (5) animal models, biospecimen repositories, and patient registries; (6) research protocols, collaborative research arrangements, and plans for clinical trials; and (7) dissemination of conference results to targeted professionals and voluntary health organizations.

The ORDR continues to be a key supporter of these conferences but believes that there are additional steps to be taken after conferences conclude. For most conferences, specific and well-defined outcomes are expected to occur. One need expressed by many of the meeting participants is to define the next steps and future plans for research of specific diseases leading to the development of products for prevention, diagnosis, or treatment. This next step is important if we are to observe more rapid advances in research and development. This activity requires careful planning involving the numerous partners as part of the coordination efforts. These scientific conferences remain a springboard to future actions, many of which are suggested at the conclusion of the conference. ORDR has supported more than 1,000 conferences on rare diseases and is willing to discuss ideas or plans for scientific meetings with the research community and other potential partners, including ICs.

GENETIC TEST–DEVELOPMENT PROGRAM

The Collaboration, Education and Test Translation (CETT) program was developed by the ORDR in 2006 to assist in the translation of genetic tests from the research laboratories to Clinical Laboratory Improvement Amendments (CLIA)-certified laboratories.[2] These collaborative efforts provide for the contributions of clinicians, researchers, laboratories, and disease-specific advocacy groups. The CETT program offers rare disease researchers the opportunity to establish collaborative efforts with PAGs and CLIA-certified laboratories. The CETT program has provided assistance for the development of new genetic tests for 64 rare diseases involving 89 genes.

The major goal of the program is to translate research in gene discovery to new genetic tests for clinical practice. This translational effort meets an unfilled need for many rare diseases for which the results of research were not translated to a clinical diagnostic test that would be available from a CLIA-certified laboratory. Currently, research laboratories are restricted from providing the results of research-laboratory tests to patients. The CETT program has assisted in the development of educational materials for families, clinicians, medical geneticists, and genetic counselors. This information accompanies the results of the genetic test analyses. Information on the availability of genetic tests can be found at Gene Tests (http://www.ncbi.nlm.nih.gov/sites/GeneTests/?db=GeneTests).

The CETT program is investigating the best mechanism to assist in the collection of de-identified clinical and genetic mutation information that will be publicly available to the clinical and research community through a partnership with the National Library of Medicine/National Center for Biotechnology Information (NLM/NCBI). The goal of the program is to facilitate the development of standard formats and terminology for the collection of clinical information associated with genomic data for comparison of results from different research laboratories and clinics.

Information that is developed for listing an individual genetic test must include the following:

- a brief description of the clinical condition;
- information to help with ordering genetic tests, including the benefits and limitations of the tests;
- indications for the test – diagnostic, carrier testing, predictive testing for family members at risk, prenatal diagnosis, or pre-implantation genetic diagnosis;
- information to help understand the test results provided by the laboratory, including mode of inheritance and implication of test results and the reason for the screening (e.g., establishing or confirming a diagnosis or identifying carriers); and
- information is provided on the implications for prognosis and treatment decisions.

The information is provided to assist in a better understanding of the inheritance of disorders and the implications of the diagnosis of a genetic disease. This lack of a current diagnosis for a rare disease is all too frequently a major difficulty encountered by patients with rare diseases and their clinicians seeking to obtain the diagnosis. The program was developed by the ORDR under the direction of Dr. Giovanna Spinella (ORDR), Mr. Andrew Faucett (CDC and Emory University), Dr. Roberta Pagon (University of Washington), Dr. Suzanne Hart (National Human Genome Research Institute [NHGRI]), Dr. William Gahl (NHGRI), and Dr. Lisa Forman (NCBI).

UNDIAGNOSED DISEASES PROGRAM

Obtaining the correct diagnosis for many rare diseases can be difficult and costly, and it often requires many years and frequent visits to physicians and clinics that find the diseases both challenging and frustrating. Not all diseases manifest themselves with characteristic symptoms at one time. In the 1989 report of the National Commission on Orphan Diseases, 15% of patients reported that it took more than five years to obtain the correct diagnosis. Another 31% reported that the time to correct diagnosis was between one and five years.[3] Approximately 6% of the questions received by the NIH's Genetic and Rare Diseases Information Center (GARD) related to information about undiagnosed diseases.

Therefore, in 2008, the NIH announced the establishment of the Undiagnosed Diseases Program (UDP) at the Warren Grant Magnuson Clinical Center.[4] The pilot program was a result of efforts by William Gahl, MD, Clinical Director at the NHGRI, John Gallin, MD, Director of the NIH Clinical Center, and Stephen Groft, PharmD, Director of the ORDR. The Clinical Center hospital is an ideal setting for such a pilot project, with the expertise from nearly 35 medical specialty areas available for participation and consultation. The goals of the program are to improve disease management for individual patients and to advance medical knowledge in general. To be considered for the program, the patient must be without a diagnosis; referred by a physician, nurse practitioner, or physician assistant; and provide all medical records and diagnostic test results requested by the NIH staff. Patients who meet the entrance criteria to the study protocol are asked to travel to the NIH and may undergo further evaluation that may take up to a week. The referring health care provider must provide a summary letter of the condition and current health status with a list of treatments and medications already tried and their outcomes. Copies of reports and results of diagnostic tests along with x-rays, magnetic resonance imaging (MRI) results, and other imaging results must be provided to the NIH for review.

The pilot program is trans-NIH in scope, with monthly meetings to review patients and their records. Decisions on entry into an existing protocol of the UDP or another study protocol at one of the ICs are generally made at the time of the review of the patient records. At the onset of the program, 100 patients per year were expected to gain entrance into the study protocol. It became apparent, after the announcement of the UDP, that program capacity was much lower than the needs of the patients. Additional resources were requested and received from the NIH to expand the program and to accept more patients. In the initial phase of the program, more than 2,200 inquiries were received from patients and their health care providers; more than 900 patients' records were received and reviewed, and 160 patients were accepted into protocols at the NIH.

The overwhelming response to the pilot program indicates current needs. The first need is for better diagnostic criteria for most rare diseases. In recent years, there has been a greater understanding and appreciation for the information developed from longitudinal or natural history of disease studies. The value of these studies is particularly important to the phenotypic differentiation of patients resulting from different genotypes. Another need is for better utilization of currently available information-technology advances to gather reliable information obtained from patients around the world with rare diseases. This information can be categorized and expressed to achieve a better understanding of the expected course of the disease over a lifetime.

Because patients with rare diseases may be spread over large geographical areas, without any natural geographical or political boundaries, it is becoming more obvious that worldwide characterization and descriptions of rare diseases are needed. Easy access to this information will provide earlier clues to diseases that evade diagnosis for too many years.

Utilization of and requests for participation in the program also point to an extreme need for centers with an emphasis on improving the diagnostic capabilities of health care providers to reduce the period of uncertainty and to gain access to approved and investigational products available for rare diseases. The establishment of diagnostic centers of excellence throughout the United States was a major recommendation of the NIH Special Emphasis Panel on the Coordination of Rare Diseases Research in 2000.

In addition to the National Organization for Rare Disorders (NORD), the Genetic Alliance, and individual disease-specific PAGs, two other organizations with an emphasis on undiagnosed diseases have emerged. In Need of Diagnosis (INOD) and Symptoms Without a Name (SWAN) support the need for more centers throughout the world to fulfill the unmet needs of patients without an appropriate diagnosis.

COLLABORATIVE RESEARCH EFFORTS

The ORDR in its efforts to foster collaborative research programs is a major participant in two existing programs, the Bench-To-Bedside Research Program and the Rare Diseases Clinical Research Network. Each of these programs provides opportunities for the extramural and intramural research communities to participate.

The Bench-To-Bedside Research Program was initiated at the NIH Clinical Center in 1999 to encourage collaboration between basic scientists and clinical investigators from different NIH institutes and laboratories. Recently the program was expanded to include research teams composed of NIH intramural and extramural collaborators and grantees from academic research centers, health care organizations, and private industry. In addition to rare diseases, other areas of interest include human immunodeficiency virus/acquired immune deficiency syndrome (HIV/AIDS), minority health and health disparities, and women's health. The National Center for Research Resources (NCRR) and its Clinical and Translational Science Award (CTSA) institutions are also eligible for collaborative research efforts with NIH intramural research programs. Selection criteria for these two-year awards include the quality of the science in the project, the promise for becoming an active clinical trial, and the potential for offering a new medical treatment or better understanding of an important disease process.

Since 1999, approximately 500 principal and associate investigators have collaborated on more than 150 research projects. Current procedures require that a letter of intent be submitted by the primary intramural investigator to the scientific director of the cofunding institute. The scientific and clinical directors determine the appropriateness of the research proposal for further consideration in the review of all submitted applications by the NIH central review team. The ORDR is able to support 8 to 10 research projects per year in collaboration with the other institutes and centers.

RARE DISEASES CLINICAL RESEARCH NETWORK

In 2003, the ORDR published a Request for Applications (RFA) with other institutes and centers including the NCRR, The National Institute of Child Health and Human Development (NICHD), the National Institute of Neurological Disorders and Stroke (NINDS), the National Institute of Arthritis and Musculoskeletal and Skin Diseases (NIAMS), the National Institute of Diabetes and Digestive and Kidney Diseases (NIDDK), and the National Heart, Lung and Blood Institute (NHLBI). This announcement resulted in awards to 10 research consortia and a data and technology coordinating center (DTCC). The purpose of the Rare Disease Clinical Research Network (RDCRN) is to facilitate clinical research in rare diseases by supporting (1) collaborative clinical research of rare diseases, including longitudinal studies of individuals with rare diseases, Phase I and II trials, and/or pilot and demonstration studies; (2) a test bed for distributed clinical data management that incorporates novel approaches and technologies for data management, data mining, and data sharing across rare diseases, data types, and platforms; (3) training programs of new clinical investigators of rare diseases; and (4) the establishment of a partnership role of PAGs in rare disease research programs.

The ten consortia, the disorders under investigation, and the DTCC that comprise the RDCRN network[5] are listed in Table 2–1.

The Pediatrics Epidemiology Center at the University of South Florida, Tampa, serves as the DTCC with Dr. Jeffrey P. Krischer as the principal investigator.

The DTCC serves as a facilitating center to (1) assist collaborators in the design of clinical protocols, data management, and analyses; (2) develop a coordinated clinical data management system for the collection storage and analysis of data from multiple diseases and multiple clinical research sites; (3) develop tools for Web-based recruitment and referral (e.g., the patient contact registry); (4) construct a portal for access and integration of public data resources; and (5) promote novel communication and coordination of RDCRN and consortia activities.

After a protocol is developed by the research investigator, accepted by the Data Safety and Monitoring Board, and approved by the local Institutional Review Board(s), patient recruitment is initiated. One of the more successful recruitment strategies provides for the use of PAGs to assist in expanding the population for participation in the studies by registration in the Patient Contact Registry. Patients in this registry are periodically informed of new information about their diseases and opportunities for participation in planned clinical studies.

The initial five-year grant period was followed by a funding opportunity announcement in 2008 requesting applications for another five-year period for consortium grant in an open competition. As observed in 2003, interest was high and, with increased collaboration of the ICs (NINDS, NICHD, NIDDK, NIAMS, the National Institute of Allergy and Infectious Diseases [NIAID], the National Institute of Dental and Craniofacial Research [NIDCR] and NHLBI), 19 research consortia will receive support from the NIH. Any concerns that research on rare diseases could not be conducted because of the small number of patients available for investigation, the distribution of patients over wide geographical areas, and/or

Table 2–1. Consortia of the Rare Disease Clinical Research Network

Name of center	Disorder	PI*
Children's National Medical Center, Washington, DC	**Urea Cycle Disorders Consortium:** Urea cycle disorders including citrullinemia, argininosuccinic aciduria, hyperargininemia, and others	Dr. Mark L. Batshaw
Baylor College of Medicine, Houston, TX	**Angelman, Rett, & Prader–Willi Syndromes Consortium:** Genetic developmental disorders, including Angelman syndrome, Rett syndrome, and Prader–Willi syndrome	Dr. Arthur L. Beaudet
Boston University School of Medicine, Boston, MA	**Vasculitis Clinical Research Consortium:** Vasculitides including Wegener's granulomatosis, Takayasu arteritis, and Churg–Strauss syndrome	Dr. Peter A. Merkel
Cleveland Clinic Foundation, Cleveland, OH	**Bone Marrow Failure Disease Consortium:** Bone marrow failure including aplastic anemia, myelodysplastic syndromes, paroxysmal nocturnal hemoglobinuria, and large granular lymphocyte leukemia	Dr. Jaroslaw P. Maciejewski
Mount Sinai School of Medicine, New York, NY	**Rare Genetic Steroid Disorders Consortium:** Rare genetic defects in steroidogenesis leading to congenital adrenal hyperplasia, androgen receptor defects, and low renin hypertension	Dr. Maria I. New
Children's Hospital Medical Center, Cincinnati, OH	**Rare Lung Diseases Consortium:** Rare lung diseases including lymphangioleiomyomatosis, alpha-1 antitrypsin deficiency, pulmonary alveolar proteinosis, and hereditary interstitial lung disease	Dr. Bruce C. Trapnell
University of Rochester, Rochester, NY	**Consortium for Clinical Investigations of Neurological Channelopathies (CINCH):** Rare lung diseases including lymphangioleiomyomatosis, alpha-1 antitrypsin deficiency, pulmonary alveolar proteinosis, and hereditary interstitial lung disease	Dr. Robert C. Griggs
University of North Carolina at Chapel Hill, NC	**Genetic Diseases of Mucociliary Clearance Consortium:** Genetic impairments in mucociliary clearance including primary ciliary dyskinesia, cystic fibrosis, pseudohypoaldosteronism, and other chronic sinopulmonary diseases	Dr. Michael R. Knowles
The Children's Hospital, Denver, CO	**Cholestatic Liver Disease Consortium (CLiC):** Genetic causes of intrahepatic cholestasis including rare liver diseases associated with alpha-1 antitrypsin deficiency, Alagille syndrome, progressive familial intrahepatic cholestasis, bile acid synthesis defects, and mitochondrial hepatopathies	Dr. Ronald J. Sokol
Duke University School of Medicine, Durham, NC	**Rare Thrombotic Diseases Consortium:** Antiphospholipid antibody syndromes, heparin-induced thrombocytopenia, paroxysmal nocturnal hemoglobinuria, catastrophic antiphospholipid antibody syndrome (thrombotic storm), thrombotic thrombocytopenic purpura	Dr. Thomas L. Ortel

* PI = principal investigator.

the lack of research interest have been addressed and are being eliminated. With the availability of research support, there are many research investigators willing to participate in these programs provided there is continued institutional commitment to support the proposed projects. This conclusion was stated clearly in the Report of the National Commission on Orphan Diseases in 1989 and verified by the extremely high level of interest in rare disease research programs announced by the NIH ICs, the Office of Orphan Products Development at the FDA, and the individual PAGs in their solicitations to the research community. Likewise, patients are willing to participate in clinical studies of rare diseases. The individual consortia were able to initiate 37 studies at 79 research sites with several sites outside of the United States and have enrolled more than 5,500 patients in these clinical studies.

The RDCRN has expanded traditional methods of recruiting patients for clinical studies by providing for the active involvement of the PAGs as research partners. The RDCRN also has an increased presence on the Internet with an informational Web site featuring the individual consortia and their research programs. In an early analysis of 4,360 inquiries from patients, 71% preferred to be contacted by e-mail, 15% by phone, and 13% by mail. The results are not too surprising, given that 43% of the patients found the registry through the Internet, and another 50% through the PAGs. Health professionals referred 8% of the patients.

NIH EMPHASIS ON PAGs AS COLLABORATORS

In recent years many of the PAGs have expanded their traditional roles as voices of support for more research for their disease, suppliers of information for the health care providers and the public, and support services for patients, family members, and caregivers. Expansion of services and increased commitment to research and development of products have occurred with the addition of strong scientific and medical advisory boards to guide their activities. The PAGs remain strong supporters of research and training programs for research investigators with an interest in their diseases. Many of the leaders of PAGs are now recognized as the knowledgeable voices of specific rare diseases and provide ready access to the media. The leaders and their staffs serve as direct links to physicians and other health care providers, patients, and families, and they are frequently asked to organize research-based conferences and meetings for the scientific and patient communities, including caregivers. In this capacity, PAGs are recognized as partners in the research program during the development of the study protocol, providing valuable insight into the feasibility of the proposed study, the clarity of the informed consent document and translation of the intent of the proposed study to their constituents, and explaining the resulting outcomes of the study for the public.

The NIH continues to consider PAGs as research collaborators and to seek their presence on the institute's advisory councils and special committees, including the Council of Public Representatives and Institutional Review Boards. They are frequently asked to provide advice on NIH research priorities and the content of disease-specific information contained in fact sheets and policy statements.

It is important that basic and clinical research investigators continue to provide the leadership of patient organizations with information about the science and clinical aspects of the disease, cutting edge scientific tools, and advances in research technology. The ORDR, through weekend leadership forums sponsored with NORD for the leaders of the PAGs, has provided interactive training programs about government and industry research and regulatory structures, procedures and requirements of research investigators, and the specific requirements at the individual research institutions and organizations. When considered a true partner, an informed patient community becomes an even stronger supporter of the research investigators.

THE GENETIC AND RARE DISEASES INFORMATION CENTER

Established by the ORDR and the NHGRI in 2002 to respond to the many different questions received about rare and genetic disorders, the Genetic and Rare Diseases Information Center (GARD) focuses on these disorders. Its information includes that provided by the NIH NLM, institutes and centers, and other PAGs and foundations and that from the pharmaceutical, biotechnology, and medical device industries.

The GARD provides information on more than 6,400 rare and genetic conditions via active links to more than 6,900 terms in the database on its Web site (Table 2–2). Particular attention is directed to the development of information that is known about the disease; what research studies are actively recruiting patients or have completed recruitment, some with study results available (see http://clinicaltrials.gov/); what genetic testing services and tests are available from CLIA-certified and research laboratories; how patients gain access to PAGs and their information; and the most recent advances and results from studies in the published literature.

The arrival of Internet services and ready access to information about rare diseases has provided patients and patient organizations with frequent informational updates and research advances. To assure the release of useful information, the GARD has embarked on a program to use their resources more effectively. Starting in 2008, responses provided to queries received from the public and health care providers are now archived and available for easy reference on the Web site. This decision reduced the number of questions to the information center but has increased dramatically the visitors to the information centers who are searching for disease-specific information. More than 65,000 visitors each month use the Web site for the GARD. The Web site for the ORDR is visited by more than 90,000 users per month. Each Web site continues to see increases in the number of visitors.

Table 2–2. Genetic and Rare Diseases Information Center (GARD)

Toll-Free Number:	1–888-205–3223
E-mail:	GARDinfo@nih.gov
Web site:	ORDR: http://rarediseases.info.nih.gov
	GARD: http://rarediseases.info.nih.gov/GARD/Default.aspx

GAINING ACCESS TO RESEARCH DISCOVERIES

The Office of Technology Transfer (OTT) at the NIH and the ORDR provide access to more than 500 research discoveries from the federal and state governments and from not-for-profit organizations worldwide, including academic research centers for rare and neglected diseases. The technologies related to these disorders are available for commercial licensing. The disorders in the rare disease categories are defined by the prevalence figure of less than 200,000 people in the United States with the disease. The term "neglected disease" agrees with that used by the World Health Organization and is defined as those diseases that are prevalent among many of the developing nations around the world. Limited access to health care, living conditions causing increased susceptibility to certain diseases, and a tropical environment contribute to the risk of these conditions over a large population in many nations. The neglected diseases are categorized into the following groups (with examples provided): (1) bacterial: leprosy, tuberculosis, cholera, trachoma; (2) helminths: hookworm, schistosomiasis, filariasis; (3) protozoan: trypanosomiasis, leishmaniasis, Chagas disease, malaria; and (4) viral: dengue fever and rotavirus. The capacity to include more discoveries from research by the not-for-profit organizations is much greater than current utilization and can include inventions for diagnostics, research materials, therapeutics, vaccines, and software. Academic research centers and other qualified organizations should consider use of this information source to provide greater public access to discoveries from their institutions. Dr. Bonny Harbinger and Mr. Ajoy Prabhu of the OTT were responsible for developing the content and the Web site for these initiatives, which are as follow:

Rare diseases: http://www.ott.nih.gov/rd
Neglected diseases: http://www.ott.nih.gov/nd

THE NIH ROADMAP FOR MEDICAL RESEARCH AND OTHER SIGNIFICANT NIH RESEARCH INITIATIVES

The NIH Roadmap for Medical Research was initiated in 2004 to address roadblocks to research and to transform the way biomedical research is conducted by overcoming barriers or filling defined knowledge gaps. Roadmap programs extend over all areas of disease research of NIH ICs. They are programs that usually would not be supported by the NIH because they are inherently risky.

Roadmap Programs are to transform how biomedical research is conducted over a shorter period of time (e.g., a 5- to 10-year period). The goal is to eliminate the major road blocks, thereby stimulating further research conducted through the ICs. Roadmap programs were initially funded by a 1% contribution from each of the NIH ICs. In 2006, Congress subsequently authorized funding the NIH Common Fund within the Office of the Director. The annual Common Fund budget was $498 million in 2008.

These programs provide the flexibility to respond quickly to novel ideas, new challenges, major gaps, and recent advances in biomedical research. Programs are selected from a planning process involving input from multiple scientific and public sources. Three areas of emphasis have been adopted by the NIH: New Pathways to Discovery, Research Teams of the Future, and Reengineering the Clinical Research Enterprise. Initiatives funded within these areas fit into one or more of the major themes and address specific road blocks or existing informational gaps to foster high-risk/high-reward research, enable the development of transformative research tools and methodologies, and change academic culture to foster collaborations within the institution and between other institutions.

The Molecular Libraries program and the Rapid Access to Interventional Development (RAID) program are initiatives representative of these activities. The research community is encouraged to consider the opportunities presented in the numerous road map initiatives and discuss their needs and opportunities for research advances with the responsible program officials at the NIH. Several of the areas of research are at preclinical stages of drug discovery and development. It is in this area that many compounds are eliminated from further research and development as possible candidates for human trials because of toxicity concerns.

MOLECULAR LIBRARIES INITIATIVE

The Molecular Libraries initiative provides researchers with access to small, organic molecules that can be used as chemical probes to study the functions of genes, cells, and biochemical pathways in health and disease. This initiative stimulates development of new drugs by providing early-stage chemical compounds to researchers so that they can find successful matches between a compound and its target and thus help validate new therapeutic targets.

The Small Molecule Repository will acquire, maintain, and distribute a collection of up to 500,000 compounds. The repository will provide these compounds, obtained from both commercial and academic sources, to the Molecular Libraries Screening Centers Network (MLSCN). The compounds will be used in high-throughput screening (HTS) of biological assays submitted by the research community. It is anticipated that screening "hits" will be further developed into optimized chemical analogs that can be used by the scientific community as bioactive probes to study molecular targets and cellular pathways, and potentially as starting points for therapeutics development of compounds outside of the MLSCN. The probes will be available to researchers via the repository, and the chemical structures of the compounds in the repository, along with the associated screening data obtained from the MLSCN, will be shared with the public through PubChem.

THE RAID PROGRAM

Potential compounds for novel therapeutic interventions encounter road blocks in efforts to move from basic research to clinical protocols. Although translation is sometimes facilitated by public–private partnerships, high-risk ideas or therapies for rare diseases and conditions do not always attract sufficient private sector or industry resources to meet the needs of product-development programs for all of the rare diseases. Where private sector capacity is limited or not available, public resources are being used to bridge the gap between discovery and clinical testing to bring about more efficient translation of promising discoveries to make them available as possible treatments. To help address this need, the NIH established a program to provide access to critical resources needed for the development of new, small molecule therapeutic agents. The NIH Rapid Access to Interventional Development (RAID) program is intended to reduce some of the common barriers between laboratory discoveries and clinical trials for new therapies. Projects in both the early and late stages of preclinical development are suitable for NIH RAID applications. The National Cancer Institute has a separate RAID program. These programs are available to the research community for potentially useful compounds. Services available from the two RAID programs are provided under the contract mechanism include scale-up synthesis, pharmacology, preclinical toxicity, material for clinical trials, and preclinical development of monoclonal antibodies, recombinant proteins, and gene therapy agents. Manufacture of non-Good Manufacturing Practices (GMP) viral and nonviral gene vectors as well as GMP-grade adeno-associated virus and lentivirus vectors can be manufactured for investigators with small businesses, academic laboratories, and not-for-profit organizations. Applicants use the NIH Resource Access (X01) award mechanism, through Grants.gov. Additional information and guidance can be found at the Web site for the NIH RAID program (http://nihroadmap.nih.gov/raid/).

THERAPEUTICS FOR RARE AND NEGLECTED DISEASES PROGRAM

The NHGRI and the ORDR created a therapeutics-development program to encourage and speed the development of new drugs for rare and neglected diseases. The Therapeutics for Rare and Neglected Diseases (TRND) program extends the incentives and provisions of the RAID program by providing resources to identify possible candidate compounds at an earlier stage in the drug-development continuum. To assist in the activities of the program, the NIH established the Trans-NIH Staff Advisory Group with NIH staff members who have expertise and experience in product-development programs. This intra-NIH group will provide ongoing consultation regarding the operation of the TRND program and help to integrate it with related or complementary efforts at the NIH. A second group assisting the ORDR in the governance is an external expert panel composed of experts in preclinical drug development and rare and neglected diseases from academia, industry, and patient advocacy communities. This group will assist TRND program staff in developing criteria to determine which compounds will be accepted for preclinical development, review the projects submitted for consideration, and develop milestones to assess project progress. Periodic assessments will be considered as projects reach time- or stage-specific milestones. The group will also give guidance to TRND program staff on when and how to transition individual projects to external partners and how long projects should continue if milestones are not met.

The NIH budget for fiscal 2009 provided $24 million to establish this initiative. The TRND program will bridge the wide gap in time and resources that often exists between basic research and human testing of new drugs. The ORDR will handle TRND program oversight and governance. The TRND program will build on the pathway of the NIH Chemical Genomics Center (NCGC). The NCGC facilitates drug development from the basic research laboratory to the preclinical stage, which is when researchers begin to lay the groundwork for possible human testing of candidate drugs. Picking up where The NCGC leaves off, the TRND program will concentrate its efforts on the preclinical stage of drug development. The aim of the TRND program will be to move candidate drugs forward in the drug-development pipeline until they meet FDA requirements for an Investigational New Drug (IND) application. After the TRND program generates enough data to support an IND application for a candidate drug, the drug will then be transferred to an experienced pharmaceutical company for clinical trials. The TRND program will encourage investigators from both inside and outside of the NIH to submit compounds for consideration of further development. The TRND program will create ongoing collaborations that will benefit researchers and, most importantly, patients with rare and/or neglected diseases.

The TRND program officials plan to support pilot projects in fiscal year 2009 in both rare and neglected diseases. These projects will include testing the feasibility of optimizing novel compounds and the possibility of repurposing drugs already approved for other diseases. The NIH has not yet chosen the exact diseases and candidate compounds to be focused on by the TRND program. Selection criteria will include the quality of the candidate drug compounds, the clarity of the path to clinical testing, and the commitment and enthusiasm of collaborating researchers.

CONCLUSION

We have neither accurate data on the prevalence of rare diseases nor a single mechanism to determine the prevalence of the disorders in the United States. The demand for diagnostics and treatments for more than 6,500 rare diseases affecting between 25 million and 30 million people in the United States alone presents a global public health problem. It has been estimated that rare diseases affect between 6 and 10% percent of the population.[6] The impact can be tremendous on families, friends, and others in the health care community and the public. Even with major efforts by the research community, federal agencies, private foundations, PAGs, and members of the pharmaceutical, biotechnology, and medical device industries, the need for interventions exceeds the financial and program capacity of the collective organizations. In recent years, new models for drug development have evolved that use the resources available from public–private partnerships. Resources and commitments from many private and public organizations are required to advance research discoveries through compound discovery leading to the development of products for the diagnosis, prevention, or treatment of rare diseases.

Several PAGs have taken on the additional responsibility of using existing resources and developing working relationships with multiple partners by moving research advances to investigational compounds for clinical trials for their diseases. There are now several successful models of PAGs directing partnerships to reach their organizational goals of providing treatments for their patients. A systematic approach to meet these needs will use the limited resources from the public and private sectors. An awareness of these resources and how to gain access to them needs to be developed by the leaders of all rare disease organizations.

The NIH recognizes and acknowledges the need for collaborative efforts among multidisciplinary research teams and the need for new approaches to drug discovery and development. The ORDR offers assistance in many areas to stimulate rare diseases research and to complement the research and training programs of the 27 ICs at the NIH. Many of the programs offered by the NIH are related to several stages of product discovery and development and are consistent with the goals of the PAGs of developing treatments for rare diseases.

REFERENCES

1. Rare Diseases Act of 2002, *Public Law 107–280*, Washington, D.C., November 2002
2. Faucett WA, Hart S, Pagon RA, Neall LF, Spinella G. A model program to increase translation of rare disease genetic tests: Collaboration, education and test translation program. *Genet Med*. 2008;10(5):343–348
3. Report of the National Commission on Orphan Diseases: *Appendices – Volume I, Publication No. HRP-0907249, 10–11*, Springfield, VA: National Technical Information Services; April 1989
4. NIH Launches Undiagnosed Diseases Program, *NIH News*, May 19, 2008. Available at: http://www.nih.gov/news/health/may2008/nhgri-19.htm
5. Griggs RC, Batshaw M, Dunkle M, Gopal-Srivastava R, Kaye E, Krischer J, Nguyen T, Paulus K, Merkel PA. Rare diseases clinical research network: Clinical research for rare disease: Opportunities, challenges, and solutions. *Mol Genet Metab*. 2009;96(1):20–26
6. Zurynski Y, Frith K, Leonard H, Elliott E. Rare childhood diseases: How should we respond? *Arch Dis Child*. 2008;93(12):1071–1074

3 Introduction to pharmacokinetics and pharmacodynamics

Juan J. L. Lertora and Konstantina M. Vanevski

INTRODUCTION

This chapter summarizes general principles of pharmacokinetics and pharmaco-dynamics (PK/PD) that are relevant to the therapeutic use of small molecules in genetic diseases. Most therapeutic drugs are small molecules (molecular weight <1,000 D, and typically between 300 and 700 D), and characterizing their

PK/PD properties is usually accomplished in the early stages of drug development (preclinical and clinical Phase "0" and Phase I studies). Defining the PK/PD profile of a drug is essential for the rational selection of effective and safe dosing regimens.

Definition of pharmacokinetics and pharmacodynamics

Pharmacokinetics is the branch of pharmacology dealing with the processes of drug absorption from the site/route of administration, distribution to tissues and organs, biotransformation (metabolic inactivation and activation), transport across cell membranes, and elimination from the body via excretory organs like the liver, kidneys, and lungs. *Pharmacodynamics* is the branch of pharmacology dealing with drug effects and the mechanisms of drug action, including drug–receptor interactions, signal transduction pathways, the concentration– or dose–response relationship, and the phenomena of pharmacologic tolerance and resistance to drug therapy. Genetic and environmental determinants contribute to the variability in drug response and can impact both pharmacokinetic and pharmacodynamic processes.

PK/PD Key abbreviations

PK/PD	Pharmacokinetics and pharmacodynamics
AUC	Area under the curve
C_{max}	Maximum concentration
T_{max}	Time needed to reach C_{max}
FDA	U.S. Food and Drug Administration
Cl	Clearance
VD	Volume of distribution
Co	Initial plasma concentration of drug
$T_{1/2}$	Elimination half-life
C_{ss}	Steady-state drug concentration
GFR	Glomerular filtration rate
CYP450	Cytochrome P450 enzyme system
LD10	Lethal dose in 10% treated mice
FIH	First-in-human (drug dose)
MTD	Maximum tolerated dose
PGDE	Pharmacologically guided dose escalation scheme
IND	Investigational new drug
PET	Positron emission tomography
TBW	Total body water
ABC	ATP-binding cassette
OATP	Organic anion-transporting polypeptide
OAT	Organic anion transporter
OCT	Organic cation transporter
PGT	Prostaglandin transporter
NTCP	Na^+-taurocholate cotransporting polypeptide

GENERAL PRINCIPLES OF PHARMACOKINETICS

Drug absorption and bioavailability

Absorption

Drugs are absorbed primarily from the small intestine given the large surface area provided by the intestinal mucosa. Absorption usually involves passive drug diffusion driven by a concentration gradient, but many examples exist where drugs are absorbed via facilitated diffusion or through active membrane transport mechanisms that translocate small molecules from the lumen of the intestine into cells and from the cytoplasm to the interstitial fluid space via transporters in the basolateral cell membranes. From there drugs are carried via the portal circulation to the liver, and then they reach the systemic circulation for distribution across the body. Small intestinal mucosal cells also possess efflux drug transporters, like P-glycoprotein, that counteract absorption and transport drug back into the intestinal lumen, as well as drug-metabolizing enzymes like CYP3A4, that biotransform drugs before they reach the portal circulation, a process known as *intestinal first-pass metabolism* (e.g., ocetaxel, midazolam, nifedipine, verapamil).[1] Drugs can also undergo *hepatic first-pass metabolism* that limits systemic drug availability after oral administration (e.g., nitrates, morphine, lidocaine).

Because of their physicochemical properties some drugs are poorly absorbed if given orally, and the parenteral route is required (subcutaneous, intramuscular, or intravenous injections). Drugs can also be given by the sublingual (buccal mucosal absorption of nitroglycerin), inhalational (nasal, pulmonary; e.g., β-adrenergic agonists, vasopressin), or transdermal routes (e.g., nitroglycerin, progesterone, nicotine, scopolamine). Less frequently, intrathecal, intraperitoneal, or intraarterial (selective organ perfusion) administration is required for effective drug delivery to a site of action.

Bioavailability

Bioavailability is defined as the fraction of the administered dose that reaches the systemic circulation unchanged and the rate at which this occurs. If the drug is given by the intravenous route, the full dose reaches the systemic circulation directly, so the bioavailability is 100%. Using this as a reference, the *absolute oral bioavailability* of a drug is defined as the fraction of the same dose given orally that reaches the systemic circulation unchanged (Figure 3–1). If no intravenous formulation of the drug is available for comparison, absolute bioavailability can be inferred only from total drug excretion as parent drug and/or metabolites in urine and feces (if the agent is volatile, elimination via the lungs also needs accounting). Otherwise, only *relative bioavailability* can be established when comparing different formulations of the same drug given orally at equal doses. *Bioavailability studies* (Figure 3–1) usually determine the area under the plasma concentration versus time curve (AUC) after dosing, the maximum (peak) concentration achieved (C_{max}), and the time to reach C_{max} (T_{max}).

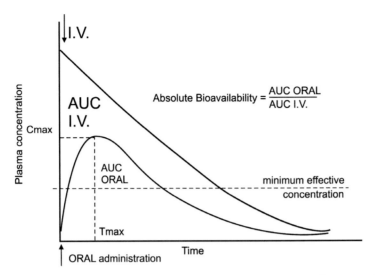

Figure 3–1: Pharmacokinetic profile with typical plasma concentration versus time curves after an intravenous (I.V.) and oral administration of equal doses of a drug. This example indicates reduced oral bioavailability for the drug.

Bioavailability and bioequivalence studies are essential to characterize generic formulations of drugs. Two drugs are said to be bioequivalent if they show analogous (comparable) bioavailability and achieve peak blood concentrations within similar time ranges.

The U.S. Food and Drug Administration (FDA)[2] defines bioequivalence as "The absence of a significant difference in the rate and extent to which the active ingredient or active moiety in pharmaceutical equivalents or pharmaceutical alternatives becomes available at the site of drug action when administered at the same molar dose under similar conditions in an appropriately designed study."

According to the FDA, two products are bioequivalent if the 90% confidence interval (90% CI) of the relative mean C_{max}, $AUC_{(0-t)}$, and $AUC_{(0-\infty)}$ of the test (e.g., generic formulation) to reference (e.g., innovator brand formulation) is within 80.00–125% in the fasting state.

Drug distribution, elimination, and the concept of clearance

Two primary (basic) pharmacokinetics parameters are (1) volume of distribution (VD), the measure of the apparent physical space in the body available to contain the drug, and (2) clearance, the measure of the ability of the body to eliminate the drug.

Drug distribution and apparent VD

After reaching the systemic circulation (blood/plasma compartment), drugs are distributed to tissues and organs. The extent and rate of distribution are a function of the drug's physicochemical properties, degree of protein and tissue binding, tissue perfusion rate, and the anatomic features of tissue capillary blood vessels (continuous or fenestrated endothelial surface). From the intravascular space drugs first enter the interstitial fluid space and may or may not enter the intracellular space. Unless drugs are very lipid soluble (thiopental, propofol, lidocaine), their distribution may be blocked at physiological barriers like the blood–brain barrier, blood–cerebrospinal fluid barrier, and blood–testicle barrier. Efflux pumps like P-glycoprotein play a role in impeding drug transfer to these organs, as well as limiting placental–fetal drug distribution (e.g., anticancer drugs such as vincristine, vinblastine, anthracyclines, etoposide, paclitaxel, and mithramycin; cytotoxic agents such as colchicine and emetine;[3] and human immunodeficiency virus (HIV) protease inhibitors such as saquinavir, indinavir, and ritonavir).[4] The *apparent volume of distribution* is a primary pharmacokinetic parameter estimated in relation to the initial plasma concentration of drug (Co) obtained after administering a dose (amount) of drug intravenously, such that VD = Dose/Co. It is a theoretical estimation of the volume of plasma needed to explain the observed Co and to account for the full amount (dose) that was administered based on the dilution principle, assuming instantaneous distribution throughout the body and no drug elimination (one compartment model). Thus, the VD usually does not represent physiological body fluid compartments, although some molecules have apparent VDs equivalent to the extracellular fluid (inulin, aminoglycoside antibiotics, d-tubocurarine) and total body water (caffeine, urea, alcohol). If the *tissue:plasma partition ratio* for the drug is high, the apparent VD will greatly exceed total body water (e.g., digoxin, amiodarone). Estimation of the proper loading dose needed to obtain a target plasma drug concentration requires knowledge of the VD. Pharmacokinetic data tables usually report VD normalized to body weight (L/kg).

Concept of half-life

For drugs exhibiting first-order kinetics of elimination, the parameter of elimination half-life ($T_{1/2}$) is often used as a descriptor of drug elimination rate. It is important to note, however, that elimination $T_{1/2}$ is a dependent parameter determined by both the VD and the elimination clearance (CL), such that $T_{1/2} = 0.693\ VD/CL$.[5] Elimination $T_{1/2}$ is related to the first-order elimination rate constant (k) such that $T_{1/2} = 0.693/k$.

Concept of clearance

Clearance (CL) is also a primary pharmacokinetic parameter, and it represents either the drug-transfer rate from a central distribution compartment to a peripheral compartment or the drug elimination rate from the body via organs of elimination (liver, kidneys, lungs), in each case *normalized* to the simultaneous plasma concentration of the drug. We therefore distinguish between *intercompartmental clearance* (distribution clearance) and *elimination clearance* parameters. Elimination clearance is also known as systemic plasma clearance and it is the sum of available organ clearances for a given drug (renal and nonrenal components). Clearance has units of flow (L/h or mL/min). Elimination clearance is a determinant of *steady-state* drug concentration (C_{ss}) with continuous dosing (constant intravenous infusion or repeated oral or parenteral dosing), such that $C_{ss} = $ Dosing rate/CL. Pharmacokinetic data tables also report clearance normalized to body weight (L/h/kg).

Mechanisms and determinants of renal drug clearance

Renal drug elimination occurs by glomerular filtration of parent drug and/or metabolites and also by renal tubular secretion of drugs. Some drugs are both secreted and reabsorbed, so that the net urinary excretion is the result of both mechanisms operating. Generally, if the renal clearance for the drug exceeds the estimated glomerular filtration rate (GFR), secretion also plays a role. Likewise, if the renal clearance is less than GFR, reabsorption is taking place. There are multiple drug transporters in renal tubular cells. These transporters are saturable (T_{max}) and can also be inhibited by pharmacological agents. Renal drug clearance can also be conceptualized using the Fick principle [(CL = Q × E), where Q = organ blood flow, and E = (A – V)/A (the extraction ratio)]. Glomerular filtration is limited if the drug is extensively protein bound, but renal clearance may occur by renal tubular secretion (e.g., furosemide). Some drugs are rapidly extracted and secreted by renal tubular cells such that their clearance approaches renal blood flow. Dose adjustments are necessary for drugs that are eliminated by the kidneys in patients with impaired renal function (digoxin, aminoglycosides, metformin).

Mechanisms and determinants of hepatic drug clearance

Drugs must first be delivered to the eliminating organ through the systemic circulation, such that hepatic blood flow is a determinant of clearance. Clearance across the liver can also be conceptualized with the Fick equation (CL = Q × E). On the basis of empirical observations, Rowland developed a modified equation (CL = Q × f × Cl_{int}/Q + f × Cl_{int}), with limiting cases being CL = Q for highly extracted drugs and CL = f × Cl_{int} for drugs that are poorly extracted by the liver. The term "f" is the fraction of unbound drug in plasma, and "Cl_{int}" (intrinsic clearance) is the maximum clearance rate possible in the absence of flow and protein binding limitations. Highly extracted drugs usually undergo extensive first-pass hepatic metabolism when given orally and are impacted by changes in *liver blood flow* (congestive heart failure, orthostatic hypotension, shock), whereas clearance of poorly extracted drugs is sensitive to both, changes in *extent of protein binding* (displacement of one drug from its protein binding site by an interacting drug or by endogenous substances in uremia, or decreased binding capacity due to hypoalbuminemia secondary to malnutrition, advanced liver disease, or proteinuria), and changes in *intrinsic clearance* (enzyme induction or inhibition, hepatocellular disease). Poorly extracted drugs typically do not undergo first-pass metabolism.

Drug metabolism and transport

Kinetics of drug metabolism

Most drugs used clinically exhibit *apparent first-order kinetics* of elimination (a constant fraction of drug remaining in the body is eliminated per unit time), and drug concentrations in plasma and tissues change in proportion to changes in dose and dosing rate. For drugs that undergo metabolic biotransformation, this implies high enzymatic capacity in the therapeutic range of concentrations. Some drugs (phenytoin, aspirin, alcohol), however, exhibit *saturable kinetics of the Michaelis–Menten type*, resulting in nonlinear changes in plasma– and tissue–drug concentrations with changes in dose. These changes are often associated with dose-related drug toxicity and require cautious dose escalation.

Reactions of drug metabolism

Drug-metabolizing enzymes are found primarily in the liver but also in the intestinal mucosa and the kidney parenchyma, and they catalyze a variety of reactions generally classified as Phase I (oxidation, reduction, hydrolysis, etc.) and Phase II (conjugation with glucuronic acid, acetylation, sulfation, etc.).[6]

Phase I reactions convert lipophilic molecules into more polar molecular entities and thus provide for efficient renal drug elimination. The cytochrome P450 (CYP450) enzyme system is membrane bound in the endoplasmic reticulum and quantitatively represents the major pathway for drug metabolism. Multiple isoenzymes with varying substrate specificity have been characterized (CYP3A, CYP2C, CYP2B, CYP1A, CYP2D, CYP2E, etc.).

Some drugs require active transport into hepatic cells to be available as substrates for CYP enzymes and may also be substrates for transport from the hepatic cell into the bile. CYP isoenzymes are important targets for pharmacokinetic drug interactions because there are many compounds that can either induce (phenobarbital, rifampin, carbamazepine, dexamethasone, phenytoin) or inhibit (omeprazole, erythromycin, ketoconazole, ritonavir, and selective serotonin reuptake inhibitors [SSRIs]: paroxetine, fluoxetine, sertraline) the activity of the CYP450 system (both of a single and/or several isoenzymes) and as a result lead to serious adverse events.

Other enzyme systems are cytoplasmic (soluble, not membrane bound) and involve amine oxidation, alcohol dehydrogenation, and hydrolysis. Additionally, there are multiple specialized drug-transport mechanisms in hepatocytes, such as transporter proteins located in the basolateral (sinusoidal) membrane of hepatocytes (e.g., organic anion transporting polypeptides [OATPs], organic anion transporters [OATs], organic cation transporters [OCTs], prostaglandin transporters [PGTs], and Na^+-taurocholate cotransporting polypeptide [NTCP]) and adenosine triphosphate (ATP)-binding cassette (ABC) transporter proteins in the canalicular membrane of hepatocytes.[6,7] Upregulation (induction) of drug transporters can also occur, as seen with clofibrate-induced upregulation of carnitine transport via the organic cation transporter OCTN2 in liver and small intestine, resulting in increased intestinal absorption of carnitine and higher carnitine concentrations in the liver.[8]

Pharmacogenetics/Genomics

Variant alleles of CYP enzymes and drug transporters (Table 3–1) have been described that have functional consequences and can alter drug elimination rate and hepatic drug clearance.[9] These alleles allow distinction between "poor,"

Table 3–1. Drug-metabolizing enzymes

Affected reaction	Enzyme involved	Drug and therapeutic use	Clinical consequences in poor metabolizers
Oxidation	CYP2D6	Metoprolol (β-adrenoceptor blocker)	Exacerbation of β-blockade, nausea
Oxidation	CYP2D6	Codeine (analgesic)	Reduced analgesia
N-Acetylation	N-Acetyl transferase	Hydralazine (antihypertensive)	Lupus erythematosus-like syndrome
N-Acetylation	N-Acetyl transferase	Isoniazid (antitubercular)	Peripheral neuropathy
Oxidation	CYP2C19	Mephenytoin (antiepileptic)	Overdose toxicity
S-Methylation	Thiopurine methyltransferase	Mercaptopurines (cancer chemotherapeutic)	Myelotoxicity
Oxidation	CYP2D6	Nortriptyline (antidepressant)	Toxicity
O-Demethylation	CYP2C19	Omeprazole (proton pump inhibitor)	Increased therapeutic efficacy
Ester hydrolysis	Plasma cholinesterase	Succinylcholine (neuromuscular blocker)	Prolonged apnea
Oxidation	CYP2C9	S-Warfarin (anticoagulant)	Bleeding
Oxidation	CYP2C9	Tolbutamide (hypoglycemic)	Cardiotoxicity
Oxidation	CYP2D6	Tamoxifen (breast cancer treatment and prevention)	Reduced efficacy with resulting increase in cancer recurrence rates
Glucuronidation	UGT 1A1	Irinotecan (colon cancer treatment)	Severe neutropenia and diarrhea

"extensive," and "ultrarapid" metabolizer phenotypes for some drugs. For example, CYP2D6 poor metabolizers are unable to convert codeine to morphine and do not experience analgesia, whereas CYP2D6 ultrarapid metabolizers treated with codeine generate high levels of morphine with the risk of toxicity in breastfeeding infants. The frequency of these variant alleles varies with the population studied. For example, the prevalence of CYP2D6 poor metabolizers is 8% in white and 1% in black American populations, and a 30% prevalence of CYP2D6 ultrarapid metabolizers is seen in black Ethiopians.[9,10]

Also, there is high prevalence of CYP2C19 poor metabolizers in Asian populations (e.g., omeprazole therapy results in higher cure rates for peptic ulcer disease as a result of increased drug exposure).[11,12]

Variant alleles also have been characterized for conjugating enzymes, such as: N-acetyltransferase (NAT), uridine 5′-diphospho-glucuronosyltransferase (UGT), and thiopurine methyltransferase (TPMT). Both subtherapeutic and toxic drug levels may result from the operation of these variant alleles. Genetically determined quantitative and qualitative changes in receptor function can also contribute to variability in drug response.

Routes of drug elimination

Removal of a drug from the body primarily occurs through the kidneys into the urine, but also through the bile, intestines, and lungs. Drugs can be eliminated in unchanged form (parent drug) or can be converted first to metabolites and then excreted.

Mechanisms and determinants of renal drug elimination

Renal drug elimination involves three distinct processes: glomerular filtration, active tubular secretion, and passive tubular reabsorption. Changes in overall renal function will thus affect the rate of drug elimination.[13]

GFR and plasma protein binding are the main determinants of the amount of filtered drug (i.e., the amount of drug that will enter the tubules). Only unbound drugs can be filtered through the glomeruli, and this process follows first-order kinetics.

The process of *active tubular secretion* takes place in the proximal tubules, is carrier mediated (e.g., involves transporters such as P-glycoprotein and the multidrug-resistance–associated protein type 2 [MRP2]), and follows Michaelis– Menten elimination kinetics.

Passive tubular reabsorption occurs in the distal tubules, where drug is highly concentrated, and if uncharged may leave the tubular lumen and diffuse back into the systemic circulation. Manipulating the pH of the urine will help increase the ionized portion of the drug and minimize back-diffusion ("trapping"), hence increasing drug excretion rate.

DRUG-DOSING REGIMEN – DEPENDENT KINETICS

The discussions in this section assume a single body compartment distribution following administration of the drug.[13,14]

The plateau principle

Under conditions of first-order kinetics of elimination and continuous drug administration at a constant dosing rate, drug concentration in plasma will increase exponentially until reaching a plateau (steady state) at a time when the dosing rate and the elimination rate are equal.[15] The time to reach any fraction of the steady-state concentration can be estimated, and the time to reach 90% of steady state is often estimated as $t_{0.90} = 3.3 \, T_{1/2}$. Therefore, it will take longer to reach the steady-state concentration for drugs with longer $T_{1/2}$ values. Likewise, if the elimination clearance for the drug is impaired by renal or hepatic disease and these result in prolonging the elimination $T_{1/2}$, it will take longer to reach steady state as well with continuous drug administration. The latter scenario may lead to "unexpected" toxicity as drug accumulates over time.

Determinants of steady-state drug concentration

Steady state is achieved when the amount of drug administered per unit time equals the amount of drug eliminated per unit time. The time required to reaching a steady state is solely dependent on the elimination half-life, and independent of the drug's dose, frequency, or route of administration:

$$C_{ss} = R/k_e V_d = R/CL_{(total\ body\ clearance)}$$

where

$\quad\quad\quad C_{ss}$ = steady state,

$\quad\quad\quad R$ = rate of infusion (mg/min or mg/hr),

$\quad\quad\quad k_e$ = first-order elimination rate constant (min^{-1} or hr^{-1}), and

$\quad\quad\quad V_d$ = volume of distribution (L).

From this equation, two main variables that determine steady state can be derived.

- The steady-state concentration is *directly proportional* to the rate of drug infusion (administration) (i.e., faster rate of infusion will not change the time needed to achieve the steady state; it will only affect the steady-state concentration of the drug).
- The steady-state concentration is *inversely proportional* to the clearance of the drug, thus any factor that leads to decreased drug clearance (aging, renal or liver disease) will lead to increased steady-state concentration. With intermittent dosing, peak and trough concentrations will be constant at steady state given an unchanged VD.

Continuous infusion

This dosing regimen implies a constant rate of drug administration and (most often) first-order elimination (i.e., a constant fraction of the drug is eliminated per unit time). As a result, and irrespective of rate of infusion, it will take the same amount of time to reach the steady state. The rate at which the drug will achieve steady state entirely depends on its $T_{1/2}$ and/or factors that influence this parameter. When the infusion is stopped the plasma drug concentration will decline following the same exponential pattern observed in approaching the steady state (Figure 3–2).

Single- and multiple-dose regimens (fixed time interval)

Assuming one body compartment and instantaneous mixing, the *single intravenous bolus* will rapidly achieve maximum plasma concentration, followed by an exponential rate of elimination.

Multiple-dose regimens are more common than single-dose regimens but must take into consideration time-dependent fluctuations of the plasma drug concentration in a dosing interval. Most drugs are given at intervals that are either a fraction or multiple of their plasma $T_{1/2}$, and are eliminated exponentially with time. Although with such intermittent dosing plasma levels oscillate through peaks and troughs, there is net accumulation until, within a dosing interval, the

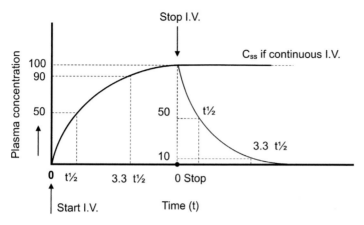

Figure 3–2: Model of attainment of C_{ss} with continuous intravenous (I.V.) dosing and the washout phase after stopping the infusion.

rate of drug elimination balances the rate of drug administration, at which point a steady state has been achieved (Figure 3–3).

When designing a rational dosage regimen, it is crucial to consider the pharmacokinetic variables that determine the dose–concentration relationship, such as dosing frequency, loading and maintenance doses, and individual drug-elimination parameters (e.g., clearance).

GENERAL PRINCIPLES OF PHARMACODYNAMICS

Effective pharmacologic therapy requires delivery of drugs to their site of action. Drugs typically interact with specific receptors (macromolecules) at the cell

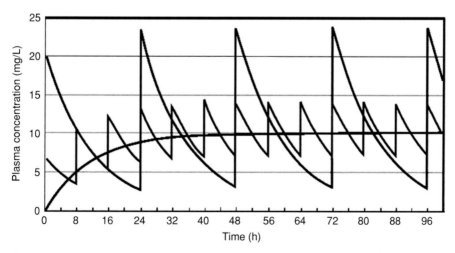

Figure 3–3: Relationship between frequency of dosing and maximum and minimum plasma concentrations when a steady-state theophylline plasma level of 10 mg/L is desired. The smoothly rising black line shows the plasma concentration achieved with an intravenous infusion of 28 mg/h. The doses for 8-hourly administration (lower-intensity peaks and troughs) are 224 mg; for 24-hourly administration (higher-intensity peaks and troughs), 672 mg. In each of the three cases, the mean steady-state plasma concentration is 10 mg/L.

surface or intracellularly (cytoplasm, nucleus, organelles). When activated, these receptors elicit signal transduction and the pharmacological effect through alterations of cell, tissue, and organ functions. Drugs can also interact with soluble and membrane-bound enzymes in critical biochemical pathways such that the pharmacological effect results from enzyme inhibition. Indirectly, drugs can also increase enzymatic activity (enzyme induction).

Drug–receptor interactions

Drugs bind to their receptors reversibly with variable affinity and kinetics according to mass action. Binding alone, however, does not elicit a pharmacological response. Thus, we distinguish between pharmacological agonists, partial agonists, and antagonists (blockers) depending on the intrinsic activity of the compound (Figure 3–4). An agonist has affinity for binding and can elicit the maximal intensity of the pharmacological effect as the drug concentration is increased. A partial agonist binds the receptor but elicits only a partial response (the effect plateaus at a lower intensity) and can act as an antagonist in the presence of a full agonist. An antagonist binds to the receptor but does not elicit a pharmacological response while it prevents the access of an agonist to the receptor-binding site. A pure antagonist has no intrinsic pharmacological activity. Some antagonists bind a site different from the agonist-binding site but can elicit a conformational change in the receptor such that the binding of the agonist is impaired (allosteric inhibition). There are also examples of agonists and antagonists that bind irreversibly (covalently) to the receptor sites. When this is the case, an agonist can act only when new receptors are synthesized by the target cells.

Dose–response relationship

The concept of a dose– (or concentration–) response relationship is central to pharmacology. It signifies that the intensity of the pharmacological effect varies with the dose (amount of drug administered) or, more specifically, with the concentration of drug in the immediate vicinity of the target receptor population. The same concept applies when dealing with the adverse effects of drugs, either as an extension of the primary pharmacological effect or due to interactions with other receptor populations that mediate the adverse effects and/or toxicity.

The relationship between drug concentration and effect intensity is usually log linear, and the graded concentration–response relationship has a sigmoid shape. The plateau of this curve defines the drug *efficacy* (Figure 3–4). Pharmacologically, efficacy is defined by the maximal intensity (plateau) of the effect of a given agonist. (In a therapeutic context, the efficacy of a drug is defined in comparison with a placebo or another active agent in terms of the degree of change in a clinical endpoint.) Two or more drugs in the same class may differ in potency but have parallel concentration–response curves that reach the same plateau of effect and thus have the same pharmacological efficacy. A competitive antagonist will shift the concentration–response curve to the right, but if enough agonist

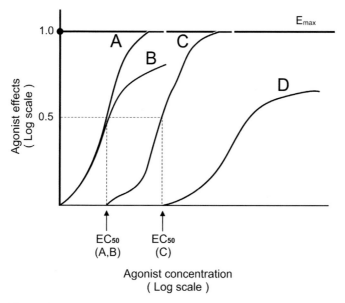

Figure 3–4: Logarithmic transformation of the dose axis. **Curve A** shows agonist response in the absence of antagonist. Treatment with partial agonist (**curve B**) will not change the value of EC_{50} (median effective concentration), but the maximum response (E_{max}) will not be reached. After adding a competitive antagonist (**curve C**), the curve is shifted to the right and maximal responsiveness is preserved. An irreversible antagonist (**curve D**) causes both a shift to the right and a reduction in E_{max}.

is present the maximal effect intensity can still be achieved. A noncompetitive (irreversible) antagonist may cause both a shift to the right and a lower plateau for the agonist's concentration–response curve.

Synergism, antagonism, and tolerance

One drug may enhance the pharmacological effect of another by a variety of mechanisms. If the resulting effect is more than additive, the drugs are said to be synergistic. As described earlier in this chapter, one drug may antagonize the effect of another by blocking access to a receptor population but also by eliciting an opposite physiological response. Repeated administration of an agonist may result in tolerance, such that increasing doses of the drug are required to obtain a similar effect intensity (opioid analgesics, nitrates). If tolerance develops over a short time period, it is termed *tachyphylaxis* (tyramine).

CLINICAL DRUG DEVELOPMENT

Phase I (safety and pharmacokinetics) and Phase II (efficacy and proof of concept) studies in the clinical stage of drug development are part of the learning phase that ideally defines the target clinical population and the dose or dose range to be used in Phase III randomized, controlled clinical trials in the confirming phase of the learn and confirm paradigm of drug development. Safety continues to be evaluated throughout and includes postmarketing surveillance (Phase IV) after FDA approval and marketing.

How to estimate the first-in-human (FIH) drug dose

The traditional approach, commonly used in oncology, is to start at one-tenth of mouse LD10 (lethal dose in 10% of treated mice),[16] because empirical observations have shown that the mouse LD10 is approximately equivalent to the maximal tolerated dose (MTD) in humans. Other approaches based on estimations of equivalent drug exposure (AUC) in several animal species may be more predictive, however.

Dose-escalation schemes

The goals of Phase I clinical trials are to determine MTD, toxicity profile, safety limits, pharmacokinetics for the drug and, based on these parameters, recommend Phase II dose levels.[17] Several drug escalation schemes have been developed for these purposes.

Fibonacci scheme

The most frequently used scheme for more than two decades was derived from the original Fibonacci number sequence and is referred to as the *Modified Fibonacci Search*.[18]

The fundamental principle of this dose–escalation scheme is to provide *decreasing increases* (2n, 3.3n, 5n, 7n, 9n, 12n, 16n) as multiples of the initial dose (n), which translates into a percent increase over the previous dose (100%, 65%, 52%, 40%, 29%, 33%, and 33%, respectively). The major limitation of this scheme is the fact that it takes too long and too many patients to determine the Phase II dose.

Pharmacologically guided dose escalation scheme

This approach bridges preclinical and clinical development and is based on both the PK/PD hypothesis ("When comparing animal and human doses, expect equal toxicity for equal drug exposure")[19] and the fundamental pharmacological principle that drug effects are caused by the circulating concentrations of the free (unbound) drug molecules. As a result, an alternative to the fixed dose escalation scheme was developed in which the magnitude of each dose-escalation step is based on two variables (Figure 3–5): (1) current concentration of the drug measured in human blood and (2) target concentrations established in preclinical (animal) studies (e.g., MTD in mice).

The advantages of the pharmacologically guided dose escalation (PGDE) scheme lies in the fact that the dose escalation is modified (adjusted) throughout the study and thus it substantially decreases the number of patients at risk and hastens the time to identifying the appropriate Phase II dose.

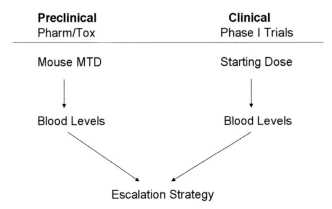

Figure 3–5: Bridge between preclinical and clinical development: Pharmacologically guided dose escalation (adapted from Jerry M. Collins: Phase I Clinical Studies; AJ Atkinson Jr., DR Abernethy, CE Daniels, RL Dedrick, SP Markey. *Principles of Clinical Pharmacology*, 2nd edition (2007), Academic Press; Burlington, MA; pp. 473–478).

Other methods used are *statistically based methods* (e.g., Escalation With Overdose Control [EWOC] and the modified Continual Reassessment Method [CRM]).[20]

Exploratory trials with "nonpharmacological" doses

Minimal drug-exposure trials geared at comparing the pharmacokinetic profile of several candidate lead compounds have recently been designated as Phase "0" trials as a reference to the exploratory, first-in human trials conducted in accordance with the FDA 2006 Guidance on Exploratory Investigational New Drug (IND) Studies.[21,22] They are also referred to as "microdosing" studies, and their purpose is to accelerate the development of compounds that have shown promising results during the preclinical development through establishing very early if the compound of interest behaves in human subjects as expected from preclinical studies.

Phase "0" trials involve a small number of human subjects (10–15) and are characterized by administration of subtherapeutic doses to collect preliminary data pertinent to PK/PD properties of the investigated compound(s) and do not address safety or efficacy because the dose is too low to have any therapeutic effect. Yet, the preliminary data that a Phase "0" trial produces aids the "go/no go" decision-making process and the ranking of candidate drugs.

Biomarkers in drug development

Clinical biomarkers have increasingly proven invaluable in clinical drug development as it has been shown that their use reduces the attrition of new drugs, thereby decreasing the overall cost of drug development.[23]

The value of biomarkers is that they can reveal drug targets and optimize the selection of molecules that interact with these targets for further development. These applications can accelerate the progression from Phase I to Phase II studies and possibly be more predictive of drugs' success during Phase III trials.

Use of positron emission tomography scanning in human pharmacology

In the past few years there has been an increased utilization of positron emission tomography (PET) scanning in the process of drug development. PET is a noninvasive tool that has enabled us to study drug distribution, drug–target interactions (e.g., receptor occupancy), and disease process/progression, and it has proven particularly useful in studies of underlying disease processes affecting the central nervous system (CNS) and in the field of oncology.

Longitudinal PET studies can certainly facilitate the selection of both the drug candidate and its dose, as well provide a tool for decision making ("go–no go" and "proof of concept").[24] Moreover, these studies can help elucidate underlying pathophysiologies of the studied entity (target disease), follow its progression, and monitor the outcomes of treatment. Finally, a combination of genomic knowledge with PET imaging will certainly lead to identifying more specific phenotypes, which in turn will help identify genetic (molecular) predictors of drug response.[25]

CLINICAL APPROACH

In clinical practice, therapy is best individualized to minimize toxicity and maximize the likelihood of therapeutic benefit, and these depend on the conceptual understanding and application of principles of PK/PD at the bedside. Individual variation in drug response should be expected based on both environmental and genetic determinants that impact drug metabolism, transport, and the effect of drugs at the target receptor population. Dose adjustments should be implemented accordingly, with attention to organ clearance mechanisms in patients with compromised renal and hepatic function. Chronic renal failure (CRF) can also lead to alterations in drug metabolism and transport, such that drugs not primarily eliminated via the kidneys may also require dose adjustments in this patient population.[26] For example, CYP2C9, UGT2B7 (glucuronosyltransferase), and NAT-2 (N-acetyltransferase) activity is reduced in CRF, potentially increasing the plasma levels and effects of warfarin, morphine, and isoniazid due to decreased metabolic clearance.

The *Cockroft–Gault* (CG) equation:

$$\text{GFR (mL/min)} = (140 - \text{age}) * \text{weight (kg)}/[72 * \text{SCr (mg/dL)} * (0.85 \text{ if female})]$$

is commonly employed for estimation of creatinine clearance and to guide dose adjustments.[27] Other equations, such as the Modification of Diet in Renal Disease

(MDRD) Study equation, have been proposed to estimate GFR. Although the MDRD Study equation is reportedly more accurate, it is not without bias and does not perform well at higher levels of GFR. Both equations apply under conditions of stable renal function and should not be used in patients with acute renal failure. The MDRD equation has not been validated in elderly subjects (older than 70 years). Advanced renal disease and uremia may also result in impaired metabolic (nonrenal) clearance of drugs and impaired drug transport. Finally, these equations are not suited for estimating GFR in children. For that purpose, several formulae have been developed, such as the Schwartz equation, which utilizes the proportionality between GFR and height/serum creatinine[28] and thus provides clinically useful estimates of GFR.

The Schwartz equation is

$$\text{GFR (mL/min/1.73m}^2) = k * \text{Height (cm) / Serum Cr (mg/dL)},$$

where k = constant with the following values:

k = 0.33 in preterm infants,
k = 0.45 in term infants up to one year old,
k = 0.55 in children from 1 to 13 years old, and
k = 0.70 in adolescent males (not females because of the presumed increase in male muscle mass; the constant remains 0.55 for females).

Developmental changes in body fluid compartments, hepatic drug metabolism, and renal excretory mechanisms should be considered in the pediatric patient population (all depicted in Table 3–2).[30]

As discussed previously in this chapter, factors that impact drug distribution include protein binding and body composition, especially water and fat content among others. These factors are highly age dependent, thus warranting careful adjustments in drug administration regimens (e.g., highly protein bound drugs [promethazine] or water-soluble drugs [sulfisoxazole]).

The capacity of the liver to metabolize drugs is lower at birth and has a different degree of maturation of the respective metabolizing pathways postnatally. Moreover, this development can be affected by drugs both *in utero* and in the postnatal period.

As a result, drug metabolism may differ in both its degree of development and type of primary metabolic pathways during various stages of postnatal growth and development (e.g., glucuronide conjugation is very low at birth and reaches adult levels by age three, whereas sulfate conjugation is active *in utero* and in infancy, but declines with age [acetaminophen metabolism]).[30]

Kidneys are anatomically and functionally immature at birth with very low corresponding GFR (5–10 mL/min/m^2 in premature infants, 10–15 mL/min/m^2 in term infants) and a functional glomerular/tubular imbalance, both of which greatly delay the renal clearance process, thus warranting careful dose reductions in these populations. Renal excretion rate becomes comparable to that of older children by age 8–12 months and may even exceed that of adults.[30]

Table 3–2. Important pharmacokinetics parameters in respective pediatric populations

FDA stratification (29)	Body composition as percentage of TBW* (30)	Distribution volume L/kg (e.g., sulfisoxazole) (30)	Metabolism (CYP450 selective liver expression of isoforms) (30)	Renal clearance of zidovudine (mL/min/kg) (30)
Preterm newborn infant	ECF 60% ICF 25% Protein 10% Fat < 5%	N/A	N/A	2.5–4.4 (5.5. days to 17.7 days of age, respectively)
Term newborn infant (0–27d)	ECF ~ 40% ICF ~ 40% Protein ~10% Fat ~ 15%	~0.5 L/kg	CYP4A CYP3A7	10.9–19 (14 days of age)
Infants and toddlers (28 d–23 mo)	ECF ~ 30% ICF ~ 30% Protein ~ 15% Fat ~ 25%	~0.375 L/kg	CYP1A2 CYP3A4	24 (after the first year of life)
Children (2–11 y)	ECF ~ 20% ICF ~ 40% Protein ~ 20% Fat ~ 20%	~0.2 L/kg	CYP2D6 CYP2E1 CYP3A4 CYP1A2	24 (1–13 years old)
Adolescents (12–16 y)	ECF ~ 20% ICF ~ 40% Protein ~ 20% Fat ~ 15%		*Same as adult population	21 (values as in adult population)
Adult population	ECF ~ 20% ICF ~ 40% Protein ~ 20% Fat ~ 15%	~0.25 L/kg	CYP4A CYP2D6 CYP2E1 CYP3A5 CYP3A4 CYP2C CYP1A2	21

* TBW: total body weight; ECF: extracellular fluid; ICF: intracellular fluid; N/A: not applicable.

Another important factor affecting pharmacokinetic variables in children is their larger organ size (e.g., kidneys, liver, and CNS) relative to their body surface area (as compared to that of adults), which in turn requires careful dose adjustments (e.g., methotrexate and its cerebrospinal fluid concentrations).[30]

REFERENCES

1. Thummel KE. Gut instincts: CYP3A4 and intestinal drug metabolism. *J Clin Invest.* 2007;117:3176–3179
2. Food and Drug Administration (FDA). (March, 2003). Bioavailability and bioequivalence studies for orally administered drug products – General considerations. Rockville, MD: FDA. http://www.fda.gov/downloads/Drugs/GuidanceComplianceRegulatory Information/Guidances/ucm070124.pdf (Last accessed August 13, 2009)

3. Ganapathy V, Prasad PD, Ganapathy ME, Leibach FH. Placental transporters relevant to drug distribution across the maternal–fetal interface perspectives in pharmacology. *J Pharmacol Exp Ther*. 2000;294:413–420

4. Ambudkar SV, Dey S, Hrycyna CA, Ramachandra M, Pastan I, Gottesman MM. Biochemical, cellular, and pharmacological aspects of the multidrug transporter. *Annu Rev Pharmacol Toxicol*. 1999;39:361–398

5. Arthur J. Atkinson, Jr. Clinical pharmacokinetics. AJ Atkinson Jr., DR Abernethy, CE Daniels, RL Dedrick, SP Markey. *Principles of Clinical Pharmacology, Second Edition* (2007), Academic Press; Burlington, MA; p. 11–23

6. Gonzalez Frank J, Tukey Robert H. Drug metabolism. LL Brunton, JS Lazo, KL Parker. *Goodman & Gilman's The Pharmacological Basis of Therapeutics, 11e.* (2006), McGraw Hill; New York; p. 71–91

7. Jones PM, George AM. The ABC transporter structure and mechanism: Perspectives on recent research. *Cell Mol Life Sci*. 2004;61(6):682–699

8. Ringseis R, Posel S, Hirche F, Eder K. Treatment with pharmacological peroxisome proliferator-activator receptor alpha agonist clofibrate causes upregulation of organic cation transporter 2 in liver and small intestine of rats. *Pharmacol Res*. 2007;56:175–183

9. Flockhart DA, Bertilsson L. Clinical pharmacogenetics. AJ Atkinson Jr., DR Abernethy, CE Daniels, RL Dedrick, SP Markey. *Principles of Clinical Pharmacology*, 2nd edition (2007), Academic Press; Burlington, MA; p. 179–195

10. Aklillu E, Persson I, Bertilsson L, Johansson I, Rodrigues F, Ingelman-Sundberg M. Frequent distribution of ultrarapid metabolizers of debrisoquine in an Ethiopian population carrying duplicated and multiduplicated functional CYP2D6 alleles. *J Pharmacol Exp Ther*. 1996;278(1):441–446

11. Wang JH, Li PQ, Fu QY, Li QX, Cai WW. Cyp2c19 genotype and omeprazole hydroxylation phenotype in Chinese Li population. *Clin Exp Pharmacol Physiol*. 2007;34(5–6):421–424

12. Desta Z, Zhao X, Shin JG, Flockhart DA. Clinical significance of the cytochrome P450 2C19 genetic polymorphism. *Clin Pharmacokinet*. 2002;41:913–958

13. Holford Nicholas H, "Chapter 3. Pharmacokinetics & Pharmacodynamics: Rational Dosing & the Time Course of Drug Action" (Chapter). *Katzung BG: Basic & Clinical Pharmacology*, 11th edition: http://www.accessmedicine.com/content.aspx?aID=4513158.

14. Buxton I.L.O. Pharmacokinetics and pharmacodynamics: The dynamics of drug absorption, distribution, action, and elimination. LL Brunton, JS Lazo, KL Parker. *Goodman & Gilman's The Pharmacological Basis of Therapeutics*, 11th edition., (2006), McGraw Hill; New York; p. 1–39

15. Atkinson AJ Jr. Clinical pharmacokinetics. AJ Atkinson Jr., DR Abernethy, CE Daniels, RL Dedrick, SP Markey. *Principles of Clinical Pharmacology*, 2nd edition (2007), Academic Press; Burlington, MA; p. 11–23

16. Collins JM. Phase I clinical studies. AJ Atkinson Jr., DR Abernethy, CE Daniels, RL Dedrick, SP Markey. *Principles of Clinical Pharmacology*, 2nd edition (2007), Academic Press; Burlington, MA; p. 473–478

17. Food and Drug Administration (FDA). (July, 2005). Estimating the Maximum Safe Starting Dose in Initial Clinical Trials for Therapeutics in Adult Healthy Volunteers. Rockville (MD): FDA. Last accessed August 13, 2009, from: http://www.fda.gov/downloads/Drugs/GuidanceComplianceRegulatoryInformation/Guidances/ucm078932.pdf

18. Omura GA. Modified Fibonacci search. *J Clin Oncol*. 2003;21:3177

19. Collins JM, Zaharko DS, Dedrick RL, Chabner BA. Potential roles for preclinical pharmacology in phase I clinical trials. *Cancer Treat Rep*. 1986;70(1):73–80

20. Eisenhauer EA, O'Dwyer PJ, Christian M, Humphrey JS. Phase I clinical trial design in cancer drug development. *J Clin Oncol*. 2000;18:684–692

21. Food and Drug Administration (FDA). (January, 2006). Exploratory IND Studies. Rockville (MD): FDA. Last accessed August 13, 2009, from: http://www.fda.

gov/downloads/Drugs/GuidanceComplianceRegulatoryInformation/Guidances/ucm078933.pdf

22. Collins JM. Phase 0 clinical studies in oncology. *Clin Pharmacol Ther.* 2009;85:204–207

23. Woodcock J. Chutes and ladders on the critical path: Comparative effectiveness, product value, and the use of biomarkers in drug development. *Clin Pharmacol Ther.* 2009;86:12–14

24. Uppoor RS, Mummaneni P, Cooper E, Pien HH, Sorensen AG, Collins J, Mehta MU, Yasuda SU. The use of imaging in the early development of neuropharmacological drugs: A survey of approved NDAs. *Clin Pharmacol Ther.* 2008;84:69–74

25. Collins JM. Imaging and other biomarkers in early clinical studies: One step at a time or re-engineering drug development? *J Clin Oncol.* 2005;23:5417–5419

26. Dreisbach AW, Lertora JJL. The effect of chronic renal failure on drug metabolism and transport. *Expert Opin Drug Metab Toxicol.* 2008;4:1065–1074

27. National Kidney Foundation. KDOQI Clinical Practice Guidelines for Chronic Kidney Disease: Evaluation, Classification, and Stratification. Last accessed August 13, 2009, from: http://www.kidney.org/professionals/kdoqi/guidelines_ckd/p5_lab_g4.htm

28. National Kidney Disease Education Program: GFR Calculators for Children. Last accessed August 13, 2009, from: http://www.nkdep.nih.gov/professionals/gfr_calculators/gfr_children.htm

29. Food and Drug Administration (FDA). (November, 1998). Guidance for Industry: General Considerations for Pediatric Pharmacokinetic Studies for Drugs and Biological Products. Rockville (MD): FDA. Last accessed August 13, 2009, from: http://www.fda.gov/downloads/Drugs/GuidanceComplianceRegulatoryInformation/Guidances/ucm072114.pdf

30. Fox E, Balis FM. Drug therapy in neonates and pediatric patients. AJ Atkinson Jr., DR Abernethy, CE Daniels, RL Dedrick, SP Markey. *Principles of Clinical Pharmacology*, 2nd edition (2007), Academic Press; Burlington, MA; p. 359–373

SECTION II
COFACTORS

4 Biotin and biotin-responsive disorders

Kirit Pindolia and Barry Wolf

OVERVIEW OF THE BIOTIN CYCLE AND BIOTIN-RESPONSIVE DISORDERS

In 1971, a child with a deficiency of β-methylcrotonyl-coenzyme A (COA) carboxylase (MCC), a biotin-dependent enzyme, was described who improved clinically and metabolically following administration of the water-soluble B vitamin, biotin. Individuals who improved with biotin therapy were considered biotin-responsive. Further study revealed that this child also had deficient activity of propionyl-CoA carboxylase (PCC), another biotin-dependent carboxylase. Subsequently, other children were reported who had biochemical profiles consistent with deficiencies of all three mitochondrial carboxylases – PCC, MCC, and pyruvate carboxylase (PC) – or multiple carboxylase deficiency (MCD). All children with MCD have improved when treated with pharmacological doses of biotin.[1] These biotin-responsive MCD disorders were subsequently classified into three groups based on their underlying genetic defects: biotin holocarboxylase synthetase (HCS) deficiency (Online Mendelian Inheritance in Man [OMIM] 253260), biotinidase deficiency (OMIM 253260), and, most recently, biotin-responsive basal ganglia disease (OMIM 607483).

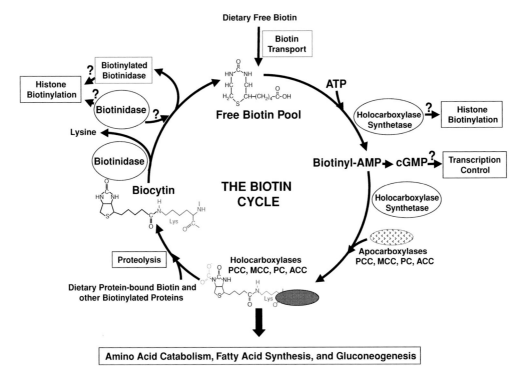

Figure 4–1: The biotin cycle: known and putative pathways involving biotin. Dietary free biotin enters the free biotin pool via biotin transport. After biotin is transported in the cell, HCS can attach biotin (two-step reaction) to inactive apocarboxylases forming active holocarboxylases. The holocarboxylases can subsequently participate in amino acid catabolism, fatty acid synthesis, and gluconeogenesis. HCS can biotinylate histones and possibly participate in the cGMP-mediated signaling pathway. Biotin may have a role in transcription regulation. Biotinidase releases biotin from biocytin or proteolytically degraded holocarboxylases and biotin-bound dietary peptides. The released biotin can recycle to the free biotin pool. Biotinidase may posttranslationally modify histones by biotinylating them in the presence of biocytin and removing biotin from histones.

To gain a better understanding of these biotin-responsive disorders, it is important to consider the metabolism of biotin.[2] Humans cannot synthesize biotin. Although biotin is widely found in the diet, it is not readily found in the free, unbound form. As shown in Figure 4–1, only free biotin, not bound to protein or other moieties, enters the biotin pool through intestinal absorption. Although biotin is synthesized by flora in the large intestine, it does not contribute to the biotin pool because the usual site of absorption of biotin is in the sterile duodenum.

Cells use one or more mechanisms to transport biotin from the extracellular biotin pool into the cytosol.[3] These mechanisms include both active and passive transport in addition to carrier protein–mediated pinocytosis. Upon free biotin translocation into the cells, HCS converts inactive apocarboxylases into functionally active holocarboxylases by covalently attaching biotin to ε-amino groups of specific lysyl residues of each of the four biotin-requiring carboxylases (see Figure 4–1). Biotinylation of apocarboxylases proceeds in a two-step reaction. In the first step, biotin is activated to 5′-biotinyl adenosine monophos-phate (5′-biotinyl-AMP), and in the second step, the biotin moiety from 5′-biotinyl-AMP gets transferred to the biotin-binding domain of the carboxy-lases.[1,4] These holocarboxylases have important roles in gluconeogenesis, fatty acid synthesis, and the catabolism of several branched-chain amino acids and odd-chain fatty acids. PC converts pyruvate to oxaloacetate, the initial step in gluconeogenesis. PCC catabolizes several branched-chain amino acids and odd-chain fatty acids, whereas MCC is involved in the catabolism of leucine. The fourth carboxylase, acetyl-CoA carboxylase (ACC), converts malonyl-CoA to acetyl-CoA, the first step in the biosynthesis of fatty acids. PCC, MCC, and PC are located in the mitochondria, whereas ACC is located mainly in the cytosol and to a lesser extent in mitochondria.

Holocarboxylases and other biotinylated proteins are proteolytically degraded to biotinylated peptides and biocytin (biotinyl-ε-N-lysine) (see Figure 4–1). These biotinylated peptides and biocytin are subsequently cleaved by biotinidase to free biotin, thereby recycling the vitamin.[1,5] In addition, the proximal tubular epithelia of the kidneys reabsorb some excreted biotin and return it to the body's free biotin pool.

Clinical presentation

There is considerable variation and overlap in the clinical findings of children with the various biotin-responsive disorders.[1] Because untreated children with HCS deficiency usually exhibit symptoms in the neonatal period, the disorder was initially known as early-onset or neonatal MCD. Children with biotinidase deficiency usually did not show symptoms until several months of age, some not until adolescence; therefore, the disorder was known as late-onset or juvenile MCD. However the age of onset of symptoms became less important in discrim-inating the two disorders after the determination that biotinidase deficiency was responsible for causing the late-onset MCD. Individuals with biotin-responsive basal ganglia disease defects usually first become symptomatic when they are several years old.[6,7]

Biotin HCS deficiency
Untreated, children with HCS deficiency usually exhibit breathing abnormal-ities, such as tachypnea, hyperventilation, and apnea. Many children present with feeding difficulties, including continuous vomiting. Neurological problems in these children include irritability, lethargy, hypotonia or hypertonia, and seizures. Some develop skin rashes and complete or partial alopecia. Essentially all affected children have metabolic ketoacidosis, organic aciduria, and hyper-ammonemia, and some will have thrombocytopenia. In rare cases children may exhibit developmental delay and may ultimately become comatose and die if not treated in a timely manner. Most children with HCS deficiency respond well to biotin supplementation, but a small number require a higher dose of the vitamin and still fail to entirely resolve their metabolic abnormalities.[1,8]

Biotinidase deficiency

Similar to children with HCS deficiency, untreated children with biotinidase deficiency usually exhibit breathing abnormalities, such as hyperventilation, stridor, and apnea. Common neurological symptoms include seizures, hypotonia, lethargy, ataxia, hearing loss, optic atrophy, and loss of vision.[9] Skin rash and alopecia are also common. Some affected children have defective cellular immunity manifested by episodes of fungal infection. Developmental delay is a problem only in those children who were not ascertained and treated early. Most untreated children will ultimately exhibit metabolic acidosis, organic aciduria, and mild hyperammonemia. Most of the symptoms can be reversed or ameliorated, and essentially all of the metabolic abnormalities will resolve with biotin therapy, whereas the hearing loss, optic atrophy, and developmental delay are frequently irreversible. Adolescents with biotinidase deficiency usually exhibit different clinical features, including sudden loss of vision (scotomas) with progressive optic neuropathy and spastic paresis.

Biotin-responsive basal ganglia diseases

Untreated individuals with biotin-responsive basal ganglia disease usually exhibit neurological symptoms, including subacute encephalopathy, confusion, dysarthria, dysphagia, and sometimes supranuclear facial nerve palsy and/or external ophthalmoplegia.[6,7] If untreated, the symptoms can progress to severe cogwheel rigidity, dystonia, and quadriparesis. Residual paresis, mild mental retardation, or dystonia is seen in the individuals whose diagnosis and treatment are delayed. Fortunately, the majority of symptoms disappear within a few days after biotin treatment is begun; however, some patients may continue to have residual paresis, mild mental retardation, or dystonia.

Pathophysiology

Acquired biotin deficiency is rare. It may occur if an individual ingests large quantities of avidin, an egg white protein that strongly binds biotin. Prolonged total or near total intravenous feedings that lack biotin can also cause biotin deficiency. Secondary biotin deficiency can occur in biotinidase deficiency (but not in HCS deficiency) due to failure to recycle the vitamin. Defective biotin transport in biotin-responsive basal ganglia disease causes cellular biotin deficiency and its unavailability for cellular functions.

Biotin deficiency, biotinidase deficiency, and HCS deficiency can all alter the function of the carboxylases that subsequently results in organic acidemia/uria and metabolic acidosis.[10,11] These metabolites likely interfere with other biochemical pathways and may adversely affect immune and neurological functions.

Untreated children with HCS and biotinidase deficiencies usually have elevated concentrations of β-hydroxyisovalerate, β-methylcrotonylglycine, β-hydroxypropionate, methylcitrate, and/or lactate in serum and urine. Considerable variability in the expression of the diseases has been observed, however, even within the same family. Therefore, the absence of organic aciduria or metabolic ketoacidosis, especially in symptomatic children with biotinidase deficiency, should not be considered an absolute criterion to exclude the disorder.

Untreated children with biotinidase deficiency can have serum biotin concentrations that are low, whereas their biocytin concentrations are elevated. These determinations are impractical and expensive, and interpretation is dependent on the method of analyte determination used. In HCS deficiency, however, the serum biotin and biocytin concentrations are in the normal ranges. Although the determination of biotin concentrations may be used to assess compliance with treatment, measuring biotin and/or biocytin is of little clinical value.

Biotinidase activity in cerebrospinal fluid and in the brain is low suggesting that the brain is not capable of recycling biotin and, therefore, must depend on biotin that is transported across the blood–brain barrier, as implicated in biotin-responsive basal ganglia disease. Supportive evidence also comes from several symptomatic children with biotinidase deficiency who had elevations of organic acids and lactate in their cerebrospinal fluid but did not have these metabolites in their blood or urine. This compartmentalization of the biochemical abnormalities may explain why neurological symptoms usually occur first.

Brain imaging performed on several affected children with HCS and biotinidase deficiencies reveals a broad range of abnormal findings.[12,13] In HCS deficiency, these findings include diffuse cerebral atrophy with or without low attenuation of the white matter, basal ganglia calcifications, cerebral edema, subacute necrotizing encephalopathy, enlargement of the ventricles, and even cysts. Brain studies of children with biotinidase deficiency reveal cerebral degeneration and atrophy. Gliosis of the white matter and dentate nucleus is seen, but the brainstem and cerebral peduncles are normal. Defective myelination has been noted in some children. Brain-imaging studies of individuals with basal ganglia disease may show variable abnormalities of the brain, such as bilateral necroses in the central part of the caudate heads with partial or complete involvement of putamen and white matter edema during acute crisis.

The hearing loss in biotinidase deficiency is usually irreversible, although several young, affected children have shown some improvement with therapy.[14] Biotin therapy appears to stop further hearing loss. The precise mechanism causing the hearing loss and alopecia still remains elusive.

Immunological abnormalities vary among children with HCS and biotinidase deficiencies and are absent in individuals with basal ganglia disorders. This variation may be due to the effects of abnormal organic acid metabolites or low concentrations of biotin on immune cell proliferation. Specific organic acids may have toxic effects on both T- and B-lymphocyte functions affecting the innate and adaptive immune system.

As shown in Figure 4–1, biotin may have a role in regulating gene transcription and translation on a cellular level. Biotinylation of histones has also been proposed as one of several posttranslational histone modifications, collectively called histone codes, thereby causing epigenetic changes due to chromatin structural changes.[15,16] HCS has been shown to biotinylate various histones, acting as a histone code writer. Biotinidase, as a biotin transferase, may transfer biotin from biocytin, thereby biotinylating histones. Also, biotinidase may remove the biotin from histones, erasing the biotin code.

In addition, biotin has been shown to enhance cyclic guanosine monophosphate (cGMP) activity, thereby modifying cell-cycle regulation. Biotinylated-AMP, which is generated by HCS, is also proposed to play an important role in the activation of a nuclear signal transduction cascade, which involves guanylate cyclase and cGMP and regulates the gene expression of sodium-dependent multivitamin transporter (SMVT), HCS, PC, PCC, MCC, and ACC. Future investigations in this area may help to explain the neurocutaneous pathology in children with biotin-responsive disorders.

Newborn-screening programs to ascertain children with inherited metabolic disorders have been instrumental in identifying presymptomatic children with various enzyme deficiencies. Biotin-responsive MCDs, especially biotinidase deficiency, meet the major criteria for inclusion in such screening programs, particularly because of the simple and effective treatment and the inexpensive method of screening. A colorimetric assay for determining biotinidase activity in the same blood spots on filter-soaked cards used for other newborn-screening tests was developed and is being used by most screening programs. Although HCS deficiency may be identified by finding the characteristic metabolites of the disorder in blood, it likely will not identify all enzyme-deficient children. Often it is the metabolic acidosis and organic aciduria in the symptomatic child that lead to the diagnosis of HCS deficiency. Unfortunately, there are likely no metabolic abnormalities in newborns that can be used to identify children with basal ganglion disorders.

Molecular genetics and inheritance

HCS deficiency is inherited as an autosomal recessive trait. The HCS gene has been mapped to chromosome 21q22.1. Enzyme-activity analyses in many children with HCS deficiency have revealed elevated K_m values for biotin, ranging from 3 to 70 times that of the normal value. The age of onset of symptoms in these children correlates negatively with the K_m values for biotin. Although HCS activity usually increases to normal or near normal after biotin treatment, in several children with HCS deficiency the carboxylase activities increased to only half the lower normal range with as much as 200 milligrams of biotin per day. Children with HCS deficiency and altered K_m values readily respond to biotin therapy, whereas those with normal K_m values respond to biotin to a lesser extent.

Multiple mutations have been identified in the HCS gene that can cause HCS deficiency.[17] Enzyme activity in Japanese children with various mutations is severely affected in comparison to that in non-Japanese children. Many of the mutations are localized within the HCS biotin-binding domain. Mutations within the biotin-binding region of the enzyme result in an enzyme with increased K_m values of biotin, whereas those outside of this region result in enzymes with normal K_m values, but with reduced V_{max} values. Children with mutations in the N-terminal region, outside the biotin-binding domain, show severe clinical phenotype and partial responsiveness to biotin supplementation. Differences in the stability of the mutant enzymes suggest biochemical heterogeneity for the disorder. The 780delG, L237P, and 665insA mutations are unique to Japanese children, whereas the R508W, G581S, and V550M mutations are found in both Japanese and non-Japanese populations. Mutation analyses of children with this disorder may be useful in predicting phenotype.

Biotinidase deficiency is inherited as an autosomal recessive trait. The biotinidase gene maps to human chromosome location 3p25. Individuals with profound biotinidase deficiency have less than 10% of mean normal activity in serum, and individuals with partial deficiency have between 10 and 30% activity. Multiple mutations have been described in symptomatic children and in those with profound biotinidase deficiency identified by newborn screening.[18] When mutations among children identified by newborn screening were compared with those of children ascertained by exhibiting symptoms, four mutations comprised approximately 60% of the abnormal alleles. Two of the most common mutations in symptomatic children are the deletion/insertion mutation, G98del3ins7, and the missense R538C. Two other missense mutations; Q456H and A171T:D444H (the compound allelic missense mutation) are commonly seen in children with profound biotinidase deficiency identified by newborn screening. The most common mutation, D444H, results in a 50% decrease in biotinidase activity. The D444H mutation on one allele with a second mutation for profound biotinidase deficiency on the second allele is responsible for essentially all cases of partial biotinidase deficiency. More than 100 mutations that cause biotinidase deficiency and their predicted effect on the enzyme's hydrolase and transferase activity have been reported.[18,19]

Biotin-responsive basal ganglia disease, inherited as an autosomal recessive trait, was first described in 1998 in a cluster of families in Saudi Arabia.[6,7] By using linkage analysis and positional cloning, it was determined that mutations in the SLC19A3 gene were responsible for the disorder. The gene for SLC19A3 maps to chromosome 2q36.3 and encodes a transporter related to the reduced-folate and thiamine transporter. Each child with the disorder was homozygous for one of two missense mutations. Biotin deficiency reduces the expression of SLC19A3 in leukocytes, suggesting that either the vitamin has a role in regulating biotin transport or that biotin is a sensory molecule in a positive feedback loop for the expression of the SLC19A3 protein. In vitro analysis using an overexpression strategy did not find any increase in biotin transport, suggesting tighter control of biotin transport.

Recently, a three-year-old boy with encephalopathy and organic aciduria consistent with MCD improved with biotin therapy.[20] Biotinidase and HCS activities were normal, and nutritional biotin deficiency was excluded. The rate of biotin uptake was significantly lower in blood lymphocytes, suggesting a defect in cellular transport of biotin. Intestinal biotin absorption mediated by sodium-dependent multivitamin transporter may also play a significant role in establishing a free biotin pool. Although no mutations in sodium-dependent multivitamin transporter gene had been identified, suggesting altered regulation of sodium-dependent multivitamin transporter at gene expression level.

OVERVIEW OF BIOTIN

Biotin, designated "bios or bios IIB," was originally extracted from egg yolk in 1901.[21] In 1936, Kögl crystallized the bios IIB and called it biotin. The structure of biotin was described by du Vigneaud in 1942 followed by its chemical synthesis in 1943. Stereo-controlled chemical synthesis processes for biotin – starting with cysteine, cystine, and carbohydrates – have been described. Biotin has a chemical formula of $C_{10}H_{16}N_2O_3S$, has a molecular weight of 244.31 daltons, and is a crystalline, colorless material that is fairly stable under ambient conditions. Biotin contains a bicyclic ring structure with both imidazolidone and thiophane rings. Having three asymmetrical carbon atoms allows biotin eight possible stereoisomers; however, only the dextrorotatory isomer, d-biotin, is bioactive and found in nature. The side chain length as well as the structure of the imidazolidone ring is important in the biotin-dependent carboxylation reaction catalyzed by carboxylases. Biotin is covalently bound to carboxylases through an amide bond to ε-amino groups of evolutionarily conserved lysine residue of the carboxylases. The total bond length of 1.4 nanometers of this amide bond makes it flexible so that it can simultaneously alternate between the two catalytic centers of the carboxylases.

The bioactivity of biotin is adversely affected by exposure to ultraviolet (UV) light and heating in strong acid or base. The solubility of biotin in water is approximately 200 μg/mL, but it remains insoluble in most organic solvents because of its negatively charged hydroxyl group. Even though biotin is present in most plant and animal tissues and can be isolated from plant cells in small quantities, it is usually found in the protein-bound form.

Biosynthetic pathways of biotin and its regulation in microorganisms have been described in detail. Biotin biosynthesis in most microorganisms uses pimelic acid as the starting compound and is regulated at the transcription level in *Escherichia coli*, where biotin itself acts as a strong repressor for the operon consisting of all the enzymes involved in its biosynthesis. Interest in biotin increased when it was shown that biotin was involved in carboxyl group transfer, including carboxylation, transcarboxylation, and decarboxylation, and it was the curative factor of skin lesions caused by feeding individuals a prolonged diet of raw eggs. Various microbial and enzyme assays, in addition to the tests based on other properties of biotin, have been described to measure biotin content.

Biotin preparations and dosage

Biotin is considered a nutrient supplement and is available over the counter in most pharmacies and health-food stores. Although biotin preparations may be found in varying doses and forms, capsules or tablets, most of the biotin in these preparations is obtained from the same original manufacturer. The doses of biotin used to treat profound and partial biotinidase deficiencies are usually 5–10 mg/d and 2.5–5 mg/d, respectively. The dose for those with profound biotinidase deficiency may be increased to 10–20 mg/d when children go through puberty or reach adolescence. The dose of biotin for individuals with HCS deficiency varies depending on the molecular defect. Most enzyme-deficient children have mutations affecting the K_m of biotin; therefore, in general, the higher the K_m value the larger the dose, varying from 10 milligrams, adequate for most children, up to 100 milligrams or more per day in some individuals.

Although biotin is a water-soluble vitamin, it is not readily soluble in water, other liquids, or syrups, especially when in combination with filler compounds. In addition, when biotin is chilled it is even less soluble. Therefore, when the biotin in a capsule or crushed tablet is mixed with milk, it rarely dissolves, but is a slurry or suspension that will settle with time. Much of the biotin, when dispensed in large volumes of liquid, is likely not in solution and settles and sticks to the inside plastic or glass surface. In addition, biotin sitting in liquids or syrup for long periods of time is prone to promote growth of bacteria.

Fortunately, the dosage of biotin used to treat these disorders is usually in excess of that actually required. For the administration of a consistent daily dose to a neonate or infant, however, it is recommend that the contents of the biotin capsule or the crushed tablet first be added to a small volume of milk (expressed or formula) or water to make a slurry. This slurry is then placed into the mouth of the baby. Then small amounts of milk can be used to wash the biotin down, thereby delivering a consistent dose. As the child gets older, the biotin can be added to applesauce or other similar foods that allow the entire dose to be taken consistently and at once. Eventually, the child will be old enough to swallow the entire capsule or tablet.

Side effects of biotin

There are no reports of biotin toxicity in humans.[22] Children with HCS deficiency have tolerated doses of 100–200 mg/d for long periods of time without exhibiting adverse effects. Individuals with biotinidase deficiency excrete large quantities of biocytin in their urine; however, to date there is no study showing evidence of accumulation of this metabolite in the tissues. It remains to be determined whether biotin therapy increases the concentration of biocytin in these children and if there are long-term consequences.

U.S. Food and Drug Administration recommendation for biotin

Biotin, like many other vitamins, is an essential nutrient supplement for humans. The U.S. Recommended Dietary Allowances (U.S. RDA) for biotin is 50 µg/d for infants, 150 µg/d for children, and 300 µg/d for adults. Because biotin is considered a nutrient, and there are no known adverse effects of this vitamin in humans, even over extended periods of time, there are no U.S. Food and

Drug Administration (FDA) guidelines or recommendations for its therapeutic use.

RESULTS OF BIOTIN THERAPY

All symptomatic children with biotinidase deficiency clinically and metabolically improve within hours or days of beginning biotin therapy. In general, the symptoms that these children exhibited will resolve, and lost milestones will be regained, with the exception of optic atrophy, hearing loss, and some cognitive deficits. Biotin therapy initiated at birth following identification by newborn screening or because a prior sibling had the disorder prevents the development of symptoms. Most children with HCS deficiency and basal ganglion disease will respond markedly to biotin therapy, but some children with specific genotypes require higher doses of the vitamin. These latter individuals benefit from the therapy but may continue to have neurological deficits.

FUTURE DEVELOPMENTS

Although biotin therapy can ameliorate the majority of symptoms due to HCS and biotinidase deficiencies, some aspects are irreversible. Newborn screening and a greater awareness of the symptoms of these disorders have greatly improved the identification of children with MCDs before they become symptomatic. Early presymptomatic identification and treatment of children with these disorders can prevent the irreversible symptoms. Better methodologies of screening for HCS deficiency are needed. Unlike many genetic diseases in which the correction of genetic defects is considered the ultimate goal, gene therapy for biotin-responsive disorders is not being considered because biotin treatment is so simple and effective.

REFERENCES

1. Wolf B. Disorders of biotin metabolism. C. Scriver, A. Beaudet, W. Sly, D. Valle, eds. *The Metabolic and Molecular Bases of Inherited Disease*, 8th edition, McGraw Hill, 5085–5108, 2001
2. McMahon RJ. Biotin in metabolism and molecular biology. *Annu Rev Nutr.* 2002;22:221–239. Epub 2002 Jan 4
3. Said HM. Recent advances in carrier-mediated intestinal absorption of water-soluble vitamins. *Annu Rev Physiol.* 2004;66:419–446
4. Chapman-Smith A, Cronan JE Jr. The enzymatic biotinylation of proteins: a post-translational modification of exceptional specificity. *Trends Biochem Sci.* 1999;24(9):359–363
5. Hymes J, Fleischhauer K, Wolf B. Biotinidase in serum and tissues. *Methods Enzymol.* 1997;279:422–434
6. Zeng WQ, Al-Yamani E, Acierno JS Jr, Slaugenhaupt S, Gillis T, MacDonald ME, Ozand PT, Gusella JF. Biotin-responsive basal ganglia disease maps to 2q36.3 and is due to mutations in SLC19A3. *Am J Hum Genet.* 2005;77(1):16–26

7. Ozand PT, Gascon GG, Al Essa M, Joshi S, Al Jishi E, Bakheet S, Al Watban J, Al-Kawi MZ, Dabbagh O. Biotin-responsive basal ganglia disease: a novel entity. *Brain*. 1998;121(Pt 7):1267–1279

8. Baumgartner ER, Suormala T. Multiple carboxylase deficiency: inherited and acquired disorders of biotin metabolism. *Int J Vitam Nutr Res*. 1997;67(5):377–384

9. Wolf B. Disorders of biotin metabolism: treatable neurologic syndrome. R. N. Rosenberg, S. DiMauro, H. L. Paulson, L. Ptácek, eds. *The Molecular and Genetic Basis of Neurologic and Psychiatric Disease*, 4th edition, Lippincott Williams & Wilkins, 705–710, 2007

10. Wolf B, Heard GS. Biotinidase deficiency. *Adv Pediatr*. 1991;38:1–21

11. Wolf B, Feldman GL. The biotin-dependent carboxylase deficiencies. *Am J Hum Genet*. 1982;34(5):699–716

12. Suchy SF, McVoy JS, Wolf B. Neurologic symptoms of biotinidase deficiency: possible explanation. *Neurology*. 1985;35(10):1510–1511

13. Bousounis DP, Camfield PR, Wolf B. Reversal of brain atrophy with biotin treatment in biotinidase deficiency. *Neuropediatrics*. 1993;24(4):214–217

14. Wolf B, Spencer R, Gleason T. Hearing loss is a common feature of symptomatic children with profound biotinidase deficiency. *J Pediatr*. 2002;140(2):242–246

15. Pérez-Monjaras A, Cervantes-Roldán R, Meneses-Morales I, Gravel RA, Reyes-Carmona S, Solórzano-Vargas S, González-Noriega A, León-Del-Río A. Impaired biotinidase activity disrupts holocarboxylase synthetase expression in late onset multiple carboxylase deficiency. *J Biol Chem*. 2008;283(49):34150–34158

16. Jenuwein T, Allis CD. Translating the histone code. *Science*. 2001;293(5532):1074–1080

17. Suzuki Y, Yang X, Aoki Y, Kure S, Matsubara Y. Mutations in the holocarboxylase synthetase gene HLCS. *Hum Mutat*. 2005;26(4):285–290

18. Hymes J, Stanley CM, Wolf B. Mutations in BTD causing biotinidase deficiency. *Hum Mutat*. 2001;18(5):375–381

19. Pindolia K, Jensen K, Wolf B. Three dimensional structure of human biotinidase: computer modeling and functional correlations. *Mol Genet Metab*. 2007

20. Mardach R, Zempleni J, Wolf B, Cannon MJ, Jennings ML, Cress S, Boylan J, Roth S, Cederbaum S, Mock DM. Biotin dependency due to a defect in biotin transport. *J Clin Invest*. 2002;109(12):1617–1623

21. Visser CM, Kellogg RM. Biotin. Its place in evolution. *J Mol Evol*. 1978;11(2):171–187

22. US FDA Drug Watch url: http://www.fda.gov/medwatch/SAFETY/2001/apr01.htm

5 Cobalamin treatment of methylmalonic acidemias

Hans C. Andersson

CLINICAL CHARACTERISTICS OF METHYLMALONIC ACIDEMIAS

Methylmalonic acidemias (MMAs) result from enzymatic deficiency in the catabolism of methylmalonyl-coenzyme A (CoA) leading to acid–base imbalance and growth failure,[1] mitochondrial dysfunction,[2] and, in some disorders, an increased incidence of birth defects.[3] These conditions can result from (1) genetic abnormality in synthesis of the enzyme methylmalonyl-CoA mutase, (2) genetic deficiency of the enzyme's cofactor, adenosylcobalamin (AdoCbl), or (3) dietary deficiency of cobalamin. The clinical characteristics of these conditions vary considerably, and treatment is variably effective depending on disease etiology. Therapy in genetic deficiency with oral or intramuscular cobalamin is intended to enhance residual enzyme activity in patients whose mutations result in stably transcribed proteins.

The classic cases of MMA were first described in children who developed a severe, sometimes life-threatening, metabolic acidosis with an increased anion gap. In these children, methylmalonic acid was markedly elevated in the urine and blood.[4,5] Whereas these cases appeared not to benefit from cobalamin supplementation, later cases with MMA were observed to benefit from pharmaco-logic doses of cobalamin.[6–8] Many clinical reports, paired with careful cell biolog-ical investigation, have provided a rudimentary understanding of the important components of methylmalonic acid metabolism and the clinical manifestations attendant to functional deficiencies of these components.[1,2]

Methylmalonic acid results from intramitochondrial metabolism of propionate in the catabolism of certain amino acids and fats.[1,6] In a two-step conversion, carboxylation of propionate yields D-methylmalonyl-CoA, which is converted by methylmalonyl-CoA racemase to L-methylmalonyl-CoA. The AdoCbl-dependent enzyme methylmalonyl-CoA mutase converts methylmalonyl-CoA to its iso-mer, succinyl-CoA. Mutase activity is markedly impaired in cobalamin deficiency states, leading to MMA even when the enzyme is otherwise normal in structure and concentration.

Cobalamin metabolism

Cobalamin (B12) is composed of a central cobalt (Co) atom, capable of existing in at least three redox states, within a planar corrin ring with a variety of complex side chains that may be bound to the Co.[1] Cobalamin exists in several natural and pharmacological forms determined by the side chain attached to the Co: The most common natural forms are methylcobalamin (MeCbl), AdoCbl, and hydroxocobalamin (OHCbl), whereas the most common pharmacologic form is cyanocobalamin (CNCbl), a form not normally found in nature. Recent studies have demonstrated that the MMACHC protein, which in the deficient state causes cobalamin C (CblC) disease, is responsible for decyanation and dealkylation of CNCbl, MeCbl, and AdoCbl.[9,10] This finding explains the inefficacy of CNCbl supplementation in CblC patients.[11]

Cobalamin is an essential vitamin in humans that is derived from dietary sources. Its bioavailability to methylmalonyl-CoA mutase and methionine syn-thase, the only known human enzymes for which cobalamin acts as a coenzyme, requires a complex set of binding proteins and transporters mediating gastroin-testinal absorption and intracellular processing.[12] Briefly, dietary cobalamin binds with gastric intrinsic factor (IF) and then with cubilin to become transcytosed into ileal epithelial cells. It then arrives to the portal blood bound to transcobalamin II, which allows cellular endocytosis and encapsulation within lysosomes. A recently identified lysosomal transporter for cobalamin explains the egress of cobalamin from within the lysosome and its appearance in the cytoplasm.[13] Cobalamin is further processed within the cytoplasm, at least partly involving MMACHC,[10] to yield MeCbl, which either binds to cytosolic methionine synthase or is trans-ported into the mitochondrion, where it is processed to AdoCbl, the cofactor for methylmalonyl-CoA mutase.

Mutase deficiency

Patients with mutations in methylmalonyl-CoA mutase (MUT), usually inherited as an autosomal recessive condition, typically present in infancy with severe

Table 5–1. Features of methylmalonic acidemias

Disorder	Gene name	Serum cobalamin levels	Cobalamin therapy
Methylmalonyl-CoA mutase deficiency	MUT	Normal	CNCbl,OHCbl
Cobalamin biosynthesis defects			
CblA	MMAA	Normal	OHCbl
CblB	MMAB	Normal	OHCbl
CblC	MMACHC	Normal	OHCbl
CblD	MMADHC	Normal	OHCbl
CblF	LMBRD1	Normal*	OHCbl
Cobalamin deficiency (dietary or acquired)		Low	OHCbl

* Only one case reported serum B12 levels.

metabolic acidosis.[1] Newborn screening by tandem mass spectrometry detects the marked elevation of the C3 acylcarnitine, suggestive of propionic acidemia or MMA, and offers the potential for detection and initiation of therapy before full-blown disease ensues.[14] Classic MMA patients develop massive increases in tissue, plasma, and urine methylmalonic acid in the first week of life, leading to feeding intolerance, lethargy, profound anion gap metabolic acidosis, central nervous system dysfunction and, eventually, coma. The condition is easily diagnosed by the presence of a massive elevation of methylmalonic acid in serum or urine by organic acid analysis (see Table 5–1). A categorization among patients with a complete absence of mutase protein (mut°) and more severe, earlier-onset disease and those with some residual protein (mut⁻) who generally present somewhat later has provided some correlation with outcome: Although mut⁻ patients are less common, the outcome in this group appears in some cases to be significantly improved when compared with that in mut° patients.[15] The massive elevation of methylmalonic acid leads to hyperglycinemia and hyperammonemia, which are related to organic acid interference with the glycine-cleavage enzyme and the proximal steps of the urea cycle, respectively. Generalized mitochondrial dysfunction and severe acid–base imbalance lead to multiorgan damage and, if not aggressively treated, death. Long-term outcomes are highly variable in survivors with growth delay, psychomotor retardation,[16] and progressive renal disease.[17] The suggestion that liver transplantation may benefit mutase-deficiency patients has not been borne out with clearly beneficial outcomes, owing most likely to the intramitochondrial disease within remaining tissues, especially brain and kidney.[18]

Treatment for mutase-deficiency patients begins with prompt and aggressive reversal of the overwhelming metabolic acidosis with short-term protein restriction, efforts to reverse any catabolic processes, oral (100 mg/kg/d) or intravenous (50 mg/kg/d) carnitine supplementation, and intramuscular OHCbl (1 mg/d). Responsiveness to OHCbl may be difficult to determine clinically during the acute illness and should be evaluated when the patient is well. At that time, a trial of intermittent (every other day) OHCbl administration and daily urine or serum organic acid analysis may be performed to assess any increase in methylmalonic acid over baseline (while on daily therapy). If no changes are noted, mutase-deficiency patients may be considered for a trial of twice weekly or weekly OHCbl injections, oral CNCbl, or discontinuation of cobalamin supplementation. Each patient must be individually evaluated. Additional approaches may include in vitro fibroblast studies to assess responsiveness to cobalamin. No absolute target ranges for serum or urine methylmalonic acid levels exist, as each patient has unique residual methylmalonic acid metabolism capacity.

Cobalamin-processing defects

Several defects in cobalamin processing, inherited as autosomal recessive conditions, have been identified and have given insight into the normal processing steps for AdoCbl and MeCbl. These defects were classified by their ability to complement a known defective fibroblast cell line; cells that did not complement a cell line with a known defect (e.g., CblC) were considered to manifest the same defect, whereas cells that corrected a known defect were assumed to have a defect other than the known cell line.[19] In this way, distinct cobalamin defects with MMA were identified and are now being more carefully defined. The great majority of patients with a cobalamin-processing defect have CblC defect that results in deficient synthesis of both AdoCbl and MeCbl and concomitant deficient enzyme activity for methylmalonyl-CoA mutase and methionine synthase, respectively.

CblA

CblA patients typically present with nonlethal metabolic acidosis and/or developmental delay, and are often responsive to cobalamin therapy.[6,15] Long-term outcome has not been reported presumably because of the paucity of cases. It is interesting that a single case of an affected fetus treated by high-dose administration of cobalamin to the mother during the third trimester, with marked decrease in maternal urine methylmalonic acid and only minimal elevations present in the baby at birth, showed normal development at a few months of age.[20] The gene for CblA disease (MMAA) has been cloned and numerous mutations defined, making prenatal diagnosis and carrier ascertainment possible.[21]

CblB

A handful of patients have been described with a phenotype generally similar to other patients with nonlethal MMA who are generally less responsive to cobalamin therapy than are CblA patients.[22] The gene for CblB (MMAB) has been cloned and mutations identified.[22,23]

CblC

This condition has been well-described (>100 patients reported) as variably affecting newborns or older infants sometimes with or without severe acidosis and occasionally associated with megaloblastic anemia, lacunar retinitis pigmentosa, an increased incidence of structural anomalies (e.g., congenital microcephaly, hydrocephalus, congenital heart disease), and invariable developmental delay.[3,24,25] Early onset of therapy and good compliance do not predict good neurologic outcomes, most likely owing to the prenatal onset of brain dysplasia. Occasional cases of late-onset CblC disease have been described, with milder symptoms involving neurologic abnormalities and with improved survival.[25–27] The MMACHC gene responsible for CblC disease was cloned, and a common mutation, among more than 40 found, was seen in 40% of alleles analyzed.[23] Because these patients have homocystinemia (-uria) in addition to MMA, they must be treated for both disorders.[3,24]

CblD

This condition is rare, presenting with combined MMA and homocystinemia. In some variant patients, only one of these biochemical phenotypes is present. Patients typically have growth and developmental delay. Once thought to be caused by an allelic form of CblC, a gene was recently identified in this condition (MMADHC) with multiple mutations described in affected patients.[28]

CblF

The lysosomal transporter defect that allows egress of intralysosomal cobalamin into the cytoplasm was shown to cause this disorder resulting in methylmalonic acid and homocystinuria causing growth and developmental delay.[29] Recent cloning of the CblF gene (LMBRD1) confirmed homology to a membrane receptor and described disease-causing mutations.[13]

Cobalamin deficiency

Diets deficient in cobalamin and defects in intestinal cobalamin absorption cause tissue cobalamin deficiencies and can create symptoms of MMA, hyperhomocysteinemia, and (occasionally) neurologic abnormalities. Vegetarian diets are often deficient in cobalamin, and infants drinking cobalamin-deficient mother's breast milk become ill with typical manifestations of cobalamin deficiency. Autoimmune thyroiditis with antibodies to IF-producing cells prevent normal absorption of cobalamin leading to MMA and (occasionally) hyperhomocysteinemia. Treatment with parenteral cobalamin often rapidly remedies the symptoms of cobalamin deficiency.

COBALAMIN

Pharmaceutical formulations

The most readily available form of cobalamin is oral CNCbl, which is available as a powder or tablets but also as an injectable liquid (usually 1 mg/ml). As described in the "Cobalamin metabolism," section, CNCbl is not metabolized normally in certain metabolic defects and should be avoided unless clinical and biochemical efficacy has been demonstrated. A preferable agent in a critically ill patient with CblC disease is parenteral OHCbl, which comes in an injectable liquid (1 mg/ml).

Mechanism of action

Oral CNCbl is absorbed as described (see "Cobalamin metabolism") and acts either as a chaperone for a nascent enzyme or as a stabilizing agent for defective enzyme. No clear demonstration of the mechanism of action has been described. Because no significant complications are typically seen, administration of OHCbl in a patient with MMA is always advised during the acute episode and until a lack of efficacy has been demonstrated in a patient.

THERAPEUTIC RESULTS

Dosage/adverse effects

Treatment of all forms of MMA during acute illness should include 1 mg of OHCbl daily. No common side effects have been reported in patients with this dosage and administration other than mild transient diarrhea and mild local irritation.

Clinical effects

In mutase deficiency and cobalamin defect patients who are cobalamin-responsive, a rapid (12- to 24-hour) decrease in serum and urine methylmalonic acid and plasma hyperhomocysteinemia may be observed. As these critically ill patients have many interventions simultaneously, the independent effects of OHCbl are difficult to quantify. Long-term studies have been few in number, but some small patient-cohort studies have described the effects of CNCbl and OHCbl in CblC patients.[3,13] In patients with dietary deficiency of cobalamin, rapid improvement after a single injection of 1 mg of OHCbl is observed (author's personal experience). Improvement in growth and development is associated with improvement in metabolic control and normalization of acid–base status. Patients with mutase deficiency and cobalamin-synthesis defects will always have increased levels of MMA, although CblC patients will often normalize plasma free homocystine values after being treated with OHCbl.

Long-term outcome studies of cobalamin-responsive MMA patients are lacking. Long-term outcome in eight CblC patients demonstrated marked improvement in growth for most patients, although developmental delay was noted in all patients, even after an average of 5.7 years of therapy.[3] A study of MMA patients showed improved survival but invariable neurocognitive delays in those patients who survived infancy.[14] Mortality is still high in infants with MMA, and the effects of early detection by newborn screening have not been quantified.

FUTURE DEVELOPMENTS

Expanded newborn screening offers the hope of identification of affected patients prior to full-blown disease expression and an opportunity to initiate lifesaving and potentially brain-protecting therapy. No studies have described such a benefit, but, in many states, screening for MMA has been in use for only a few years. With a disease incidence of approximately 1:90,000 live births,[30] such a study may require more time. The opportunity to treat pregnancies and newborns in women with previously affected patients may significantly improve the outcomes. The recent elucidation of MMACHC function and description of the cblF transporter offers the first chance to fully understand the pathophysiology of cobalamin biosynthesis defects.

REFERENCES

1. Fenton WA, Gravel RA, Rosenblatt DA. Disorders of propionate and methylmalonate metabolism. C Scriver, A Beaudet, W Sly, D Valle, eds. *The Metabolic and Molecular Bases of Inherited Disease, 8th edition*. McGraw Hill, 2165–2193, 2001
2. Chandler RJ, Zerfas PM, Shanske S, Sloan J, Hoffmann V, DiMauro S, Venditti CP. Mitochondrial dysfunction in mut methylmalonic acidemia. *FASEB J.* 2009;23:1252–1261
3. Andersson HC, Marble M, Shapira E. Long-term outcome in treated combined methylmalonic acidemia and homocystinemia. *Genet Med.* 1999;1:146–150
4. Oberholzer VG, Levin B, Burgess EA, Young WF. Methylmalonic aciduria: An inborn error of metabolism leading to chronic metabolic acidosis. *Arch Dis Child.* 1967;42:492–504
5. Stokke O, Eldjarn L, Norum KR, Steen-Johnsen J, Halvorsen S. Methylmalonic acidemia. A new inborn error of metabolism which may cause fatal acidosis in the neonatal period. *Scand J Clin Lab Invest.* 1967;20:313–328
6. Rosenberg LE, Lilljeqvist AC, Hsia YE. Methylmalonic aciduria: Metabolic block localization and vitamin B12 dependency. *Science.* 1968;162:805–807
7. Rosenberg LE, Lilljeqvist AC, Hsia YE. Methylmalonic aciduria: An inborn error leading to metabolic acidosis, long-chain ketonuria and hyperglycinemia. *N Engl J Med.* 1968;278:1319–1322
8. Lindblad B, Lindblad BS, Olin P, Svanberg B, Zetterström R. Methylmalonic acidemia. A disorder associated with acidosis, hyperglycinemia, and hyperlactatemia. *Acta Paediatr Scand.* 1968;57(5):417–424
9. Kim J, Gherasim C, Banerjee R. Decyanation of vitamin B12 by a trafficking chaperone. *Proc Natl Acad Sci USA.* 2008;105:14551–14554
10. Hannibal L, Kim J, Brasch NE, Wang S, Rosenblatt DS, Banerjee R, Jacobsen DW. Processing of alkylcobalamins in mammalian cells: A role for the MMACHC (cblC) gene product. *Mol Genet Metab.* 2009;97:260–266
11. Andersson HC, Shapira E. Biochemical and clinical response to hydroxocobalamin versus cyanocobalamin treatment in patients with methylmalonic acidemia and homocystinuria (cblC). *J Pediatr.* 1998;132:121–124
12. Seetharam B, Bose S, Li N. Cellular import of cobalamin (Vitamin B-12). *J Nutr.* 1999;129:1761–1764
13. Rutsch F, Gailus S, Miousse IR, Suormala T, Sagné C, Toliat MR, Nürnberg G, Wittkampf T, Buers I, Sharifi A, Stucki M, Becker C, Baumgartner M, Robenek H, Marquardt T, Höhne W, Gasnier B, Rosenblatt DS, Fowler B, Nürnberg P. Identification of a putative lysosomal cobalamin exporter altered in the cblF defect of vitamin B12 metabolism. *Nat Genet.* 2009;41:234–239

14. Dionisi-Vici C, Deodato F, Röschinger W, Rhead W, Wilcken B. "Classical" organic acidurias, propionic aciduria, methylmalonic aciduria and isovaleric aciduria: Long-term outcome and effects of expanded newborn screening using tandem mass spectrometry. *J Inherit Metab Dis.* 2006;29:383–389

15. Matsui M, Mahoney MJ, Rosenberg LE. The natural history of inherited methylmalonic acidemia. *N Engl J Med.* 1983;308:857–861

16. Deodato F, Boenzi S, Santorelli FM, Dionisi-Vici C. Methylmalonic and propionic aciduria. *Am J Med Genet C Semin Med Genet.* 2006;142:104–112

17. Rutledge SL, Geraghty M, Mroczek E, Rosenblatt D, Kohout E. Tubulointerstitial nephritis in methylmalonic acidemia. *Pediatr Nephrol.* 1993;7:81–82

18. Kasahara M, Horikawa R, Tagawa M, Uemoto S, Yokoyama S, Shibata Y, Kawano T, Kuroda T, Honna T, Tanaka K, Saeki M. Current role of liver transplantation for methylmalonic acidemia: A review of the literature. *Pediatr Transplant.* 2006;10(8):943–947

19. Gravel RA, Mahoney MJ, Ruddle FH, Rosenberg LE. Genetic complementation in heterokaryons of human fibroblasts defective in cobalamin metabolism. *Proc Natl Acad Sci USA.* 1975;72:3181–3185

20. Ampola MG, Mahoney MJ, Nakamura E, Tanaka K. Prenatal therapy of a patient with vitamin-B12 responsive methylmalonic acidemia. *N Engl J Med.* 1975;293:313–317

21. Lerner-Ellis JP, Dobson CM, Wai T, Watkins D, Tirone JC, Leclerc D, Dore C, Lepage P, Gravel RA, Rosenblatt DS. Mutations in the MMAA gene in patients with the cblA disorder of vitamin B12 metabolism. *Hum Mut.* 2004;24:509–516

22. Dobson CM, Wai T, Leclerc D, Kadir H, Narang M, Lerner-Ellis JP, Hudson TJ, Rosenblatt DS, Gravel RA. Identification of the gene responsible for the cblB complementation group of vitamin B12-dependent methylmalonic aciduria. *Hum Mol Genet.* 2002;11:3361–3369

23. Lerner-Ellis JP, Gradinger AB, Watkins D, Tirone JC, Villeneuve A, Dobson CM, Montpetit A, Lepage P, Gravel RA, Rosenblatt DS. Mutation and biochemical analysis of patients belonging to the cblB complementation class of vitamin B12-dependent methylmalonic aciduria. *Mol Genet Metab.* 2006;87:219–225

24. Bartholomew DW, Batshaw ML, Allen RH, Roe CR, Rosenblatt D, Valle DL, Francomano CA. Therapeutic approaches to cobalamin-C methylmalonic acidemia and homocystinuria. *J Pediatr.* 1988;112:32–39

25. Rosenblatt DS, Aspler AL, Shevell MI, Pletcher BA, Fenton WA, Seashore MR. Clinical heterogeneity and prognosis in combined methylmalonic aciduria and homocystinuria (cblC). *J Inherit Metab Dis.* 1997;20:528–538

26. Goodman SI, Moe PG, Hammond KB, Mudd SH, Uhlendorf BW. Homocystinuria with methylmalonic aciduria: Two cases in a sibship. *Biochem Med.* 1970;4:500–515

27. Bodamer OAF, Rosenblatt DS, Appel SH, Beaudet AL. Adult-onset combined methylmalonic aciduria and homocystinuria (cblC). *Neurology.* 2001;56:1113

28. Coelho D, Suormala T, Stucki M, Lerner-Ellis JP, Rosenblatt DS, Newbold RF, Baumgartner MR, Fowler B. Gene identification for the cblD defect of vitamin B12 metabolism. *N Engl J Med.* 2008;358:1454–1464

29. Rosenblatt DS, Hosack A, Matiaszuk NV, Cooper BA, Laframboise R. Defect in vitamin B-12 release from lysosomes: Newly described inborn error of vitamin B-12 metabolism. *Science.* 1985;228:1319–1321

30. Frazier DM, Millington DS, McCandless SE, Koeberl DD, Weavil SD, Chaing SH, Muenzer J. The tandem mass spectrometry newborn screening experience in North Carolina: 1997–2005. *J Inherit Metab Dis.* 2006;29:76–85

6 Sapropterin treatment of phenylketonuria

Barbara K. Burton

NATURAL HISTORY OF PHENYLKETONURIA

Phenylketonuria (PKU) was first described in 1934 by the Norwegian physician Asbjorn Folling, who noted a strange odor in the urine of two mentally retarded siblings.[1] He studied the chemical composition of the urine and identified the presence of phenylpyruvic acid, a phenylketone, and recognized its relationship to phenylalanine levels in body fluids. Over the subsequent 20 years, many other cases of PKU were identified and the possibility of treatment with dietary protein restriction was suggested. It was not until the mid-1950s that a patient with PKU was treated by a German physician, Horst Bickel, by using a low phenylalanine protein drink that he had developed. Although the patient already had irreversible developmental disabilities, clinical improvement was observed and blood phenylalanine levels declined. At about this same time, it was demonstrated that the underlying biochemical defect in PKU is a deficiency of the hepatic enzyme phenylalanine hydroxylase (PAH). In the mid-1960s, Dr. Robert Guthrie developed the first test for PKU that could be applied to general population screening of all newborns.[2] For many years to follow, newborn screening was conducted using this bacterial inhibition assay or "Guthrie test."

Patients with PKU appear normal at birth. Although blood phenylalanine levels begin to rise shortly after birth, symptoms are not observed in the neonatal period. Persistent severe elevations of the blood phenylalanine level are toxic to the brain and impair brain growth. Over time, developmental delay, behavioral problems, and acquired microcephaly become evident. Many affected individuals develop a seizure disorder. In the absence of treatment, severe mental retardation develops. A musty odor may be noted in the urine. Dry skin and eczema are common. High levels of phenylalanine and its metabolites lead to inhibition of the enzyme tyrosinase resulting in hypopigmentation of the skin and hair. Adults with untreated PKU may exhibit abnormal neurologic findings, such as spasticity or tremor. Severe psychiatric disturbances are often seen.

PAH deficiency, like most other metabolic disorders, represents a spectrum of severity. At the most severe end of the spectrum are patients with classical PKU who, if untreated, exhibit the characteristic features of the disorder and have blood phenylalanine levels greater than 1,200 μmol/L. (The mean normal level in unaffected individuals is approximately 60 μmol/L.) Several different classification schemes have been used to describe patients with less severe defects in phenylalanine metabolism and greater residual PAH activity. The National Institutes of Health (NIH) Consensus Development Conference Statement[3] categorized all patients with untreated blood phenylalanine levels greater than normal but less than 1,200 μmol/L as having hyperphenylalaninemia. A European multicenter group of experts proposed classifying patients with PKU based on their phenylalanine tolerance.[4] In this classification scheme, patients with classical PKU are those who tolerate less than 250–350 milligrams of dietary phenylalanine per day to keep blood phenylalanine levels in a safe range less than 300 μmol/L. Patients with moderate PKU tolerate 350–400 milligrams whereas those with mild PKU tolerate 400–600 milligrams. Patients with mild hyperphenylalaninemia in this classification system have untreated blood phenylalanine levels of less than 600 μmol/L. In practice, many physicians refer to patients with blood phenylalanine levels high enough to warrant treatment but less than 1,200 μmol/L as having mild to moderate or variant PKU and reserve the term "non-PKU hyperphenylalaninemia" for those patients whose untreated levels are below the threshold that would trigger intervention. Although that threshold was originally defined as 600 μmol/L, many clinics in the United States have lowered that threshold to either 360 or 480 μmol/L. The risks of adverse outcomes associated with untreated blood phenylalanine levels less than 600 μmol/L appear to be low, and mental retardation does not occur,[5] but there is debate with regard to whether more subtle neurocognitive consequences may be observed.

Newborn screening for PKU became widespread in the United States and in the United Kingdom by the mid- to late-1960s and in the rest of the developed world by the early 1970s. It was conducted initially using the Guthrie method, but later some laboratories adopted an automated fluorometric method, and, most recently, many laboratories have converted to screening by tandem mass spectrometry, which allows testing for a wide range of other metabolic disorders simultaneously. Since the initiation of newborn screening, almost all cases of PKU have been diagnosed following a positive newborn-screening test. A blood phenylalanine level on newborn screening in excess of 120 μmol/L is considered elevated and requires further testing with quantitative plasma amino acid analysis for confirmation of diagnosis. Tests to rule out a defect in tetrahydrobiopterin synthesis or recycling as the cause of hyperphenylalaninemia are also essential. Treatment using dietary phenylalanine restriction and supplementation with phenylalanine-free amino acid mixtures (medical foods, "formulas") is ideally initiated before 10 days of age with the goal in the United States of maintaining blood phenylalanine levels less than 360 μmol/L. There is some variation in target blood phenylalanine levels in other countries. Dietary therapy has been effective in preventing the severe mental retardation associated with untreated classical PKU. Nonetheless, the outcome in treated patients with PKU is not comparable to that observed in their unaffected siblings or in the general population. Mean IQ is decreased, and there is an increased incidence of attention-deficit/hyperactivity disorder[6] and of school problems.[7] In the adult, psychiatric disorders – such as depression, anxiety, and phobias – are seen with increased frequency.[8] There is evidence of decreased autonomy and difficulty in forming stable social relationships. To a large extent, these adverse outcomes can be attributed to poor control of blood phenylalanine levels. As patients grow older, compliance with the restricted diet typically becomes more difficult. Studies show that the majority of adolescents and adults have blood phenylalanine levels higher than the recommended target range. Many adults abandon the restricted diet altogether. In the early years following the initiation of newborn screening, it was common for treating physicians to discontinue dietary therapy at the age of four to six years. Subsequently, it was demonstrated through the U.S. Collaborative Study that IQ declined in patients who discontinued dietary therapy. For the past several decades, the recommendation has been to continue the restricted diet for life. There is considerable debate, however, regarding the appropriate target for blood phenylalanine levels in the adult.

Patients who are treated from the early weeks of life for PKU with initial good metabolic control but who lose that control in later childhood or adult life experience both reversible and irreversible neuropsychiatric consequences. If blood phenylalanine levels remain elevated for a prolonged period, a decline in IQ may be observed, particularly if this elevation occurs in early childhood. The decline is unlikely to be reversible. Attentional deficits, defects in working memory, deficits in executive functioning, and psychiatric symptoms are often reversible with improvements in metabolic control. White matter abnormalities may be observed in patients with PKU and are correlated with the most recent blood phenylalanine level; the clinical significance of these changes is unclear. Even severely mentally retarded adults with late-diagnosed PKU may show improvements in challenging behavior with the lowering of the blood phenylalanine level.[9]

Pregnancy represents a difficult problem in treating patients with PKU. Affected women are at relatively low risk of having a fetus with PKU, but high levels of phenylalanine are extremely toxic to the brain of the developing fetus and can have other teratogenic effects as well. The abnormalities observed in infants born to women with PKU are referred to as the maternal PKU syndrome and include prenatal and postnatal growth retardation, microcephaly, congenital heart disease, and a variety of other major and minor anomalies.[10] The frequency of these abnormalities increases with increasing maternal blood phenylalanine level and is correlated with the time in gestation at which metabolic control is achieved. Several large studies have documented that if women with PKU achieve and maintain blood phenylalanine levels less than 360 μmol/L prior to conception

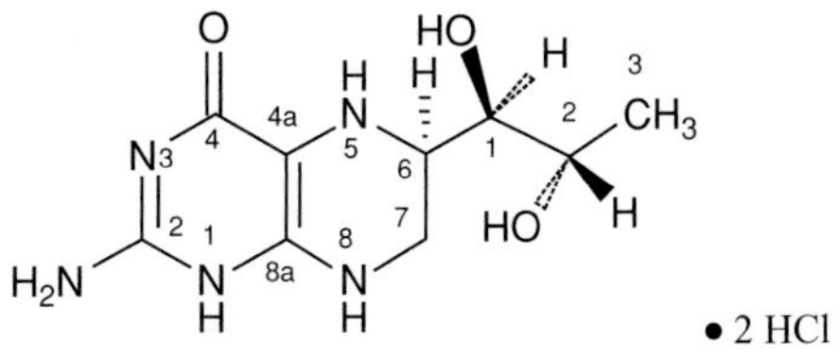

Figure 6–1: Chemical structure of sapropterin.

and throughout pregnancy, the outcome is generally good. Unfortunately, many pregnancies are unplanned and occur in patients whose disorder is not under good metabolic control. In these circumstances, if the patient is able to achieve control by eight weeks gestation, cognitive outcome can be good although a high incidence of congenital heart defects is still observed.

The pathophysiology of central nervous system dysfunction in PKU is unclear. The prevailing view is that phenylalanine itself is the primary toxic metabolite, adversely affecting a number of biochemical pathways in the brain and impairing brain growth. In addition to the neurotoxic effect of phenylalanine, it has recently been suggested that a deficiency of large neutral amino acids in the brain could also contribute to the adverse neuropsychiatric consequences of the disorder.[11] It has been demonstrated that high concentrations of phenylalanine in the blood decrease the blood–brain transport of other large neutral amino acids and that a deficiency of these amino acids could adversely impact cerebral protein synthesis, which has been shown to be decreased in a mouse model of PKU.

PAH deficiency is an autosomal recessive disorder. The gene is located on chromosome 12 at 12q24.1. More than 500 different mutations in the PAH gene have been described.[12] Most are point mutations, but deletions, duplications, and insertions are also observed. Most missense mutations result in abnormal folding of the PAH enzyme, increased protein turnover, and decreased activity. Although genotype–phenotype correlations are imperfect, genotype is clearly the best predictor of severity in PAH deficiency. In compound heterozygotes, the less severe mutation predominates. Many patients with non-PKU hyperphenylalaninemia have a severe (null) mutation on one chromosome with a milder mutation on the other that modifies the phenotype. PAH deficiency is most common in whites in whom the overall incidence is 1 in 10,000 live births. It is particularly common in the Irish and the Turks who have an incidence of 1 in 4,500 and 1 in 2,600, respectively. It is uncommon in individuals of Japanese, Finnish, and Ashkenazi Jewish descent. It is also relatively uncommon in Africans, although precise estimates of incidence are not available.

SAPROPTERIN DIHYDROCHLORIDE

Sapropterin dihydrochloride (6-R-L-erythro-5,6,7,8-tetrahydrobiopterin; BH4) is a pharmaceutical form of the naturally occurring cofactor, tetrahydrobiopterin. The chemical structure of sapropterin dihydrochloride is shown in Figure 6–1. Tetrahydrobiopterin is synthesized in the body through a series of enzymatic reactions and recycled through the action of dihydropteridine reductase. It serves as a cofactor for PAH, tyrosine hydroxylase, tryptophan hydroxylase, and nitric oxide synthase. Although not deficient in endogenous tetrahydrobiopterin, a subset of patients with PKU respond to administration of exogenous BH4 with an increase in the metabolism of phenylalanine to tyrosine. In some cases, this increase may occur because the mutant enzyme has a higher K_m or because the BH4 acts as a pharmacologic chaperone leading to improved folding and increased stability of the mutant protein. In this sense, PKU is much like other cofactor-responsive inborn errors of metabolism, such as methylmalonic acidemia and homocystinuria. It is estimated that approximately 40–50% of patients with PAH deficiency are BH4 responsive. Patients at the mild end of the spectrum are most likely to respond because some residual enzyme activity is required. Nonetheless, responsive patients are identified even among those with classical PKU.

Sapropterin dihydrochloride (Kuvan; BioMarin Pharmaceutical, Novato, CA) was approved by the U.S. Food and Drug Administration in December 2007 for the treatment of BH4-responsive PKU. It was given orphan drug status. It is marketed in Japan, where it was approved in July 2008 as Biopten (Asubio Pharma Co., Ltd., Tokyo). It is marketed by Merck Serono in the European Union and was granted approval by the European regulatory authority in December 2008. Pharmacokinetic studies have documented a mean half-life of 6.69 hours and maintenance of reduced blood phenylalanine levels over a 24-hour period.[13] The drug is therefore given once a day at a dose of 5–20 mg/kg/d. The most commonly used dose is 20 mg/kg/d. Doses greater than 20 mg/kg/d have not been studied.

During clinical trials, no serious side effects of sapropterin were identified. The adverse events that were reported were generally mild, self-limited, and similar to those observed in a placebo group. The most commonly observed side effects that appear to be related to drug administration are gastrointestinal and include gastric distress, nausea, and diarrhea – symptoms that are typically mild and self-limited. Most gastrointestinal side effects can be avoided by taking the medication with food. If side effects are still observed, the once-a-day dose can be divided and given twice a day or the dose of the drug can be reduced and then gradually increased until the desired dose is reached.

RESULTS OF THERAPY

Before treatment with sapropterin can be initiated, a responsiveness test must be conducted to determine if the patient has BH4-responsive PKU. Diet should remain constant throughout the test so that any decline in the blood phenylalanine level observed can be reasonably attributed to the exposure to the drug. In the United States, this testing is most commonly done by obtaining a baseline blood phenylalanine level and then starting the patient on a single daily dose of sapropterin at 20 mg/kg/d. Additional blood phenylalanine levels are then

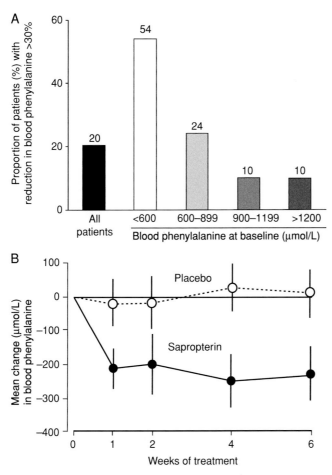

Figure 6–2: Efficacy of sapropterin dihydrochloride in the management of PKU. (A) Response rates (%) according to blood phenylalanine levels before treatment with sapropterin 10 mg/kg/d over eight days. (B) Comparison of the effect of sapropterin dihydrochloride at 10 mg/kg/d and placebo on blood phenylalanine levels in BH4-responsive PKU patients over a period of six weeks. Reprinted with permission from Blau et al.[16]

obtained at 24 hours, one week, and two weeks.[14] The product labeling recommends testing responsiveness initially at a dose of 10 mg/kg/d and subsequently increasing the dose to 20 mg/kg/d if no response is observed. Figure 6–2A demonstrates the likelihood of response to sapropterin at 10 mg/kg/d as documented in clinical trials.[15] A significantly greater rate of response is observed using a dose of 20 mg/kg/d. Responsiveness to the drug is often defined as a decline in the blood phenylalanine level of 30% or greater by two weeks of treatment. It is important that physicians use clinical judgment in assessing responsiveness, however. Occasional slow responders are encountered who have only a modest decline in the blood phenylalanine level by two weeks but a much greater decline by four weeks of therapy. In addition, there are patients who have a decrease in the blood phenylalanine level that is less than 30% but still judged to be significant either because of the absolute blood phenylalanine level achieved or because the

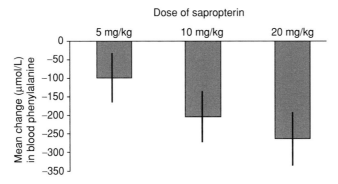

Figure 6–3: Effect of increasing doses of sapropterin dihydrochloride on blood phenylalanine levels in patients with BH4-responsive PKU. Reprinted with permission from Blau et al.[16]

patient reports an improvement in symptoms. BH4-responsive PKU patients who start responsiveness testing with a baseline phenylalanine level of 120 μmol/L or lower rarely show a significant decline in blood phenylalanine level. In these patients, responsiveness must be documented by the demonstration of increased phenylalanine tolerance in the diet. In Europe, responsiveness testing has been commonly done using a 48-hour protocol in neonates and young infants with a baseline blood phenylalanine level and multiple levels throughout the 48-hour period, beginning at four hours. This protocol came into common practice in Europe recently when an unregistered BH4 product was available and increasingly used; it has since been recommended that a similar protocol be used with commercial sapropterin.[16]

The primary benefit of treatment with sapropterin is a lowering of the blood phenylalanine level with improved metabolic control of the disorder (Figure 6–2B). The lowering of blood phenylalanine observed is dose-dependent (Figure 6–3). Because neurocognitive consequences of PKU are linked to elevations of blood phenylalanine, it is anticipated that lowering the blood phenylalanine level will result in improved outcome of the disorder. Clinical trials confirmed that the decline in blood phenylalanine levels observed in patients treated with sapropterin is statistically significant.[17] There is no evidence that the efficacy of the drug in lowering blood phenylalanine deceases over time. Patients with PKU have been treated continuously for periods of up to two years without serious adverse events and with no loss of efficacy.

Many adolescents and adults with elevated blood phenylalanine levels who are started on sapropterin and achieve improved metabolic control have already self-liberalized their phenylalanine intake as a result of the difficulty in maintaining the phenylalanine-restricted diet over the long term. The diet is restrictive, and the phenylalanine-free protein supplements that are an essential component are often viewed as being unpalatable. As a result, more than 75% of adolescents and adults have blood phenylalanine levels greater than the recommended range. For these patients, diet liberalization is not the primary goal of sapropterin therapy. In contrast, patients who are well controlled on diet but exhibit responsiveness to the medication may experience a significant increase in phenylalanine tolerance. An occasional patient will be able to completely abandon the phenylalanine-restricted diet and will achieve good control of the blood phenylalanine level on sapropterin therapy alone. A study of 4- to 12-year-old children with well-controlled blood phenylalanine levels demonstrated that phenylalanine tolerance was significantly increased in those patients who were responsive to the drug.[18] This finding was confirmed by evidence gathered in a European study using an unregistered form of BH4 in which patients increased their dietary phenylalanine intake from a mean of 498 to 1,475 mg/d while still maintaining good metabolic control.[19] In some infants with mild PKU, sapropterin therapy can adequately control blood phenylalanine levels, precluding the need to ever initiate dietary restrictions.

FUTURE DEVELOPMENTS

Aside from the traditional phenylalanine-restricted diet, a number of other treatment options for PKU have recently become available or are under development. A pegylated form of phenylalanine ammonia-lyase (PAL) is currently in Phase I clinical trials in the United States as a form of enzyme-substitution therapy. PAL is an enzyme found in bacteria and yeast that metabolizes phenylalanine to trans-cinnamic acid and trace amounts of ammonia. In a mouse model of PKU, it was shown to be highly effective in reducing blood phenylalanine levels to near normal.[20] If this form of therapy proves to be effective in humans, without serious immunologic consequences or side effects, it could be effective in any patient with elevated blood phenylalanine levels.

Large neutral amino acids, marketed as a dietary supplement, have been shown in preliminary studies to be effective in reducing blood phenylalanine levels in older patients with PKU under poor metabolic control. It has been theorized that they compete with phenylalanine for absorption in the gastrointestinal tract, effectively reducing the amount of phenylalanine entering the bloodstream.[21] A different formulation of large, neutral amino acids may reduce transport of phenylalanine across the blood–brain barrier, reducing the adverse neuropsychiatric consequences of elevated blood phenylalanine levels.[22] Further studies are necessary to assess the efficacy of these dietary products and to identify any adverse effects.

Gene therapy is a continuing subject of interest for investigators in the field of PKU. This is being studied in animal models and, although there are many issues that must be addressed before human trials could be considered, the progress of the work is promising.[23]

REFERENCES

1. Centerwall SA, Centerwall WK. The discovery of phenylketonuria: The story of a young couple, two affected children and a scientist. *Pediatrics*. 2000;105:89–103

2. Guthrie R, Susi A. A simple phenylalanine method for detecting phenylketonuria in large populations of newborn infants. *Pediatrics*. 1963;32:338–343
3. National Institutes of Health Consensus Development Panel: National Institutes of Health Consensus Development Conference Statement: Phenylketonuria: Screening and Management, Oct. 16–18, 2000. *Pediatrics*. 2001;108:972–982
4. Guldberg P, Rey F, Zschocke J, Romano V, François B, Michiels L, Ullrich K, Hoffmann GF, Burgard P, Schmidt H, Meli C, Riva E, Dianzani I, Ponzone A, Rey J, Güttler F. A European multicenter study of phenylalanine hydroxylase deficiency: Classification of 105 mutations and a general system for genotype-based prediction of metabolic phenotypes. *Am J Hum Genet*. 1998;63:71–79
5. Weglage J, Pietsch M, Feldmann R, et al. Normal clinical outcome in untreated subjects with mild hyperphenylalaninemia. *Pediatr Res*. 2001;49:532–536
6. Arnold GL, Vladutiu CJ, Orlowski CC, Blakely EM, DeLuca J. Prevalence of stimulant use for attentional dysfunction in children with phenylketonuria. *J Inherit Metab Dis*. 2004;27:137–143
7. Gassio R, Fuste E, Lopez-Sala A, Artuch R, Vilaseca MA, Campistol J. School performance in early and continuously-treated phenylketonuria. *Pediatr Neurol*. 2005;33:267–271
8. Sullivan JE, Chang P. Emotional and behavioral functioning in phenylketonuria. *J Pediatr Psychol*. 1999;24:281–289
9. Lee PJ, Amos A, Robertson L, Fitzgerald B, Hoskin R, Lilburn M, Weetch E, Murphy G. Adults with late diagnosed PKU and severe challenging behavior: A randomised placebo-controlled trial of phenylalanine-restricted diet. *J Neurol Neurosurg Psychiatry*. 2009;80(6):631–635
10. Levy HL, Ghavani M. Maternal phenylketonuria: A metabolic teratogen. *Teratology*. 1996;53:176–184
11. van Spronsen FJ, Hoeksma M, Reijngoud DJ. Brain dysfunction in phenylketonuria: Is phenylalanine toxicity the only possible cause? *J Inherit Metab Dis*. 2009;32:46–51.
12. Mitchell JJ, Scriver CR. Phenylalanine hydroxylase deficiency. *Gene Reviews*. 2007. Available from: www.genetests.org
13. Feillet F, Clarke L, Meli C, Lipson M, Morris AA, Harmatz P, Mould DR, Green B, Dorenbaum A, Giovannini M, Foehr E; for the Sapropterin Research Group. Pharmacokinetics of sapropterin in patients with phenylketonuria. *Clin Pharmacokinet*. 2008;47:817–825
14. Levy HL, Burton B, Cederbaum S, Scriver C. Recommendations for evaluation of responsiveness to tetrahydrobiopterin (BH4) in phenylketonuria and its use in treatment. *Mol Genet Metab*. 2007;92:287–291
15. Burton BK, Grange DK, Milanowski A, Vockley G, Feillet F, Crombez EA, Abadie V, Harding CO, Cedarbaum S, Dobbelaere D, Smith A, Dorenbaum A. The response of patients with phenylketonuria and elevated serum phenylalanine to treatment with oral sapropterin dihydrochloride (6R-tetrahydrobiopterin): A phase II, multicentre, open-label, screening study. *J Inherit Metab Dis*. 2007;30:700–707
16. Blau N, Belanger-Quintana A, Demirkol M, Feillet F, Giovannini M, Macdonald A, Trefz FK, Sponsen FV. Optimizing the use of sapropterin (BH4) in the management of phenylketonuria. *Mol Genet Metab*. 2009;96:158–163
17. Levy HL, Milanowski A, Chakrapani A, Cleary M, Lee P, Trefz FK, Whitley CB, Feillet F, Feigenbaum AS, Bebchuk JD, Christ-Schmidt H, Dorenbaum A, Sapropterin Research Group. Efficacy of sapropterin dihydrochloride (tetrahydrobiopterin, 6R-BH4) for reduction of phenylalanine concentrations in patients with phenylketonuria: A phase III randomised placebo-controlled study. *Lancet*. 2007;370:504–510
18. Trefz FK, Burton BK, Longo N, Casanova MM, Gruskin DJ, Dorenbaum A, Kakkis ED, Crombez EA, Grange DK, Harmatz P, Lipson MH, Milanowski A, Randolph LM, Vockley J, Whitley CB, Wolff JA, Bebchuk J, Christ-Schmidt H, Hennermann JB, Sapropterin Study Group. Efficacy of sapropterin dihydrochloride in increasing phenylalanine tolerance in children with phenylketonuria: A phase III, randomized double-blind, placebo-controlled study. *J Pediatr*. 2009;154:700–707

19. Burlina A, Blau N. Effect of BH(4) supplementation on phenylalanine tolerance. *J Inherit Metab Dis*. 2009;32:40–45
20. Sarkissian CN, Gamez A. Phenylalanine ammonia lyase, enzyme substitution therapy for phenylketonuria, where are we now? *Mol Genet Metab*. 2005;86(Suppl 1):S22–S26
21. Matalon R, Michals-Matalon K, Bhatia G, Burlina AB, Burlina AP, Braga C, Fiori L, Giovannini M, Grechanina E, Novikov P, Grady J, Tyring SK, Guttler F. Double blind placebo control trial of large neutral amino acids in treatment of phenylketonuria: Effect on blood phenylalanine. *J Inherit Metab Dis*. 2007;30:153–158
22. Schindeler S, Ghosh-Jerath S, Thompson S, Rocca A, Joy P, Kemp A, Rae C, Green K, Wilcken B, Christodoulou J. The effects of large neutral amino acid supplements in PKU: An MRS and neuropsychological study. *Mol Genet Metab*. 2007;91:48–54
23. Harding C. Progress toward cell-directed therapy for phenylketonuria. *Clin Genet*. 2008;74:97–104

7 L-carnitine therapy in primary and secondary carnitine deficiency disorders

Susan C. Winter, Brian Schreiber, and Neil R. M. Buist

INTRODUCTION

L-carnitine (L-3-hydroxy-4-aminobutyrobetaine) is a naturally occurring substance required for the bidirectional transport of acyl groups across the mitochondrial membrane. It is an essential part of this system because the inner mitochondrial membrane is impermeable to coenzyme A (CoA) or to compounds attached to CoA, such as long-chain fatty acids. Free fatty acids are transported in plasma and attached to albumin. They cross cellular plasma membranes via yet-to-be-completely-delineated channels, where they are converted by fatty acyl-CoA synthases to fatty acyl-CoA derivatives. These derivatives, in turn, have to enter mitochondria as fuel for beta oxidation. Because the mitochondrial membrane is impermeable to CoA, the fatty acyl-CoA is esterified to carnitine and transported into the mitochondrial matrix. This esterification of acyl groups to carnitine and subsequent transport into the mitochondrial matrix requires three enzymes: carnitine acyltransferases I and II and carnitine acyltranslocase. This process allows for the delivery of fatty acyl groups to the inner mitochondrial matrix for beta oxidation and adenosine triphosphate (ATP) generation. A reverse process by which acyl-CoA groups (including acetyl-CoA) within the mitochondrion are exported also requires the formation of carnitine esters via carnitine acetyltransferase II (Figure 7–1).

Because CoA cannot cross the inner mitochondrial membrane, any accumulation of acyl-CoAs (bound CoA) can affect the availability of free CoA that is essential to the maintenance of mitochondrial function. Any disruption of the acyl (bound)-CoA/free CoA ratio alters the redox system and can profoundly disrupt the metabolism of amino acids, organic acids, and fatty acids and the generation of energy. Under normal homeostatic conditions, acylcarnitines formed within

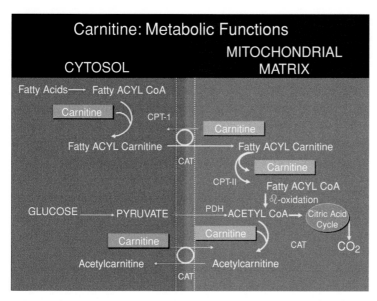

Figure 7–1: This figure includes those inborn errors of metabolism with intramitochondrial pathways resulting in accumulation of specific and toxic acyl groups depending on the enzymatic defect. Carnitine can form an acylcarnitine with these accumulating acyl groups and allow for excretion in the urine. Loss of the carnitine molecule attached to the acyl group will result in secondary carnitine deficiency if dietary intake and endogenous synthesis cannot restore adequate amounts of carnitine as needed to clear the acyl load.

the mitochondria are exported into the cytosol and either used within the cells or passed into the blood. Any extra or unused acyl-CoAs are then filtered by the kidney and excreted.

If additional amounts of acyl-CoAs accumulate in the mitochondria, they are removed by the same mechanism, thus resulting in increasing losses of carnitine from within the mitochondria. The acylcarnitines are mostly excreted by the renal tubules, resulting not only in a diminution of the toxic radicals but also in an increased loss of the carnitine that is bound to them. With each acyl group eliminated, one carnitine molecule is lost.[1,2] Free carnitine is selectively reabsorbed by the renal tubules, a transport system with evolutionary significance, but one that cannot compensate for increased losses of bound carnitine.

The accumulation of specific acylcarnitines in the plasma that occurs in many inborn errors of metabolism, particularly in fatty acid and amino acid metabolism, forms the basis of a newborn screening test that can detect as many as 30 disorders with a single assay using a double mass spectrometry assay (tandem mass spectrometry, MS/MS).

The primary sources of carnitine are either diet (mainly from red meat and dairy products) or endogenous hepatic synthesis from trimethylated lysine derivatives cleaved during muscle protein catabolism. These sources allow for maintenance of normal free carnitine levels in blood, muscle, and other tissues during states of metabolic equilibrium (Figure 7–1).[3]

In clinical conditions in which there is abnormal accumulation of acyl-CoAs, the normal homeostatic mechanisms that maintain a sufficient concentration of tissue and plasma free carnitine for the performance of its metabolic functions can be overwhelmed. Because of the central role that carnitine plays in energy generation, such insufficiency can lead to severe physiological consequences. Under such circumstances, carnitine becomes a critical compound that must be supplied to deficient patients in pharmacological doses. Because the active carnitine isomer is the levo form, carnitine needs to be replaced using that L-isomer. The existence of carnitine deficiency, as well as the successful use of pharmacological doses of L-carnitine, has been well documented in the medical literature. There are a number of specific forms of carnitine deficiency.

In primary carnitine deficiency, there is an absolute decrease in both plasma free as well as acylcarnitines due to a genetically inherited abnormality in the OCTN2 carnitine transporter that is responsible for both the transport of carnitine into tissues as well as the renal reabsorption of free carnitine necessary to maintain adequate levels of carnitine in the plasma.

Secondary carnitine deficiency is defined as carnitine deficiency resulting from loss of acylcarnitines in certain inborn errors of metabolism or drug therapies (e.g., valproic acid), dietary deficiency, increased loss of free carnitine during dialysis or with renal tubular dysfunction and decreased synthesis due to liver disease. In certain metabolic errors, massive formation and subsequent excretion of acylcarnitines, leads to profound plasma and tissue secondary carnitine deficiency. The evidence for the existence of both primary and secondary carnitine deficiency, as well for their successful treatment with pharmacological doses of L-carnitine, is presented in the following sections.

In the early years after the recognition of symptomatic carnitine deficiency, all cases were thought to be some form of a primary genetic deficiency. It was not until after the recognition of the mitochondrial carnitine transporter defect in 1988 that it became evident that deficiency could also arise secondary to other metabolic perturbations. This situation led to many years of confusion and to fierce disputes regarding the role of carnitine in intermediary metabolism and the need to replace it during periods of increased loss.[4]

PRIMARY CARNITINE DEFICIENCY

In an extensive review of carnitine deficiency syndromes written in 1995, Pons and DeVivo defined primary carnitine deficiency as "a decrease of intracellular carnitine content that impairs fatty acid oxidation and that is not associated with another identifiable systemic illness that might deplete tissue carnitine stores."[5]

The genetic defect in primary carnitine deficiency is loss of function of the high affinity carnitine membrane transporter, OCTN2, a sodium ion–dependent transporter protein. This transporter facilitates uptake of carnitine from the plasma into heart and skeletal muscle and reabsorption of free carnitine across the renal tubules resulting in a greatly reduced carnitine concentration in myocytes and plasma.

Earlier literature suggested a separate primary muscle carnitine deficiency characterized by low skeletal and/or cardiac muscle carnitine levels but with normal renal transport. Later studies suggest that this is not another primary genetic entitiy but secondary to leakage of carnitine out of the muscle cell as can be seen in skeletal myopathies and cardiomyopathies.

Primary systemic carnitine deficiency due to OCTN2 deficiency is an autosomal recessive disorder. Lamhonwah and colleagues described a variety of mutations in the SLCC2A5 (OCTN2) gene localized to the 5q31.1 locus.[6,7] Primary carnitine deficiency is rare. Koizumi and colleagues reported a prevalence of heterozygotes of 1.01% from a study population of 973 unrelated subjects in Akita, Japan.[8] This degree of heterozygosity would predict an estimated incidence of primary systemic carnitine deficiency of 1 in 40,000 live births.

The diagnosis is often suspected as a result of a workup following the death of a sibling or by the identification of a low free carnitine on expanded newborn screening by MS/MS. It is supported by the presence of characteristic clinical symptoms and decreased plasma and/or muscle total and free carnitine levels, normal or low acylcarnitine levels, and the absence of an inborn error of metabolism known to be associated with secondary carnitine deficiency. Confirmation is achieved by demonstrating a defective uptake of carnitine into fibroblasts or by identification of a pathogenic mutation upon sequencing of the SLCC2A5 gene. The mean age of presentation with symptoms was two years old prior to expansion of newborn screening. The most common clinical presentation is progressive cardiomyopathy in which the heart is both dilated and/or hypertrophic. The condition is resistant to usual therapeutic agents for heart failure. Progressive deterioration and death ensues if sufficient carnitine therapy is not administered. Additional problems that may occur include acute encephalopathy, skeletal weakness and hypotonia, hypoketotic hypoglycemia, hypoketonemia, hepatic dysfunction, hyperammonemia, metabolic acidosis, and hematological abnormalities.

In mild cases of primary carnitine deficiency, patients present at a later age, often in the second or third decades. Whereas serum carnitine levels may be mildly reduced, there is a severe reduction in muscle carnitine levels. Symptoms may include weakness and exercise intolerance as well as an associated cardiomyopathy.[9]

Because OCTN2 transporter deficiency is rare and the symptoms are so variable, it is not feasible to conduct large randomized trials of treatment for primary systemic carnitine deficiency. There are now, however, numerous published case reports documenting the significant benefit of treatment with L-carnitine. Cederbaum and colleagues have reported the long-term results of treatment of several cases of primary systemic carnitine deficiency. Among these cases was a male patient who first became symptomatic at the age of three months. Prior to initiation of carnitine therapy, he had spent one-third of the first three years of his life as an inpatient, having experienced 11 hospital admissions, eight episodes of cardiac arrest, and numerous hypoglycemic episodes. Following initiation of L-carnitine therapy, he remained free of hospitalizations for a 20-year period and had a normalization of cardiac and skeletal muscle function allowing for gainful employment. A second case was that of an infant girl who presented at the age of 14 months with abnormal motor development, weakness, and recurrent respiratory tract infections followed at age three by congestive heart failure with a dilated cardiomyopathy. Treatment with L-carnitine was associated with a marked improvement in exercise tolerance and weight as well as normalization of left ventricular function allowing for a physically active life as a university student at the age of 22 years. A third patient presented with recurrent episodes of hypoglycemic encephalopathy at age 2.5 years with cardiomyopathy. Treatment with oral carnitine therapy led to normalization of echocardiographic and electrocardiographic indices and improvement in muscle strength and growth. At last report at age 16, she was entirely asymptomatic and performing well in school on continued carnitine therapy. The report of these three patients included references to additional cases showing benefit for more than 20 years with L-carnitine treatment.[10]

Additional cases of primary systemic carnitine deficiency with resolution of cardiomyopathy and other manifestations following treatment with L-carnitine have been more recently reported by Hou[11] and Goa[12] using oral L-carnitine at 50–100 mg/kg/d.

Although, in general, patients who are heterozygous for OCTN2 mutations have long been thought to be asymptomatic, a recent report by Takahashi and colleagues suggests that such heterozygotes may be at risk for cardiac abnormalities when additional cardiac burdens are imposed. Eleven-week-old jvs/+ mice (models for the heterozygous form of primary systemic carnitine deficiency) were subjected to ascending aortic constriction as were normal mice. Four weeks after the surgical creation of pressure overload, the jvs/+ mice showed a worsening of cardiac hypertrophy and cardiac congestion, reduction of the myocardial phosphocreatine/ATP ratio, and higher mortality than their normal counterparts despite having only mild reductions in the plasma and myocardial total carnitine levels. Treatment after aortic constriction with a 1% L-carnitine diet prevented this clinical worsening, suggesting that the heterozygous state may be of significance in the presence of concurrent cardiac risk factors for hypertrophic cardiomyopathy or congestive heart failure.[13] An observational study by Koizumi and colleagues (1999) in which family members of patients with primary systemic carnitine deficiency were examined with echocardiography showed that heterozygotes for OCTN2 mutations were at risk for late-onset cardiac hypertrophy, with an odds ratio of 15.1 (95% confidence interval, 1.39–164).[6]

Clinical improvement with L-carnitine therapy has also been documented for the isolated myopathic form of primary carnitine deficiency. Engel and Rebouche (1984) summarized 19 cases of myopathic carnitine deficiency observed from 1973 through 1984. The index case was a young woman with an excess of intramyocellular lipid. An additional 18 cases were described in the review. Of the 19 patients described, 17 had generalized muscle weakness and 2 had exertional weakness and myalgias. In addition, the disease was complicated by cardiomyopathy in five patients and myoglobinuria in two patients. Intramyocellular lipid and reduced muscle carnitine levels were found in all cases. Of the cases reported, carnitine therapy was administered to 11 patients, 7 of whom had clinical improvement.[14]

In a recent report by Vielhaber and colleagues (2004), two adult patients with myalgia and fatigability on exertion were found to have markedly decreased skeletal muscle carnitine with a mildly decreased plasma free carnitine in one patient and a normal plasma level in the other, suggestive of primary myopathic carnitine deficiency. Serum creatine phosphokinase levels were mildly increased, and muscle biopsy showed characteristic lipid storage droplets predominantly in type 1 muscle fibers. Treatment with L-carnitine, 3 g/d, was associated with improvement in muscle histology and electromyographic parameters as well as complete resolution of clinical symptoms. The serum creatine phosphokinase level returned almost to control values in one patient but remained slightly elevated in the other. On therapy, an increase in muscle free carnitine was reported in both patients.[15]

Although, as stated earlier in this chapter, the small number of patients with primary carnitine deficiency precludes the performance of randomized controlled trials, Ashbrook performed a literature review of the clinical outcomes in patients with both systemic and myopathic carnitine deficiency and reported the results of an prospective, unblinded, nonrandomized treatment trial of carnitine replacement in patients with systemic, myopathic, and/or secondary carnitine deficiencies. Results were reported for 10 patients with primary systemic carnitine deficiency and for 5 with the myopathic form. The literature summary revealed that, of 14 patients treated with carnitine for systemic carnitine deficiency, 9 experienced clinical improvement (64%), 4 had no therapeutic response (29%), and 1 patient died (7%). The carnitine dose ranged from 1.5 to 5 g/d orally. Of the patients who did not receive carnitine supplementation, six of seven (86%) died and one patient survived but showed no clinical improvement. Two patients with myopathic carnitine deficiency showed no change in their condition, whereas five patients improved with carnitine alone as did an additional two patients with a combination of carnitine and steroids. The results from the prospective study were reported for the 15 patients who had received treatment for primary carnitine deficiency of either the systemic ($n = 10$) or myopathic ($n = 5$) variety. Of the 10 patients with systemic carnitine deficiency, significant improvement was reported for 4 patients, marginal improvement for 2, and a stable clinical condition for 4 patients. All 5 of the patients with primary myopathic carnitine deficiency were reported to have shown significant improvement in muscle function. Side effects of carnitine therapy included diarrhea in 1 of the 10 patients with systemic carnitine deficiency, and there were no evident side effects on the primary myopathic patients receiving a mean dose of 3.7 g/d.[16]

In summary, treatment with L-carnitine has been associated with dramatic improvement in the clinical status of patients with primary systemic carnitine deficiency that is maintained as long as the patient remains on L-carnitine therapy. Benefit has also been reported in the majority of patients treated for primary myopathic carnitine deficiency. Failure to treat with L-carnitine is associated with mortality and morbidity; complete resolution may be compromised by undue delay in the application of L-carnitine therapy. The recommended dose range for L-carnitine primary carnitine deficiency is 50–100 mg/kg/d. When the patient is in acute decompensation, L-carnitine is usually administered intravenously at 100 mg/kg/d in four divided doses six hours apart. After the patient has stabilized, the dose may be switched to 50–100 mg/kg/d orally with doses divided, ideally, every six hours. Frequent daily dosing is required because of the short half-life of L-carnitine because of its rapid renal elimination.

CARNITINE DEFICIENCY SECONDARY TO INBORN ERRORS OF METABOLISM

Carnitine deficiency occurs as a complication of many inborn errors of metabolism, specifically those involving acyl-CoA derivatives of fatty acid oxidation or organic acid metabolism. Indeed, in any situation in which excess acyl-CoAs accumulate, the acyl groups are removed from the mitochondria bound to carnitine, and these compounds are subsequently excreted by the kidney tubules in the form of acylcarnitines. This system is both beneficial and potentially dangerous. Removal of toxic acyl compounds is beneficial, but the accompanying loss of the carnitine can be detrimental.

Increased levels of acylcarnitine and concomitant loss of free carnitine results in an abnormal acyl/free carnitine ratio and consequent disruption in the acyl-CoA/free CoA ratio. This in turn leads to a disturbed redox equipoise in the mitochondria that can be life-threatening. Carnitine removes the toxic acyl groups, and deficiency of carnitine develops secondary to the inability of diet and endogenous synthesis to compensate for the excessive loss of the acylcarnitines in the urine. This carnitine deficiency is thus secondary to the primary genetic inborn error of metabolism.[17] Carnitine deficiencies secondary to other causes – such as malnutrition, renal or liver disease, diabetes, or drug therapy – are not considered here.

The symptoms of carnitine deficiency are identical in any situation in which carnitine has become rate-limiting. They relate to the compromised beta oxidation of fatty acids and the consequent strain on ATP homeostasis. In addition, in secondary deficiencies, symptoms of the underlying causative condition vary depending on the primary diagnosis. As the situation deteriorates, there is increasing likelihood of a more general disruption of mitochondrial function with all of their activities compromised or even shutting down.

The earliest findings are as subtle as those seen in emerging iron deficiency with nonspecific complaints of mild fatigue and muscle weakness. When these are of slow onset, the patient does not even recognize them until treatment has started (and he or she notices a rapid improvement). As the deficiency becomes worse, the findings are of a generalized myopathy that is characterized by increased lipid deposits in the cytosol and can be proven by assay of the muscle carnitine. It is essential to realize that, because most of the carnitine in the body is in the

Table 7–1. Inborn errors of metabolism causing secondary carnitine deficiency

---

Fatty Acid Oxidation Disorders
  Carnitine Transport
    Carnitine palmitoyltransferase I
    Translocase
    Carnitine palmitoyltransferase II
  Beta Oxidation
    Short-chain acyl-CoA* dehydrogenase deficiency
    Medium-chain acyl-CoA dehydrogenase deficiency
    Long-chain acyl-CoA dehydrogenase deficiency
    Very-long-chain acyl-CoA dehydrogenase deficiency
    Short-chain 3-hydroxyacyl-CoA dehydrogenase deficiency
    Trifunctional protein deficiency
    2,4-Dienoyl-CoA reductase deficiency
  Organic Acidurias
    Glutaric aciduria I
    Multiple acyl-CoA dehydrogenase deficiencies – Glutaric aciduria II
    Isovaleric acidemia
    Propionic acidemia
    Methylmalonic acidemias
    3-Methylcrotonyl CoA carboxylase deficiency
    3-Methylglutaconic aciduria
  3-Hydroxymethylglutaryl CoA Lyase Deficiency
    2-Methylacetoacetyl CoA thiolase deficiency
  Mitochondrial Disorders
    Mitochondrial DNA† point mutations, deletions, and depletion
    Nuclear encoded defects of electron transport
  Other Metabolic Disorders
    5,10-Methylene tetrahydrofolate reductase deficiency
    Adenosine deaminase deficiency
    Ornithine transcarbamylase deficiency
    Carbamoyl phosphate synthase I deficiency

---

* CoA: coenzyme A
† DNA: deoxyribonucleic acid
Source: Pons R, DeVivo D. Primary and secondary carnitine deficiency syndromes.
J Child Neurology. 1995;10 (Suppl 2):S8–S24

muscles, it is possible to have a considerable deficiency in total body content even if plasma levels are still normal, a situation comparable to that seen in potassium deficiency.

As the deficiency becomes more profound, dilated cardiomyopathy, hepatic encephalopathy or Reyes-like syndrome, failure to thrive, muscular hypotonia, and/or weakness with gross motor delays in children can be seen. These most severe manifestations are likely to be accompanied by biochemical evidence of compromised activity of many metabolic pathways, including the urea cycle, gluconeogenesis, and all other intramitochondrial activities. Organic acids may reveal dicarboxylic acids as evidence of extramitochondrial omega oxidation of fats. The inborn errors of metabolism that have been reported as causes of secondary carnitine deficiency are summarized in Table 7–1. The first report of muscle carnitine deficiency was in 1973 by Engel and Angelini.[18] In 1980, DiMauro, Trevisan, and Hays[19] first suggested that "secondary" carnitine deficiency may occur in mitochondrial disorders and with carnitine palmitoyltransferase deficiency. Roe and Bohan reported on carnitine therapy of propionic acidemia in 1982.[20] By 1983, Rebouche and Engel[21] reported on at least 15 genetic disorders of intermediary metabolism associated with carnitine deficiency. Stanley and colleagues first reported medium-chain fatty acyl-CoA dehydrogenase deficiency in 1983 and documented carnitine deficiency in muscle, blood, and liver in three patients.[22] A positive response to carnitine therapy was noted in methylmalonic acidemia and 3-OH 3-methylglutaric acidemia by Chalmers and colleagues in 1984[23] and later by Stumpf, Parker, and Angelini in 1985[24] and Winter and colleagues in 1987.[25]

Engel and Rebouche reviewed the various genetic defects of intermediary metabolism giving rise to secondary metabolism in 1984,[26] and multiple articles appeared in that year documenting secondary carnitine deficiency and improved excretion of specific acylcarnitine species with carnitine treatment and improved health. These reported diseases included propionic acidemia, methylmalonic acidemia,[27,28] short-chain fatty acyl-CoA dehydrogenase deficiency,[29] glutaric aciduria type II,[30] and isovaleric acidemia.[31] A 1995 review by Pons and DeVivo[5] reported on secondary carnitine deficiency syndromes, and Table 7–1 is extracted from their article.

Treatment of the secondary carnitine deficiency due to inborn errors of metabolism with pharmacologic-grade L-carnitine allows for restoration of mitochondrial energy metabolism with the simultaneous excretion of toxic metabolites. Improvement in clinical symptoms and increased excretion of disease-specific acylcarnitine derivatives were first reported in 1982.[19,25–29] In 1992, the U.S. Food and Drug Administration approved Carnitor (L-carnitine; Sigma-Tau Pharmaceuticals, Inc., Gaithersburg, MD) for secondary carnitine deficiency due to inborn errors of metabolism. Because of the small number of patients available and great variability both genetically and clinically within each specific disorder, double-blind/placebo studies were felt to be unreliable and possibly unethical due to the published cases of symptomatic carnitine deficiency. New Drug Approval was therefore based on evidence from a retrospective analysis of 90 patients by using both clinical and biochemical evidence of efficacy and by comparing them to an historical cohort of patients treated conventionally without carnitine therapy.

The results of the analysis showed that there was a significant decrease in hospitalization frequency for L-carnitine–treated patients and resolution of failure to thrive. The mortality rate in carnitine-treated patients was 2/48 versus 18/18 of the historical, untreated cohort. The biochemical evidence of efficacy included an increased excretion of disease-specific acylcarnitine species in 12 patients and restoration of ketosis indicative of improved beta oxidation in 3 medium-chain fatty acyl-CoA dehydrogenase patients with carnitine deficiency when treated with an oral carnitine load of 100 mg/kg. Normalization of the cardiac ejection fraction after 10 days of carnitine therapy was associated with increased excretion of glutarylcarnitine in a patient with glutaric aciduria II. Increased hippuric acid excretion with benzoic acid administration was demonstrated in three urea cycle disorder patients on carnitine therapy versus a baseline without carnitine treatment. Because benzoic acid must be converted to benzoyl CoA within the mitochondria to be further converted to hippuric acid, the addition of carnitine was felt to reflect an increased availability of mitochondrial free CoA. Adverse events for the treated patient cohort included vomiting in 37%, diarrhea in 23%, abdominal pain in 12%, fishy odor due to trimethylamine formation by bowel bacteria from undigested carnitine in 12%, and one patient with transient alopecia and rash. Two patients died from their disorders.[32]

A recent meta-analysis by The Cochrane Group[33] found that there were *no* randomized controlled studies on the efficacy of carnitine therapy for disorders secondary to inborn errors of metabolism. It was opined that clinicians should base therapeutic decisions on clinical experience. They did not recommend or discourage the use of carnitine for any disorder but stated that controlled trials should be done with the caveat that such trials might not be ethical in view of the risk of placebo use in potentially lethal conditions.

The Cochrane report does little to resolve a contentious situation. The use and value of L-carnitine for the treatment of secondary deficiency is not universally accepted; indeed, fierce controversy still exists in certain quarters. Many clinicians wish to practice evidence-based medicine whereas others, with extensive experience in the management of metabolic disorders, have seen the beneficial effects of therapy on many occasions and do not hesitate to use carnitine when clinically appropriate.

The recent development of expanded newborn screening by MS/MS around the world has shown that the overall incidence of disorders in which abnormal levels of CoA metabolites accumulate is approximately 1 in 5,000 births. These patients are adding a new complexity to the carnitine debate. As always, the early descriptions of these disorders were of serious cases for whom any potential therapy was justified. As has happened for every disorder detected by newborn screening, milder examples and more "variant" cases of all of these disorders are now being recognized. The natural history of such mild cases is unknown as indeed is their need for therapy. Newborn screening may open the door to the possibility of reasonably well-controlled studies of efficacy of treatment, but the above Cochrane caveat remains critical.[33]

In summary, carnitine deficiency is a frequent secondary complication in patients with inborn errors of fatty acid oxidation and organic acid metabolism. The excretion of specific accumulating acylcarnitine species provides a detoxification mechanism at the expense of loss of free carnitine. Treatment with pharmacologic doses of L-carnitine not only prevents carnitine deficiency, but allows for the excretion of toxic metabolites. Route of administration (intravenous or oral) and dosage (50–300 mg/kg/d) depend on the clinical severity of presentation, ability to absorb oral medications, and severity of the underlying metabolic disturbance. Carnitine treatment during metabolic crisis has been reported on numerous occasions to be lifesaving and has become the state-of-the-art therapy for many metabolic disorders.[20]

REFERENCES

1. Siliprandi N, Sartorelli L, Ciman M, Di Lisa F. Carnitine: Metabolism and clinical chemistry. *Clin Chem Acta*. 1989;183(1):3–11
2. Bremer J. The role of carnitine in intracellular metabolism. *J Clin Chem Clin Biochem*. 1990;28(5):297–301
3. Rebouche CJ, Paulson DJ. Carnitine metabolism and function in humans. *Annu Rev Nutr*. 1986;6:41–66
4. Treem WR, Stanley CA, Finegold DN, Hale DE, Coates PM. Primary carnitine deficiency due to a failure of carnitine transport in kidney, muscle and fibroblasts. *N Engl J Med*. 1988;319(20):1331–1336
5. Pons R, DeVivo D. Primary and secondary carnitine deficiency syndromes. *J Child Neurology*. 1995;10(Suppl 2):S8–S24
6. http://www.ncbi.nlm.nih.gov/entrez/dispomim.cgi?id=212140
7. Lamhonwah AM, Olpin SE, Pollitt RJ, Vianey-Saban C, Divry P, Guffon N, Besley GT, Onizuka R, De Meirleir LJ, Cvitanovic-Sojat L, Baric I, Dionisi-Vici C, Fumic K, Maradin M, Tein I. Novel OCTN 2 mutations: No genotype-phenotype correlations: Early carnitine therapy prevents cardiomyopathy. *Am J Med Genet*. 2002;111:271–284
8. Koizumi A, Nozaki J, Ohura T, Kayo T, Wada Y, Nezu J, Ohashi R, Tamai I, Shoji Y, Takada G, Kibira S, Matsuishi T, Tsuji A. Genetic epidemiology of the carnitine transporter OCTN2 gene in a Japanese population and phenotypic characterization in Japanese population and phenotypic characterization in Japanese pedigrees with primary systemic carnitine deficiency *Hum Mol Genet*. 1999;8(12):2247–2254
9. Angelini C, Trevisan G, Isaya G, Pegolo G, Vergani L. Clinical varieties of carnitine and carnitine palmitoyltransferase deficiency. *Clin Biochem*. 1987;20:1–7
10. Cederbaum S, Koo-McCoy S, Tein I, Hsu BY, Ganguly A, Vilain E, Dipple K, Cvitanovic-Sojat L, Stanley C. Carnitine membrane transporter deficiency: A long-term follow up and OCTN2 mutation in the first documented case of primary carnitine deficiency. *Mol Genet Metab*. 2002;77:195–201
11. Hou J. Primary systemic carnitine deficiency presenting as recurrent Reye-like syndrome and dilated cardiomyopathy. *Chang Gung Med J*. 2002;25:832–837
12. Goa K, Brogden R. l-Carnitine. A preliminary review of its pharmacokinetics and its therapeutic use in ischemic cardiac disease and primary and secondary carnitine deficiencies in relationship to its role in fatty acid metabolism. *Drugs*. 1987;34:1–24
13. Takahashi R, Asai T, Murakami H, Murakami R, Tsuzuki M, Numaguchi Y, Matsui H, Murohara T, Okumura K. Pressure overload-induced cardiomyopathy in heterozygous carrier mice of carnitine transporter gene mutation. *Hypertension*. 2007;50:497–502
14. Engel AG, Rebouche CJ. Carnitine metabolism and inborn errors. *J. Inher Metab Dis*. 1984;7(Suppl 1):38–43
15. Vielhaber S, Feistner H, Weis J, Kreuder J, Sailer M, Schroder, JM, Kunz WS. Primary carnitine deficiency: Adult onset lipid storage myopathy with a mild clinical course. *J Clin Neurosci*. 2004;11(8):919–924
16. Ashbrook DW. Carnitine supplementation in human carnitine deficiency. P.R. Borum, ed. *Clinical Aspects of Human Carnitine Deficiency*, Pergamon Press, New York, 120–134, 1986
17. Chalmers RA, Roe CR, Stacey TE, Hoppel CL. Urinary excretion of L-carnitine and acylcarnitines in patients with disorders of organic acid metabolism: Evidence for secondary insufficiency of l-carnitine. *Pediatr Res*. 1984;18(12):1325–1328

18. Engel AG, Angelini C. Carnitine deficiency of human skeletal muscle with associated lipid storage myopathy: A new syndrome. *Science*. 1973;179(76):899–902
19. DiMauro S, Trevisan C, Hays A. Disorders of lipid metabolism in muscle. *Muscle Nerve*. 1980;3(5):369–388
20. Roe CR, Bohan TP. L-carnitine therapy in propionicacidemia. *Lancet*. 1982;(8286): 1411–1412
21. Rebouche CJ, Engel AG. Carnitine metabolism and deficiency syndromes. *Mayo Clin Proc*. 1983;58(8):533–540
22. Stanley CA, Hale DE, Coates PM, Hall CL, Corkey BE, Yang W, Kelly RI, Gonzales EL, Williamson JR, Baker L. Medium-chain acyl-CoA dehydrogenase deficiency in children with non-ketotic hypoglycemia and low carnitine levels. *Pediatr Res*. 1983;17(11):877– 884
23. Chalmers RA, Stacey TE, Tracey BM, deSousa C, Roe CR, Millington DS, Hoppel CL. L-Carnitine insufficiency in disorders of organic acid metabolism: Response to L-carnitine by patients with methylmalonic aciduria an 3-hydroxy-3-methylglutaric aciduria. *J Inherit Metab Dis*. 1984;7(Suppl 2):109–110
24. Stumpf DA, Parker WD Jr, Angelini C. Carnitine deficiency, organic acidemias and Reye's syndrome. *Neurology*. 1985;35(7):1041–1045
25. Winter SC, Szabo-Aczel S, Curry CJ, Hutchinson HT, Hogue R, Shug A. Plasma carnitine deficiency. Clinical observations in 51 pediatric patients. *Am J Dis Child*. 1987;141(6):660–665
26. Engel AG, Rebouche CJ. Carnitine metabolism and inborn errors. *J Inherit Metab Dis*. 1984;7(Suppl 1):38–43
27. DiDonato S, Rimoldi M, Garavaglia B, Uziel G. Propionylcarnitine excretion in propionic and methylmalonic acidurias: A cause of carnitine deficiency. *Clin Chim Acta*. 1984;139(1):13–21
28. Roe CR, Millington DS, Maltby DA, Bohan TP, Hoppel CL. L-carnitine enhances excretion of propionyl coenzyme A as propionylcarnitine in propionic acidemia. *J Clin Invest*. 1984;73(6):1785–1788
29. Turnbull DM, Bartlett K, Stevens DL, Alberti KG, Gibson GJ, Johnson MA, McCulloch AJ, Sherratt HS. Short-chain acyl-CoA dehydrogenase deficiency associated with a lipid-storage myopathy and secondary carnitine deficiency. *N Engl J Med*. 1984;311(19):1232–1236
30. Mooy PD, Przyrembel H, Giesberts MA, Scholte HR, Blom W, van Gelderen HH. Glutaric aciduria type II: Treatment with riboflavin, carnitine and insulin. *Eur J Pediatr*. 1984;143(2):92–95
31. Roe CR, Millington DS, Maltby DA, Kahler SG, Bohan TP. L-carnitine therapy in isovaleric acidemia. *J Clin Invest*. 1984;74(6):2290–2295
32. Winter SC. Treatment of carnitine deficiency. *J Inherit Metab Dis*. 2003;26(2–3):171–180
33. Nasser M, Javaheri H, Fedorowicz Z, Noorani Z. Carnitine supplementation in inborn errors of metabolism. *Cochrane Database Syst Rev*. 2009;(2):CD006659

SECTION III
UTILIZATION OF ALTERNATIVE PATHWAYS

8 Cysteamine treatment of nephropathic cystinosis

Jess G. Thoene

NATURAL HISTORY OF NEPHROPATHIC CYSTINOSIS

Nephropathic cystinosis has been known as a clinical entity since the first decade of the last century.[1] Two small, pale children who died of wasting and whose organs were shown to be riddled with microscopic crystals were described by a German pathologist, Emil Abderhalden, in 1903. The condition was known as familial cystine diathesis, and for approximately 40 years the disease was conflated with the unrelated condition cystinuria. Cystinuria is now known to be an extracellular disease of renal cystine transport leading to excess cystine urinary excretion,[2] whereas cystinosis is known to be an intracellular disease of lysosomal cystine storage that results from a failure to transport cystine out of the lysosome, leading to its accumulation.[3]

Children with nephropathic cystinosis appear normal at birth but during the first year of life develop elements of the renal Fanconi syndrome. The renal Fanconi syndrome includes polyuria, sodium and potassium wasting, and an abnormal excretion of glucose, phosphate, amino acids, and carnitine.[1] The thirst mechanism in these children is intact, hence they are able to compensate for the excess salt and water wasting if provided with adequate salt and water to drink. They are at some risk for dehydration in summer months in tropical climates where oral intake does not keep up with the obligatory fluid and electrolyte losses. The first child born to a couple may suffer because the parents do not know what the normal amount of urinary excretion should be. Urinary volume of several liters per day is not unusual in such children who are less than a year of age. The diagnosis can be established definitively by measuring circulating white blood cell cystine and/or by skin biopsy and cultured fibroblast cystine measurement. Also, the diagnosis could be strongly suspected after an ophthalmologic examination in which the unique crystalline keratopathy is apparent after the first few months of life, accompanied by a pathognomonic salt-and-pepper retinopathy, which has been observed in 20-week fetuses.

After the first few months of life, and if the children are adequately treated with water and electrolyte replacement therapy including sodium, potassium, and phosphate, the children do relatively well. They fail to thrive, however, never achieving a height greater than the 50th percentile for a three year old. Renal function declines slowly from birth. At birth the creatinine clearance is approximately normal; however, by age 10 years, the creatinine clearance is essentially zero.[4] This decline is accompanied in the untreated patients by renal rickets, manifested by tenderness of the distal ends of the long bones and, on occasion, a rachitic rosary. The cystinotic phenotype – which also includes fair complexion, blonde hair, and blue eyes (in Caucasians); lighter complexion (in dark-skinned individuals); and universally short stature, photophobia, polyuria, and polydipsia – makes the diagnosis relatively easy once the entity has been considered.

Untreated children undergo renal death by approximately 10 years of age and require either chronic dialysis or renal transplantation. The results of renal transplantation are as good as those for a child transplanted at that age for other causes of renal failure. Early death may occur from salt and electrolyte imbalance, and from misdiagnoses in which the glucosuria is interpreted as a sign of diabetes.

Late complications of the disorder include (1) dysphagia due to esophageal dysmotility, and (2) progressive muscle wasting accompanied by a distal myopathy that can progress to inability to lift limbs against gravity. Intercostal muscle weakness can lead to a restrictive pulmonopathy, and children also develop hypothyroidism around the end of the first decade of life. The hypothyroidism is responsive to the usual thyroid-replacement therapy. The corneal crystals are progressive and may obliterate vision simply by being light impermeable. Corneal ulcers may occur and, in some severe cases, have required corneal transplantation. Pancreatitis may occur as a late manifestation. Many older patients develop a wizened appearance, which may be a result of lysosomal cystine storage on the epidermis.[4]

PATHOPHYSIOLOGY

The link between lysosomal cystine storage and the phenotype described earlier in this chapter is not clearly established. Early studies by A. D. Patrick proposed poisoning of SH enzymes by cystine as a mediator of the clinical findings. Numerous efforts linking phenotype and genotype and hypothesizing that cystine content or residual cystine transport capacity would correlate with the severity of phenotype have been made. Recent studies show that the link between the level of cystine storage and the severity of phenotype is weak and other mechanisms explaining phenotype development are required. Possible causes of phenotype development which have been advanced include a deficiency of reduced glutathione (GSH), failure of mitochondrial energy production, aberrant apoptosis, and pleiotropic effects of defective cystinosin gene activity.[5]

Essential to all the arguments for phenotype development is the apparent requirement to explain how lysosomal cystine, which is walled off from the cytosol, can affect cell metabolism. To date, only apoptosis provides a mechanism whereby lysosomal membranes are permeabilized, allowing cystine to exit from lysosomes. Following egress, it is hypothesized in this model that cystine interacts with thiols on cytosolic proteins leading to cysteinylated proteins[6] and, in some cases, altering their activity. Cyteinylation is accompanied by data showing a demonstrable increase in the rate of apoptosis in cystinotic cultured cells compared to normal control cells such that there is a good relationship between lysosomal cystine storage and the amount of apoptosis in cultured fibroblasts and renal tubular epithelial cells after an apoptotic stimulus. The basal apoptosis rate is normal in cystinotic fibroblasts and cultured renal proximal tubule cells. This normal apoptosis rate may be expected, as the patients are not born with dysmorphic features, and expression of the full phenotype takes more than a decade to develop. One specific proapoptotic protein, protein kinase C (PKC) delta, has been implicated in mediating the increased rate of apoptosis seen in cultured cystinotic cells. It has also been shown that, when PKC delta is depleted by using small interfering ribonucleic acid (siRNA), the increased apoptosis resulting from lysosomal cystine is also diminished.[6] Furthermore, normalizing the cystine content of cystinotic fibroblasts normalizes the apoptosis rate, and artificially increasing the lysosomal cystine content of normal fibroblasts produces an increase in the apoptosis rate to that seen in cystinotic cells. Increased programmed cell death could explain development of the phenotypic features of nephropathic cystinosis, including short stature, failure to thrive, retinopathy, proximal renal tubule failure, and, in the renal tubule, progression from narrowing of the proximal tubule (the swan neck deformity) due to inappropriate apoptosis to ultimately disconnection from the glomerulus, resulting in atubular glomeruli.[5] Atubular glomerulii have been found in a cystinotic kidney removed at renal transplantation.[7]

Aberrant energy production has been proposed as another means whereby the cystinotic phenotype may be developed. The results are not clear that such a failure in energy production exists, however. An early study by Baum[8] suggested that adenosine triphosphate (ATP) production was impaired in the presence of lysosomal cystine-loaded normal cells preexposed to cystine dimethyl ester (CDME). Subsequent studies in native cystinotic cells that were loaded to the same extent with cystine did not confirm such a deficit, however.

Studies on the defect in GSH have been equally conflicting. Some studies have found decreased GSH in cultured cystinotic cells, whereas others have shown an elevation in oxidized glutathione (GSSG) content. While the GSH content of fibroblasts is in the 10 mM range, (2) the lysosomal cystine storage in cultured cystinotic fibroblasts is quite small (3). Since lysosomes are approximately 10% of cell volume(4), and a saturating solution of L-cystine is approximately 1.6 mM in plasma, instantaneous dilution of the lysosomal cystine content into the cytosol should at most produce a diminution in GSH of between 0.005 and 5.2%. This diminution would not be expected to have a major impact on the cell's redox status.[5]

INHERITANCE

All forms of cystinosis are inherited as autosomal recessive traits. The gene (CTNS) is located on chromosome 17 P 13.3[9] and codes for a 367-amino-acid protein, called cystinosin, the function of which is to transport cystine out of lysosomes. The gene has 12 exons, and the messenger RNA (mRNA) is 2.6 kb.[3] The bulk of the patients of Western European descent possess a 57-kb deletion that ablates gene function. In a study of 108 American-based cystinosis patients, it was found that 44% were homozygous for this 57-kb deletion, two had a smaller deletion, and eleven were homozygous and three heterozygous for a 753 G→A (W 138 X) mutation. Twenty-four patients had another 21 different mutations.[10] In the two milder forms of the disease, intermediate and ocular, allelic mutations in CTNS were found. In the intermediate variant, new mutations were found: Two sibs from Taiwan were homozygous for a 1308 C→G (N 323 K) mutation, and two other sibs were heterozygous for the 753 G→A mutation and a splice site mutation (IVS 11 + 2T→C). Another intermediate patient was heterozygous for an 1178 A→G (K280R) mutation and the 57-kb deletion.[11] In the mildest or ocular form, patients had one severe mutation and one mild mutation consisting of either a 928 G→A mutation and the 57-kb deletion or a smaller deletion and a splice site mutation.[12]

CYSTEAMINE

Cysteamine, 2-aminoethanethiol, is the smallest solid aminothiol in the aliphatic series. It has a molecular weight of 78 daltons, and the hydrochloride salt is a deliquescent white substance. The hygroscopic nature of cysteamine hydrochloride renders it difficult to manufacture and greatly diminishes its stability due to the spontaneous dissolution of gelatin capsules that occurs when the capsules are stored in less than absolutely dry conditions. For this reason it is marketed as cysteamine bitartrate (Cystagon, Mylan Laboratories, Canonsburg, PA).

Cysteamine has the structure $SHCH_2CH_2NH_2$, with rotation permitted about the carbon–carbon, carbon–sulfur, and carbon–nitrogen bonds. All 14 theoretical rotamers were observed in a study of this phenomenon in cysteamine.[13]

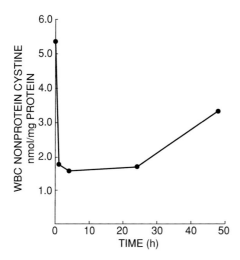

Figure 8–1: Effect of intravenous cysteamine on the cystine concentration of circulating leukocytes in a patient with cystinosis. WBC: white blood cell. Reprinted with permission from *J. Clin Invest.* 1976;58:180–189.

As noted earlier in text, the primary hallmark of cystinosis is intralysosomal cystine storage. When cysteamine is administered intravenously to a patient there is a rapid decline in the amount of leukocyte cystine, as shown in Figure 8–1.

When increasing doses of cysteamine were administered orally to a patient with cystinosis, there was a progressive drop in circulating leukocyte cystine, as shown in Figure 8–2.

Both oral and intravenous administration of cysteamine induce a decrease in the cystine content of circulating leukocytes. The maximal oral dose produced a decline from an initial value of 3.8 nmol/mg protein to a value less than 0.5 nmol/mg at a dose of approximately 115 mg/kg/d.[14] Subsequent pharmacokinetic studies demonstrate that plasma cysteamine peaks approximately one hour after administration of cysteamine hydrochloride and that, conversely, leukocyte cystine reaches a nadir at approximately the same time. Peak plasma cysteamine concentrations following a dose of 0.23 mmol/kg body weight reach values between 34 and 63 μM. This finding was correlated with a decrease in leukocyte cystine one hour after dose administration of between 54 and 75%. Similar values were found in parallel studies involving

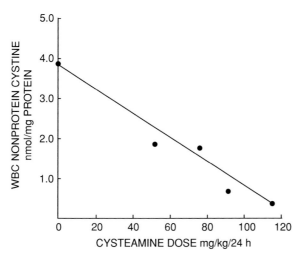

Figure 8–2: Cumulative dose–response curve of oral cysteamine on circulating leukocyte cystine content in a patient with cystinosis. Points represent measurements taken when the patient had been on a given dose on an every-six-hour schedule for 48–72 hours. WBC: white blood cell. Reprinted with permission from *J. Clin Invest.* 1976;58:180–189.

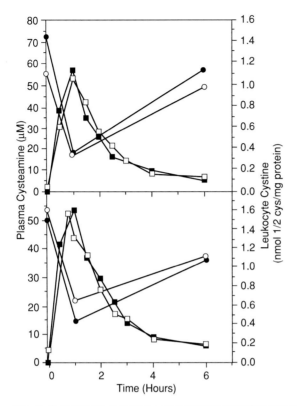

Figure 8–3: Plasma cysteamine concentration and white blood cell (WBC) content in two patients (*top* and *bottom*). Patients received an oral dose of 0.21 mmol/kg body weight of either cysteamine hydrochloride (*closed symbols*), or phosphocysteamine (*open symbols*). Cysteamine in plasma is depicted by *squares* and leukocytes cystine by *circles*. Measurements were obtained at times shown. Reprinted with permission from *Pediatr Res.* 1988;23:616–620.

phosphocysteamine, the phosphorothioester of cysteamine.[15] (Also see "Future Developments" later in the text and Figure 8–3.)

The implicit assumption in these studies is that leukocyte cystine is an adequate surrogate marker for body cystine storage, particularly renal cystine. That this assumption is correct is shown in the "Results of Therapy" section later in this chapter.

MECHANISM OF ACTION

Studies employing cystinotic fibroblasts have demonstrated that cysteamine works to remove lysosomal cystine by taking advantage of another intact lysosomal transport protein, that for lysine. Cystinosis results from failure of the lysosomal cystine transporter, cystinosin, to remove cystine from lysosomes. The transporter for lysine in the lysosomal membrane of cystinotic tissues is intact. When cysteamine reacts with cystine inside lysosome, the reaction product – a mixed disulfide, which is structurally similar to lysine – forms. This reaction product exits lysosomes on the lysine transporter and is then available for reduction to cysteine and cysteamine in the cytosol. Cysteamine may then recycle, removing

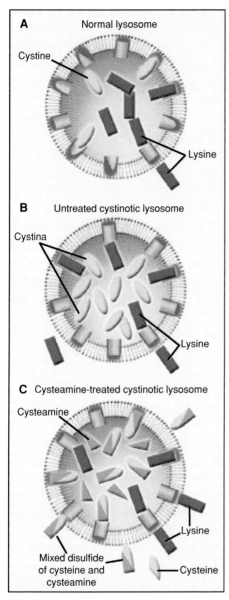

Figure 8–4: Mechanism of action of cysteamine in causing lysosomal cystine depletion. Reprinted with permission from Gahl WG, Thoene JG, Schneider JA. Cystinosis. *N Engl J Med.* 2002; 347:111–121. *See color plate.*

additional cystine. This mechanism was demonstrated by experiments from two laboratories: Gahl and colleagues at the National Institutes of Health (NIH) discovered that cysteamine treatment of leukocyte granular fractions preloaded with [35S]-cystine leads to recovery of labeled mixed disulfide inside the granules.[16] Thoene and colleagues at the University of Michigan determined that the mixed disulfide of cysteamine and cystine reduced the half time of exodus of [14C]-lysine from preloaded normal and cystinotic fibroblast lysosomes. In the presence of extracellular mixed disulfide, the half-time of lysine exodus from normal lysosomes fell from 24.6 to 13.6 minutes. In isolated cystinotic lysosomes, the half-time for [14C]-lysine exodus fell from 25.6 minutes in the presence of buffer alone to 14.7 minutes in the presence of 2 mM mixed disulfide of cystine and cysteamine.[17] This demonstration of countertransport stimulation of lysine transport by the mixed disulfide of cysteamine and cystine is strong evidence for recognition of the mixed disulfide by the lysine transporter. Taken together, these two experiments demonstrate that cysteamine causes cystine depletion of cystine from cystinotic tissues by intralysosomal reaction with cystine, leading to mixed disulfide formation followed by exit of that compound from the lysosomes via the lysine transporter. In molecular terms, the mechanism of action of cysteamine in correcting the primary biochemical defect in cystinosis is understood as well as, or better than, that for any other treatment in any disease. An illustration of this process is seen in Figure 8–4.

DOSAGE

Oral cysteamine bitartrate (Cystagon) is administered every six hours. The initial dose in patients receiving the medication for the first time is 10 mg/kg of body weight per day. After two weeks, the dosage is increased to 20 mg/kg/d (also divided every six hours) and increased sequentially every two weeks until the final dose of approximately 50–60 mg/kg of body weight per day is achieved. At this point, a white blood cell cystine determination is made. If the white cell cystine is less than 1.0 nmol of half-cystine per milligram of protein, then the dose remains at that level and the patient is followed every three months with increases in dosage as required to maintain acceptable leukocyte cystine depletion. (Half-cystine is a convention related to the way cystine is measured. Two "half-cystine" molecules equal one cystine molecule.) An increase in half-cystine above 1.0 nmol/mg of protein is a cause to increase the dose since adequate cystine depletion has not been achieved at that current dose. Patients may go as high as 90 mg/kg/ per day; however, side effects may be seen at that level. When patients approach 40 kg, the dose is recalculated using an initial dose of 1.3 g/m^2/day because maintaining the dose of 60 mg/kg/ per day at body weights greater than approximately 40 kg leads to increased side effects. As the disease has permitted growth to adulthood, the number of patients taking the maximum recommended dose (2.0 g/day) has increased. At the current dosage forms, this requires four capsules (three 150-mg capsules plus one 50-mg capsule) every six hours. Provision of a larger dosage form (e.g., 500-mg capsules) would be a great convenience for older patients.

SIDE EFFECTS

The primary side effect seen on administration of Cystagon is vomiting related to medication administration.[18,19] Vomiting was dose-related: Patients who received higher doses of Cystagon had an increased incidence of vomiting. Anorexia paralleled the incidence of vomiting. Less frequently seen side effects included weakness and/or lethargy related to drug administration. A small number of patients experienced Stevens–Johnson syndrome, and a smaller group of patients experienced impaired consciousness. The CNS complications resolved completely when the drug was discontinued and did not reappear when the drug was restarted.[18] One patient who received the drug at end-stage renal disease developed seizures attributable to cysteamine administration.[14]

Current thinking recommends a drug holiday when patients reach end-stage renal disease, with reinstitution of therapy following a successful renal transplantation or institution of hemodialysis leading to near-normal renal clearance. Under these circumstances, cysteamine appears to be well-tolerated. The continued development of late-onset disease in posttransplant patients *not* treated with cysteamine (muscle weakness, pulmonary and pancreatic involvement, esophageal dysmotility) reemphasizes the requirement for continued, lifelong administration of cysteamine in patients with cystinosis.[20] Other late, long-term effects of untreated cystinosis include delayed sexual maturation, hypothyroidism, diabetes mellitus, mild hepatomegaly, exocrine pancreatic insufficiency, and osteopenia. These late side effects can be avoided or minimized by appropriate administration of cysteamine to the transplant patient.

U.S. FOOD AND DRUG ADMINISTRATION STATUS

Cystagon received U.S. Food and Drug Administration (FDA) new drug approval on August 15, 1994. This event marked the culmination of approximately 20 years of clinical investigation by clinicians throughout the country. The efforts of Mylan Pharmaceuticals, Inc., in obtaining new drug approval for this orphan product were and are deeply appreciated by the patients, their families, and their physicians.

Cystagon is now labeled a Category C drug, and its use in pregnancy is recommended only if the benefits are thought to outweigh the risks. In pups born to pregnant rats fed 0.2–0.7 times the usual human dose, based on body surface area, there was "cleft palate, kyphosis, heart ventricular septal defects, microcephaly and exencephaly, and evidence of fetotoxicity."[21]

RESULTS OF THERAPY

Because renal death is the most severe effect of cystinosis, measurement of cysteamine's effectiveness has concentrated on that parameter. The result of cysteamine therapy in treating nephropathic cystinosis patients is shown in Figure 8–5. In this figure, the reciprocal of creatinine is plotted against age.[4] As the creatinine concentration increases, reflecting progressive renal failure, its reciprocal approaches zero, allowing extrapolation to end-stage renal function.[22] In the first line, representing 33 patients treated at the NIH between 1960 and 1990 who had not received cysteamine, the reciprocal of serum creatinine reaches the abscissa at an age slightly greater than 10 years. Twenty-eight patients who had received oral cysteamine for at least 10 years beginning before age three years with a mean age of 17 months (second line) display an intercept of the reciprocal of creatinine with the abscissa at 23 years. For these two populations, oral cysteamine produced a shift at the point at which end-stage renal disease occurs of approximately 13 years. This increase is substantial in the lifetime of the native kidney. Unfortunately, the initial hope that cysteamine would result in a normal life span with the native kidney has not been borne out, and patients now appear to approach the need for real transplantation 10–15 years later than in the untreated course of the disease. There is anecdotal evidence that the earlier patients are begun on cysteamine, the longer the native kidneys last. This hypothesis is nontestable due to ethical considerations, but institution of newborn screening for cystinosis will enable treatment to begin in infancy, hopefully allowing for the best therapeutic outcome.

There is no apparent alteration in the real Fanconi syndrome, with patients continuing to be polyuric with water, salt, and other small molecule wasting as in the untreated condition. Hypothyroidism, which is a usual pathologic finding in patients with nephropathic cystinosis,[1] also is diminished by treatment with cysteamine. Twenty-eight well-treated patients were compared to 26 partially treated and 47 poorly treated patients. There was a significantly higher probability that patients who were properly treated with cysteamine would remain

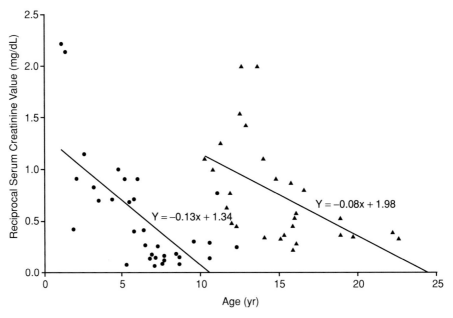

Figure 8–5: Renal function in patients with cystinosis treated with cysteamine and in untreated patients, according to age. *Circles* represent 33 patients who were seen at the NIH Clinical Center between 1960 and 1992 and who did not receive cysteamine. *Triangles* represent 28 patients who received oral cysteamine for at least 10 years, beginning before the age of three years (mean age, 17 months), and *open triangles* represent patients known to have subsequently undergone renal transplantation. Values shown are the most recent available data, and lines show the best-fit regression curves ($r = -0.67$ for the untreated group, and $r = -0.51$ for the treated group). Serum creatinine values are expressed as reciprocals (1 divided by the creatinine value, in milligrams per deciliter). To convert serum creatinine values to micromoles per liter, multiply by 88.4. Long-term cysteamine therapy has shifted the point at which serum creatinine reaches 10 mg/dL from 10 years to 23 years and has lowered the rate of decline of reciprocal serum creatinine values. Reprinted with permission from *N Eng J. Med.* 2002:111–121.

free of the need for T4 replacement therapy compared to the other two groups. Additionally, the bone age deficit was ameliorated in those patients treated with cysteamine.[23]

Thus cysteamine treatment of cystinosis is successful and provides better quality of life to patients who are diagnosed and treated early. There remain, however, significant hurdles before optimal results can be seen.

FUTURE DEVELOPMENTS

Although successful in prolonging life and function of the native kidney, oral Cystagon does not affect corneal crystals, which continue to increase, leading to obstructed vision and corneal ulcers. Cysteamine eye drops, which have been investigated for more than 15 years, have been demonstrated to diminish corneal crystals, leading to virtually normal corneae.[24] New drug approval for cysteamine eyedrops would be a great benefit for patients with cystinosis.

A major drawback to using cysteamine to treat cystinosis is the objectionable thiol odor and taste, which are intrinsic characteristics of the molecule. The free thiol smells and tastes like hydrogen sulfide. As noted earlier in this chapter, approximately 14% of children who are placed on cysteamine cannot remain on the drug because of nausea, vomiting, and sheer inability to tolerate the taste of the compound and its side effects, which include significant halitosis. In fact, some patients are known to have hidden their medicine and not taken it (except on a day when their white blood cell cystine was to be measured), leading to renal failure even though compliance (as judged by leukocyte cystine depletion and parental oversight) appeared to be acceptable. For these reasons, a better tasting formulation has been sought. Prior to new drug approval for Cystagon, the compound phosphocysteamine was tried. Phosphocysteamine is the phosphorothioester of cysteamine and, as such, does not have the objectionable thiol odor and taste.[25] In the author's personal experience, it tastes like an Alka-Seltzer (Bayer Healthcare, LLC, Morristown, NJ) solution. When phosphocysteamine reaches the gastric acidity, however, it is rapidly hydrolyzed to the parent compound, and the breath continues to smell like hydrogen sulfide. Pantethine, the disulfide of the cysteamine conjugate of the vitamin pantothenate, was assessed for cystine depletion capacity. Unfortunately, although better tolerated than cysteamine with respect to taste and odor, it did not yield adequate cystine depletion even at doses of 1,000 mg/kg/d.[26]

A product having diminished or absent thiol odor and the ability to dose less frequently is highly desirable. Every-six-hour dosing was determined based on the data shown in Figure 8–5, in which white cell cystine returns to almost pretreatment level within six hours. This schedule requires that children in school and adults at work take a dose of the drug at midday and another one at or after midnight to maintain a six-hour regimen, which is difficult to maintain. A sustained release form, which would allow 12-hour dosing, and which, by virtue of releasing cysteamine in the small bowel below the ligament of Trietz, permits a diminished thiol odor on the breath, would be a great benefit to patients.

Ultimate therapy for genetic diseases like cystinosis rests upon the hope for correction of the genetic defect. This correction may be accomplished by protein-replacement therapy, as is the case for some lysosomal storage diseases (e.g., MPS 1 and 2), or by providing the required gene in an expression vector. Finding a vector that integrates into the appropriate tissues, expresses appropriate amounts of mRNA, does not disrupt the function of other genes, and leads to amelioration of symptoms has not yet been discovered, Several groups are working with experimental animals to attempt to find such a vector.

REFERENCES

1. Gahl WA, Thoene J, Schneider J. Cystinosis: A disorder of lysosomal membrane transport. C. Scriver, A. Beaudet, W. Sly, D. Valle, eds. *The Metabolic and Molecular Bases of Inherited Disease*, 8th edition, McGraw Hill, 5085–5108, 2001

2. Palacin M, Goodyear P, Nunes V, Gasparini P. Cystinuria. C. Scriver, A. Beaudet, W. Sly, D. Valle, eds. *The Metabolic and Molecular Bases of Inherited Disease*, 8th edition, McGraw Hill, 4909–4932, 2001

3. Town M, Cherqui S, Attard M, Forestier L, Whitmore SA, Callen DF, Gribouval O, Broyer M, Bates GP, van't Hoff W, Antignac C. A novel gene encoding an integral membrane protein is mutated in nephropathic cystinosis. *Nat Genet*. 1998;18:319–324

4. Gahl WG, Thoene JG, Schneider JA. Cystinosis. *N Engl J Med*. 2002;347:111–121

5. Thoene J. A review of the role of enhanced apoptosis in the pathophysiology of cystinosis. *Mol Genet Metab*. 2007;92:292–298

6. Park M, Pejovic V, Kerisit K, Junius S, Thoene J. Increased apoptosis in cystinotic fibroblasts and renal proximal tubule epithelial cells results from cysteinylation of PKCδ. *J Am Soc Nephrol*. 2006;17:3167–3175

7. Park M, Nair R, Walker P, Thoene J. The renal proximal tubule phenotype in cystinosis results from increased apoptosis. (Abstract) *PAS*. 2005;57:1096

8. Baum M. The Fanconi syndrome of cystinosis: Insights into the pathophysiology. *Pediatr Nephrol*. 1998;12:492–497

9. McDowell GA, Gahl WA, Stephenson LA, Schneider JA, Weissenbach J, Polymeropoulos MH, Town MM, van't Hoff W, Farrall M, Mathews CG. Linkage of the gene for cystinosis to markers on the short arm of chromosome 17. *Nat Genet*. 1995;10:246–248

10. Shotelersuk V, Larson D, Anikster Y, McDowell G, Lemons R, Bernardini I, Guo J, Thoene J, Gahl W. CTNS mutations in an American based population of cystinosis patients. *Am J Hum Genet*. 1998;63:1352–1362

11. Thoene J, Lemons R, Anikster Y, Mullet J, Paelicke K, Lucero C, Gahl W, Schneider J, Shu SG, Campbell HT. Mutations of CTNS causing intermediate cystinosis. *Mol Genet Metab*. 1999;67:283–293

12. Anikster Y, Lucero C, Guo J, Huizing M, Shotelersuk V, Bernardini I, McDowell G, Iwata F, Kaiser-Kupfer MI, Jaffe R, Thoene J, Schneider JA, Gahl WA. Ocular nonnephropathic cystinosis: Clinical, biochemical, and molecular correlations. *Pediatr Res*. 2000;47:17–23

13. Giuseppe B. Conformational analysis and rotation barriers of 2-aminoethanethiol and 2-aminoethanol: An ab initio study. *Int J Quantum Chem*. 1996;59:227–237

14. Thoene J, Oshima R, Crawhall J, Olson D, Schneider J. Cystinosis: Intracellular cystine depletion by aminothiols in vitro and in vivo. *J. Clin*. Invest. 1976;58:180–189

15. Smolin LA, Clark KF, Thoene JG, Gahl WA, Schneider JA. A comparison of the effectiveness of cysteamine and phosphocysteamine in elevating plasma cysteamine concentration and decreasing leukocyte free cystine in nephropathic cystinosis. *Pediatr Res*. 1988;23:616–620

16. Gahl WA, Tietze F, Butler JD, Schulman JD. Cysteamine depletes cystinotic leucocyte granular fractions of cystine by the mechanism of disulphide interchange. *Biochem J*. 1985;22:545–550

17. Pisoni RL, Thoene JG, Christensen HN. Detection and characterization of carrier-mediated cationic amino acid transport in lysosomes of normal and cystinotic human fibroblasts. Role in therapeutic cystine removal? *J Biol Chem*. 1985;260:4791–4798

18. Corden BJ, Schulman JD, Schneider JA, Thoene JG. Adverse reactions to oral cysteamine use in nephropathic cystinosis. *Dev Pharmacol Ther*. 1981;3:25–30

19. Gahl WA, Reed GF, Thoene JG, Schulman JD, Rizzo WB, Jonas AJ, Denman DW, Schlesselman JJ, Corden BJ, Schneider JA. Cysteamine therapy for children with nephropathic cystinosis. *N Engl J Med*. 1987;316:971–977

20. Nesterova G, Gahl W. Nephropathic cystinosis: Late complications of a multisystemic disease. *Pediatr Nephrol*. 2008;6:863–878

21. http://www.drugs.com/pro/cystagon.html

22. Gahl WA, Schneider JA, Schulman JD, Thoene JG, Reed GF. Predicted reciprocal serum creatinine at age 10 years as a measure of renal function in children with nephropathic cystinosis treated with oral cysteamine. *Pediatr Nephrol*. 1990;4:129–135

23. Kimonis VE, Troendle J, Rose SR, Yang ML, Markello TC, Gahl WA. Effects of early cysteamine therapy on thyroid function and growth in nephropathic cystinosis. *J Clin Endocrinol Metab*. 1995;80:3257–3261

24. Tsilou ET, Thompson D, Lindblad AS, Reed GF, Rubin B, Gahl W, Thoene J, Del Monte M, Schneider JA, Granet DB, Kaiser-Kupfer MI. A multicentre randomised double masked clinical trial of a new formulation of topical cysteamine for the treatment of corneal cystine crystals in cystinosis. *Br J Ophthalmol*. 2003;87:28–31

25. Thoene JG, Lemons R. Cystine depletion of cystinotic tissues by phosphocysteamine (WR638). *J Pediatr*. 1980;96:1043–1044

26. Wittwer CT, Gahl WA, Butler JD, Zatz M, Thoene JG. Metabolism of pantethine in cystinosis. *J Clin Invest*. 1985;76:1665–1672

9 Nitisinone use in hereditary tyrosinemia and alkaptonuria

Wendy J. Introne, Kevin J. O'Brien, and William A. Gahl

OVERVIEW OF DISEASES

Hereditary tyrosinemia (HT) and alkaptonuria (AKU) result from enzyme deficiencies in the tyrosine degradation pathway. AKU has the distinction of being the first inborn error of metabolism described by Sir Archibald Garrod more than 100 years ago. HT (also known as hepatorenal syndrome and tyrosinemia type I) was first described in 1957 by Sakai and colleagues and is the most common and most severe of the tyrosine degradation disorders.[1,2] Although the two conditions

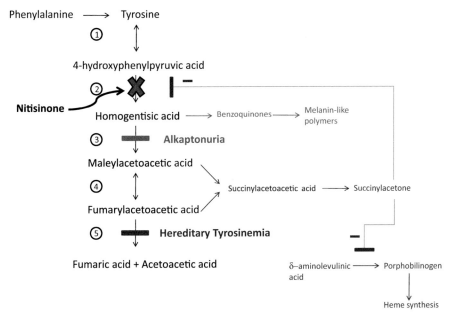

Figure 9–1: Tyrosine degradation pathway. Enzymes as labeled in the pathway. 1. Tyrosine aminotransferase. 2. HPPD. 3. HGD. 4. MAA isomerase 5. FAH. AKU results from deficiency of HGD. HGA accumulates and is converted to benzoquinones and ultimately melanin-like polymers. HT results from a deficiency of FAH. FAA and MAA accumulate and are converted to SAA and SA. SA inhibits 4-hydroxyphenylpyruvate and ALA dehydratase, leading to elevated tyrosine concentration and decreased heme synthesis. Nitisinone inhibits HPPD.

are both disorders of tyrosine catabolism, the biochemical and clinical manifestations differ widely.

HT

Deficiency of fumarylacetoacetate hydrolase (FAH), the final enzyme in the tyrosine degradation process, results in the devastating metabolic disorder HT (Figure 9–1). Worldwide, the incidence of this disease is approximately 1:100,000.[3] The incidence in Norway and Finland is 1:60,000; in Quebec, Canada, 1:16,000; and within the Saguenay–Lac-Saint-Jean area of Canada, 1:1,846.[4,5] The clinical presentation varies so much that the disease has been divided into acute and chronic forms. In the acute form, children within the first weeks to months of life present with severe, rapidly progressive liver disease. Liver transaminases are only modestly elevated, but synthetic function is markedly impaired.[4] A severe coagulopathy occurs because of decreased levels of hepatically synthesized clotting factors. Children often emit a "boiled cabbage" odor and can quickly develop ascites, jaundice, and gastrointestinal bleeding.[6] Without intervention, affected children die of liver failure within weeks to months of the initial presentation.

The chronic form of HT generally manifests with liver and kidney dysfunction, poor growth, rickets, and/or neurologic crises. Early in the course, the liver dysfunction is milder than it is in the acute form of HT, but children remain at high risk of developing cirrhosis and hepatocellular carcinoma (HCC). The kidney disease often presents as renal Fanconi syndrome, with wasting of amino acids, phosphorus, and bicarbonate, causing poor growth, rickets, and metabolic acidosis. Neurologic crises resemble porphyria episodes, with severe pain, posturing, vomiting, and muscle weakness.[7] In a study by Mitchell and colleagues,[7] 40% of children suffered neurologic crises, with 8 of 48 children requiring mechanical ventilation because of paralysis. Van Spronsen and colleagues reported that 10% of HT deaths were due to respiratory failure and the porphyria-like syndrome.[8] Cardiomyopathy has also been reported in 30% of patients with HT, but none of the children had clinical symptoms; the diagnosis was based solely on echocardiographic findings.[9] Fortunately, the cardiomyopathy generally resolves over time, and children with a normal echocardiogram initially do not develop cardiomyopathy later.

In 1994, van Spronsen and colleagues reported a correlation between age of presentation and overall prognosis. Children manifesting disease before two months of age had a two-year survival of 29%, and those developing symptoms between two and six months of age had a two-year survival of 74%. Children who presented after six months of age had a two-year survival of 96%. Even with the standard dietary restriction, long-term survival remained poor, with all children dying by the age of 12 years.[10] Dietary restriction of phenylalanine and tyrosine led to improved renal function but did little to stop the progression of liver disease. As a result, liver transplantation became the definitive treatment. Following transplantation, serum tyrosine and alpha-fetoprotein (AFP) levels, originally elevated, rapidly returned to normal. Elevated urinary succinylacetone (SA) levels were reduced, although small amounts remained in the urine, suggesting that the kidneys continued to produce the substance. Liver transplantation carries with it significant risk, including a 5–10% mortality rate secondary to transplant-related complications and a lifetime of immunosuppressive therapy.[4,11,12]

With the development of newborn screening for HT, the classification of patients' disease status into either chronic or acute for prognostic purposes became obsolete. Furthermore, the discovery of 2-(2-nitro-4-trifluoromethyl-benzoyl)-1,3-cyclohexanedione (NTBC, nitisinone, Orfadin; Swedish Orphan International AB, Stockholm, Sweden) has revolutionized the management and survival of children with HT. In fact, liver transplantation is now reserved for those individuals who have severe liver failure at presentation, who fail nitisinone therapy, or who have hepatic changes suggestive of malignancy.[4,13]

Diagnosis

In HT, plasma tyrosine levels are generally elevated at the time of presentation or when clinical symptoms occur. Several other conditions, however, can also have elevated blood tyrosine concentrations, including transient tyrosinemia of the newborn, nonspecific liver disease, and tyrosinemia types II or III. In addition, newborns with HT can have normal plasma tyrosine, so although plasma tyrosine remains a reasonable screening tool, elevated levels alone are neither necessary nor sufficient for the diagnosis. If clinical presentation is consistent with the diagnosis of HT or the plasma tyrosine is elevated, blood or urinary SA should be measured. Elevated SA is pathognomonic for HT.

Newborn-screening programs have historically measured blood tyrosine to detect HT and methionine to detect homocystinuria, but the liver disease of HT can also cause elevated methionine. Therefore, increased levels of either tyrosine or methionine should prompt additional investigations into HT. As mentioned, however, elevations in blood tyrosine and methionine are not specific for HT, and tyrosine levels may be normal or only slightly elevated in HT, particularly in the newborn. With the expansion of newborn-screening programs and the use of tandem mass spectrometry, some laboratories are developing specific assays for SA in dried blood spots.[14,15] Measurement of SA should offer high sensitivity with much improved specificity for HT.

Supporting laboratory findings include elevations of intermediates of tyrosine degradation that can be measured as urine organic acids, including *p*-hydroxyphenylpyruvate, *p*-hydroxyphenyllactate, and *p*-hydroxyphenylacetate. Children who are symptomatic with coagulopathy have prolonged prothrombin and partial thromboplastin times (PT/PTT). Serum levels of AFP are markedly elevated at an average of 160,000 ng/mL.[3] Liver transaminases may be normal or only mildly elevated, differentiating HT from other liver disorders.

Although not currently readily available, confirmatory testing previously used measurement of FAH activity within cultured fibroblasts or hepatic tissue. Today, targeted mutation analysis or direct sequencing of the FAH gene has replaced enzymatic analysis.

Pathophysiology

Deficiency of the final enzyme in the tyrosine catabolic pathway, FAH, leads to the accumulation of the precursor molecules maleylacetoacetate (MAA) and fumarylacetoacetate (FAA).[16] MAA and FAA are subsequently reduced to succinylacetoacetate (SAA) and its derivative SA.

MAA and FAA are alkylating agents promoting oxidative stress within cells, reduced levels of glutathione, and further cellular damage. Accumulation of FAA leads to apoptotic cell death in hepatocytes and renal proximal tubular cells.[17] Through mechanisms that are not well understood, FAH deficiency also appears to disrupt gene expression.[17] FAA is mutagenic, a feature further enhanced by glutathione depletion;[18] the combination may create the predisposition for HCC.

Both MAA and SA may contribute to renal Fanconi syndrome.[6,17] SA potently inhibits the second enzyme in the tyrosine degradation pathway, 4-hydroxyphenylpyruvate dioxygenase (HPPD; Figure 9–1). This inhibition likely causes elevated plasma tyrosine, which itself is not considered toxic to the liver or kidneys; patients with tyrosinemia types II and III have elevated plasma tyrosine but no liver or renal pathology. SA also inhibits aminolevulinic acid (ALA) dehydratase, an enzyme important for the production of porphyrin and ultimately heme. In HT, ALA, a known neurotoxin, accumulates and causes neurologic crises in a significant number of children.

Genetics

As with most inborn errors of metabolism, HT is inherited in an autosomal recessive fashion. FAH is the only gene the mutations of which are known to cause HT. The gene, located on chromosome 15q23–25, was cloned by Phaneuf and colleagues in 1991.[19] It contains 14 exons and is 35 kb in length, with an open reading frame of 1,260 bp coding for 419 amino acids. The enzyme functions as a homodimer with no known cofactor.

According to the Human Gene Mutation Database, 43 different mutations have been reported to date.[20] These mutations include missense, nonsense, and splice site mutations, as well as deletions and an indel. In the French Canadian population, the most frequent mutation is IVS12+5G→A. Carrier screening determined that 95% of HT heterozygotes in Saguenay–Lac-Saint-Jean bear this mutation,[21] which also has been identified frequently in Western Europe. Arranz and colleagues reported a high frequency of an additional splice site mutation, IVS 6–1G→T, in the Mediterranean region.[22] Other common mutations include P261L in the Ashkenazi Jewish population and W262X in the Finnish population.[23,24] No genotype–phenotype correlation has been established. In fact, both the acute and chronic forms of the disease have been found in two different individuals with the same genotype.[25]

In 1994, Kvittingen and colleagues reported the dramatic observation that tissue obtained from the native liver at transplant had a mosaic appearance when stained for FAH.[26] Indeed, nodules of regenerating hepatocytes staining positively for FAH enzyme were interspersed with areas that did not stain. Mutation analysis of the regenerating nodules revealed that one of the alleles had spontaneously reverted to the wild-type allele. It is hypothesized that the regenerating tissue may provide a small amount of enzyme that could account for the phenotypic differences. It is not expected that an individual could have enough regeneration to be cured, and patients remain at high risk for the development of HCC.

Finally, a pseudodeficiency allele, R341W, has been identified in otherwise normal individuals. Their fibroblasts have less than 10% of normal FAH activity, and the patients themselves have normal levels of plasma tyrosine and no hepatic symptoms.[27]

AKU

Deficiency of homogentisate 1,2-dioxygenase (HGD), the third enzyme in the catabolic pathway, results in the accumulation of its substrate, homogentisic acid (HGA) (Figure 9–1). Worldwide, the incidence of AKU is estimated at between 1:250,000 and 1:1,000,000,[28] but there are several exceptions. An increased frequency has been observed in the Dominican Republic, with 47 cases identified, whereas the incidence in Slovakia is 1:19,000.[29,30] HGA is both filtered and actively secreted by the kidney, resulting in the elimination by AKU patients of two to eight grams of HGA per day. By comparison, unaffected individuals excrete approximately 20–30 milligrams of HGA per 24-hour period. HGA is readily oxidized to form melanin-like polymers that produce the hallmark symptom of AKU (i.e., urine that turns dark upon standing or exposure to an alkalinizing agent), which is the only symptom that is present from birth and, in the current era of disposable diapers, is frequently missed. HGA that is not eliminated in the urine circulates within the body and continues to be oxidized to benzoquinones that avidly bind connective tissues, producing dark pigmentation termed "ochronosis."

Individuals with AKU remain relatively asymptomatic until their twenties or thirties when they may note pigment deposition on the sclera of the eyes at the insertion of the rectus muscles and within the helices of the ears. The degree of pigmentation is highly variable and nonuniform. Less often, pigment deposition can be appreciated as small, darkly colored, calloused lesions along the lateral surfaces of the thumb and first finger, on the web in between, on the lateral surfaces of the hands and the lateral aspects of the ankles, and under the fingernails.

The signal arthritic complaint involves low back pain, usually in the late third or fourth decade of life. Generally beginning in the lumbar spine and gradually moving into the thoracic and then cervical regions, the hallmark signs include loss of intervertebral disc height, calcification of the discs, and reactive arthritic changes including sclerosis, osteophyte formation, and, ultimately, bony ankylosis of the vertebral bodies. Plain radiographs of the spine are virtually pathognomonic for the condition.

Arthritis of the large joints generally begins in the late thirties or forties. The joints primarily affected include the hips, knees, and shoulders. Smaller joints are less often problematic. HGA deposits within connective tissues that include cartilage, meniscus, ligaments, and tendons result in dark pigmentation and the initiation of a degenerative cascade. Clinically, patients experience pain and decreased range of motion. Although swelling may be present, the joints generally do not feel warm or appear erythematous, as with rheumatoid arthritis. Radiographically, the earliest finding is loss of joint space. With time, typical arthritic features develop, including progressive loss of the joint space, sclerosis, osteophyte formation, irregularity of the articular surfaces, and subchondral cyst formation. By the age of 55 years, approximately half of the adults with AKU have had at least one joint replaced.[28] Tendons become fibrotic and can tear with minimal provocation. The Achilles tendon is particularly prone to rupture, and repair is often complicated.

Cardiac involvement includes deposition of HGA within the cardiac valves, vascular calcification, and arteriosclerosis. By the fifth decade, many individuals have aortic valve sclerosis that is visualized on echocardiogram. This thickening can progress to aortic stenosis or regurgitation. In a series of 58 patients, 3 individuals required aortic valve replacement.[28] Other valves can be affected, but to a lesser degree. Calcification of the coronary arteries, aorta, and other vessels is visualized on computed tomography (CT) scanning. In the same series of 58 patients, half had calcification apparent on CT by age 59 years.

Virtually all males over the age of 40 have prostate stones, and renal stones are seen frequently in both genders. Stones that have been analyzed contain calcium oxalate, but the stones are black in color.

Generally speaking, the life span of individuals with AKU is not reduced; however, there is a high rate of disability that progresses with age.[31] Several therapeutic modalities have been considered in attempts to reduce HGA production and deposition. The two most commonly considered options have been dietary protein restriction and vitamin C supplementation. Protein restriction theoretically lowers the phenylalanine and tyrosine load, reducing HGA production. In one study, six adult patients adhering to a self-imposed, protein-restricted diet had similar HGA excretion when compared with individuals on a regular diet.[28] Additional studies have shown a modest decrease in urine HGA levels in young children but no significant difference beyond the age of 12 years.[32,33] A tyrosine-restricted diet is difficult to maintain and unpalatable for adults, and significant protein restriction in children can lead to growth and developmental impairment. No evidence exists thus far to support long-term dietary protein limitation as a therapeutic modality in AKU.

Vitamin C is a cofactor for the enzyme HGD. It has been suggested that supplementation of large doses of ascorbic acid may drive residual enzyme activity and reduce HGA accumulation. The second enzyme in the tyrosine degradation pathway (Figure 9–1), HPPD, is also a vitamin C–dependent enzyme, so large doses of vitamin C may, in fact, promote production of HGA. In one series, ascorbic acid was administered to two adults and three infants. Although benzoquinone acetic acid was eliminated from the urine, there was no reduction in HGA excretion in the adults and a doubling of HGA excretion in the infants.[33] A second study, which evaluated 10 patients who were taking vitamin C, found urinary HGA levels in those patients comparable to levels in those patients not receiving the vitamin supplement.[28] Furthermore, ascorbic acid is degraded to oxalate, which may further predispose to renal lithiasis.

Patients with AKU are primarily treated symptomatically. Pain management is tailored to each individual's specific needs. Joint replacements are successful for severe arthritis. Implant longevity is similar to the longevity seen in individuals seeking replacement for osteoarthritis.[34] The aortic valve should be monitored regularly and valve replacement considered if aortic stenosis/insufficiency becomes severe.

Renal transplant has been performed in an individual with AKU and diabetic nephropathy.[35] Following the transplant, urinary HGA excretion was reduced, possibly because of the donor kidney supplying some HGD activity. A 47-year-old woman received a liver transplant following the development of hepatitis B cirrhosis and reportedly had "disappearance" of the AKU, presumably because of enzyme production by the donor liver that halted further progression of her disease.[36]

Diagnosis

There are two primary presentations that suggest the diagnosis of AKU. The first is the observation of dark urine, classically recognized in infancy with darkly staining diapers. The second is the presentation of early-onset, chronic back or joint disease. Often, the orthopedic surgeon discovers darkened cartilage and connective tissue during an operative procedure.

The diagnosis is easily confirmed by measuring gram amounts of HGA in urine by gas chromatography–mass spectrometry (GC-MS). Plasma tyrosine is generally not elevated, nor are other intermediates in the tyrosine catabolic pathway. Enzyme assays are no longer routinely used for diagnosis. Although not necessary for confirmation, mutation analysis can be performed to identify causative mutations.

Pathophysiology

Deficiency of HGD causes its substrate, HGA, to accumulate. HGA can be readily oxidized to benzoquinone acetic acid through the action of homogentisate polyphenol oxidase, a copper-dependent enzyme. The resulting benzoquinones form melanin-like polymers that can bind connective tissue and contribute to ochronosis. The exact mechanism through which the benzoquinones cause arthritis remains unknown.

Genetics

As with HT, AKU is inherited in an autosomal recessive fashion. HGD is the only gene the mutations of which are known to cause AKU. HGD, isolated by Fernandez-Canon and colleagues 1996, is located on 3q21–23.[37] The gene is composed of 14 exons spanning nearly 60 kb of DNA and encoding a 445 amino-acid protein. The crystal structure was determined by Titus and colleagues and was found to be a hexamer composed of a dimer of trimers with an associated iron molecule at the active site.[38]

To date, more than 60 different mutations have been identified; they include missense, nonsense, frame shift, and splice site mutations.[39] Titus and colleagues discovered that the majority of missense mutations occurred in regions of subunit association. In the Slovak region where the incidence of AKU is high, as many as 10 different mutations have been identified; 6 of the 10 mutations occurred in CCC mutational hot spots. A founder mutation, p.Cys120Trp, is likely responsible for the increased frequency of AKU in the Dominican Republic.[29] In Europe, the most frequent mutation seen outside of Slovakia is p.Met368Val.

OVERVIEW OF NITISINONE

Nitisinone has the chemical formula $C_{14}H_{10}F_3NO_5$ and a molecular mass of 329.228 g/mol. The chemical structure is shown in Figure 9–2. It is a member of a

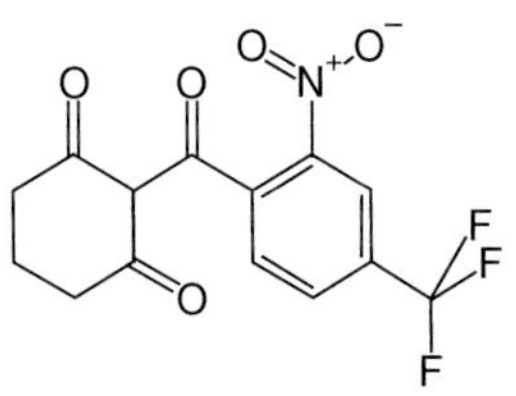

Figure 9–2: Chemical structure of nitisinone.

triketone family of herbicides.[40] The compounds in this series exert their herbicidal effect via inhibition of HPPD, which, through a series of downstream effects, results in plant bleaching.[40] Evaluation of the triketones in rats also revealed inhibition of HPPD,[41] the primary target of nitisinone in mammals. (See "Mechanism of action.")

U.S. Food and Drug Administration status

Nitisinone is commercially available as Orfadin and is marketed by Swedish Orphan International AB, based in Stockholm, Sweden. The drug is distributed in the United States through Rare Disease Therapeutics (Nashville, TN), a company that supplies the drug to the specialty pharmaceutical company Accredo Health Group Inc. (Memphis, TN). Clinicians wishing to prescribe nitisinone must complete a prescription and enrollment form with Accredo, whereupon the drug is typically mailed to the patient's home. It is available in capsules of 2, 5, and 10 milligrams and is intended only for oral administration.

Nitisinone has a different U.S. Food and Drug Administration (FDA) status for use in HT compared with use in AKU. For HT, nitisinone received FDA approval in adults and children in January 2002. Safety and efficacy have not been established in adults older than 65 years. For pregnant women, it is a category C medication.

For AKU, nitisinone was given investigational drug status in 2002. A pilot trial on AKU patients, conducted at the National Institutes of Health (NIH) from 2003 through 2005, showed promising results and led to a Phase III clinical trial that began recruiting patients in 2005; trial results are now being analyzed.

Pharmacokinetics

There is limited information on the pharmacokinetics of nitisinone in humans. Absorption kinetics, using a single dose of nitisinone in either the liquid or capsule form at a dosage of 1 mg/kg, were studied in 10 healthy male volunteers 19–39 years old. The median time to reach maximum plasma concentration was 15 minutes for the liquid and three hours for the capsule.[40] Both forms of the drug were bioequivalent. There is no other information on the absorption kinetics of nitisinone in patients with HT or in other groups of patients. No pharmacokinetic studies have been performed to determine the effect of food on absorption, but, in the treatment of HT, nitisinone is usually given one hour prior to meals.[42]

Following oral administration of radiolabeled nitisinone in rats, the drug showed a greater than 90% bioavailability with distribution to multiple organs. The greatest distribution was in the plasma, liver, and the kidneys, with selective retention in the liver and, to a lesser extent, the kidneys.[43] Radioactivity was detected for up to seven days in these organs.

Nitisinone has a half-life of 54 hours in healthy male volunteers.[40] This finding suggests that some metabolism is necessary before excretion.[40] This suggestion is supported by a metabolic study performed in HT children treated with nitisinone; their urine showed unchanged nitisinone, hydroxylated nitisinone, and, in some children, NTFA (2-nitro-4-thrifluouromethylbenzoic acid).[44] Animal and human studies indicate that excretion of nitisinone occurs through the urine and feces.[44]

Mechanism of action

The dramatic therapeutic effect and minimal side-effect profile of nitisinone reflect its affinity and specificity for, and potent antagonism of, the HPPD enzyme. Studies using animal and human liver extracts have shown that nitisinone is a reversible competitive inhibitor of the HPPD enzyme, which catalyzes the second step in the tyrosine degradation pathway, involving the conversion of 4-hydroxyphenylpyruvate to HGA (Figure 9–1).[40,43,45] Nitisinone is a structural analogue of 4-hydroxyphenylpyruvate, the substrate for HPPD, and shows great affinity for the enzyme, apparently binding in a three-step process.[46] So potent is the antagonism of the HPPD enzyme that, although nitisinone is classified as a reversible competitive antagonist, it essentially functions as an irreversible, albeit time-dependent, inhibitor. The degree of this inhibition and the affinity of nitisinone for HPPD is exhibited in various studies. Enzyme assays of liver extracts treated with nitisinone showed that the half maximal inhibitory concentration (IC_{50}) is approximately 40 nM in rat liver[47] and 5 nM in human liver.[41,47] The shape of the enzyme-inhibitor complex curve is similar to that for an irreversible inhibitor;[47] HPPD enzyme activity is virtually absent within a half hour after a dose, returning to only 25% of normal after seven days.[43]

In addition to its high affinity for HPPD, unpublished data reported by Ellis and colleagues suggest specificity of nitisinone for HPPD, a dioxygenase enzyme.[47] These data indicated that other enzymes in the tyrosine catabolic pathway were not inhibited by nitisinone at concentrations less than 100–200 μM and that nearly all other dioxygenase enzymes were also resistant.

These properties of nitisinone result in a significant reduction of all products downstream of HPPD in the tyrosine catabolic pathway and account for its therapeutic effects, but also result in a substantial increase in 4-hydroxyphenylpyruvate.[48] This compound inhibits the activity of tyrosine aminotransferase, resulting in elevations of plasma tyrosine, and accounts for some of the drug's toxicity.[43] This latter effect of nitisinone prompted the dietary restriction of tyrosine and phenylalanine recommended for HT patients receiving the drug.

In HT, inhibition of the HPPD enzyme ultimately reduces the formation of the toxic metabolites MAA, FAA, and SA. The enzyme defect in HT is FAH, which catalyzes the terminal step in the pathway (Figure 9–1). Blocking HPPD results in much less HGA being available for enzymatic conversion into MAA by HGD. Reduced levels of MAA translate into reduced levels of FAA and, ultimately, lower SAA and SA levels. The reduction of these toxic metabolites with nitisinone therapy causes a rapid and sustained clinical improvement that has drastically changed the outlook for children with HT. (See "Results of therapy" section.)

In AKU, inhibition of HPPD by nitisinone decreases the production of HGA. The enzymatic defect in AKU is at the HGD step and results in the accumulation of HGA and the subsequent formation of benzoquinone polymers (Figure 9–1). Inhibition of HPPD, one step before HGD, substantially reduces the production of HGA, the metabolite mainly responsible for the development of ochronosis.[49]

Dosage, administration, and monitoring of therapy

For HT, the starting dosage is approximately 1 mg/kg given in two divided doses, one hour before meals, in all age ranges. The doses need not be divided evenly. Dosing can be started at less than 1 mg/kg, depending on the patient's clinical situation, and then titrated upward to 1.5 mg/kg/d if normalization of biochemical parameters has not been achieved after approximately one month. The maximum dose is 2 mg/kg/d in divided doses.[42] Patients who cannot swallow the capsule can open it, then the drug can be mixed with water or formula or sprinkled on a small amount of applesauce. It can also be delivered through a gastrostomy tube. Nitisinone needs to be stored at 2–8°C (36–46°F) at all times, and patients should be instructed to keep it in a refrigerator. Patients traveling outside the home can keep the drug in a small ice cooler.

The administration of nitisinone for HT brings with it the responsibility to carefully track certain laboratory values, teach and monitor the patient for signs and symptoms of toxicity, and continually reinforce adherence to a low tyrosine and phenylalanine diet. These responsibilities are shared with the patient and family, but the clinical team must also be vigilant in observing the patient's response to therapy. Observation is best conducted in a team setting in which the prescribing clinician works in concert with:

- A dietician experienced in managing metabolic disorders. The dietician and clinician must be adept at continually manipulating the nitisinone dose and dietary restrictions, because the extent of dietary restriction varies and changes with growth and development needs. Experience becomes especially important when a patient's tyrosine level rises to worrisome levels or if signs of toxicity develop.
- A laboratory that can be trusted to produce consistently accurate results of the analysis of small molecules not commonly measured, especially when levels are markedly elevated.
- Consultants, such as ophthalmologists and hepatologists, who are familiar with nitisinone therapy and who are willing to work with the prescriber to monitor patients over time.
- Nursing staff and genetic counselors who will assess the patient at and between visits and who may notice subtle changes in the patient's condition that warrant further investigation. It can be helpful for the staff to use a checklist of questions regarding side effects and signs of toxicity that will

ensure that all areas have been covered each time the patient is assessed. This information can be stored in a database and reviewed for trends in the patient's response. The staff will also provide teaching and support to a family caring for a chronically ill patient.

After initiation of nitisinone, certain tests must be performed at regular intervals to measure response to treatment and to monitor for toxicity. Initially, laboratory tests should be checked frequently until a consistent response is seen, but the interval can be lengthened as the patient stabilizes. An excellent discussion in *Gene Reviews* provides specific information regarding the timing of blood testing. Results should also be checked more frequently if a previously stable patient becomes ill. The clinician might also develop a set of tests that needs to be checked regularly and when clinically indicated. Table 9–1 lists the studies that should be performed before and during nitisinone treatment for HT. These recommendations do not apply to AKU, for which nitisinone is not approved.

For AKU, however, a dose of 2.10 mg/d was found to be efficacious in reducing urinary HGA levels by 95% in a small treatment trial.[49] Dietary restriction has not been routinely employed. Recommendations for toxicity monitoring will follow approval of the drug.

Side effects and toxicity

Corneal injury is the most important toxicity of nitisinone therapy. It is believed to be the result of persistently elevated corneal levels of tyrosine, which can crystallize causing injury to the subepithelium.[50,51] There have been reports of keratitis, corneal opacities, ulcers, conjunctivitis, pain, and photophobia associated with nitisinone in HT, but there are no published reports of these complications in AKU.[42,50,52]

In HT, the occurrence of ocular toxicity with nitisinone treatment does not always correlate with the plasma tyrosine level. In a long-term study by Masurel-Paulet and colleagues, six patients complained of photophobia, and four had evidence of keratitis.[52] Three of those four patients had poor compliance with dietary therapy and had plasma tyrosine levels greater than 500 μmol/L. The lesions and symptoms abated after tyrosine levels decreased with proper dietary restriction. In the Gothenburg group, which studied more than 200 patients, 13 had transient and sometimes recurrent symptoms, including itching, burning, and corneal erosions and clouding. Corneal crystals were noted in one patient, but they cleared within a few days after stopping treatment.[10] The 13 patients with symptoms did not have tyrosine levels significantly different from those of the entire group. Lastly, Gissen and colleagues followed 11 patients with HT who were treated with nitisinone and dietary restriction for a mean duration of six years. Three of the 11 had mean tyrosine concentrations greater than 500 μmol/L over a two-year period, whereas the remaining eight patients had mean tyrosine concentrations ranging from 206 to 445 μmol/L. Five of the eight patients had

Table 9–1. Recommended tests to monitor response to nitisinone treatment in HT

Test	Response to therapy	Recommendations/comments
Plasma tyrosine	Will increase in a dose-dependent manner	Keep the tyrosine levels between 200 and 500 μM. Maintain patient on a low-protein diet with medical formulas low in phenylalanine and tyrosine.
Plasma phenylalanine	May increase	Increases may indicate poor compliance with diet.
Urinary SA	It will drop substantially and may fall to almost undetectable levels.	Elevated levels may indicate inadequate treatment.
AFP	AFP falls gradually but markedly during therapy. It is useful as a marker of response to therapy, as well as to screen for HCC.	After normalization, small-to-moderate increases in AFP levels during therapy may indicate inadequate treatment (especially when compared to the trend of 5-ALA and SA). Persistent and/or marked increases should prompt an investigation for HCC.
Urinary 5-ALA	May fall to almost undetectable levels	Rising levels may indicate inadequate treatment and should prompt an assessment for porphyria-like symptoms.
Total white blood cell and neutrophil counts	Transient leucopenia noted in 3%	No serious infections have been reported. Surveillance for signs and symptoms of infection should increase if counts decline.
Platelet count	Transient thrombocytopenia noted in 3%	No serious bleeding episodes have been reported. Assess for mucocutaneous signs of bleeding when counts decline.
LFTs and LEs*	LFTs and LEs will be abnormal at the initiation of therapy, and often will normalize rapidly.	Failure to normalize LFTs and LEs can indicate inadequate therapy.
Renal US	Normal morphology	Assess for evidence of renal disease.
Serum/urinary phosphate	Normalize within the first year.	Check fractional excretion of phosphate and other markers of PTD.
Eye examination	Most do not have trouble, but reports of corneal toxicity have been noted.	Examination must include slit lamp.
Liver US/CT/MRI	Slowing of the progress of cirrhosis	Check prior to treatment. Continue to monitor for signs of HCC and for any sign of cirrhosis.

* LE: liver enzyme; MRI: magnetic resonance imaging.

peak tyrosine levels greater than 500 μmol/L. No patient showed signs of toxicity on examination, and none complained of ocular symptoms.[51]

Nitisinone also has been reported to cause leukopenia and thrombocytopenia in HT patients; the mechanism remains unknown. Approximately 3% of patients with HT developed leukopenia on nitisinone, but the development was not associated with serious infections and was reversible upon cessation of the drug.

Reversible thrombocytopenia has been reported in up to 3% of HT patients on nitisinone, and there have been no reported cases of serious bleeding.[42]

In the pilot study of AKU by Suwannarat and colleagues, two patients developed a mild transaminitis after initiation of nitisinone. In these patients, other liver function tests (LFTs) remained normal and no obvious damage was noted on liver ultrasound (US). This apparent hepatotoxicity has not been reported in HT, and the mechanism of the hepatotoxicity is not known. After cessation of the drug, the patients showed a rapid resolution of the transaminitis without obvious liver sequealae.[49]

RESULTS OF THERAPY

Regarding HT, the prognosis was bleak for affected children prior to the use of nitisinone. There was no effective medical management, and, although dietary intervention was somewhat beneficial for the chronic form of the disorder, it was not very helpful for the acute form presenting with liver failure.[3] In a large survey of patients treated with diet alone, the two-year survival rate was only 29% in children presenting before two months of age. In children with an age of onset between two and six months, the two-year survival rate increased to 74%, but most had died by age 12.[8] The introduction of liver transplantation in the 1980s improved the prognosis for HT patients, yielding a two-year survival rate of 83% in a series of 51 transplanted patients.[52] Still, patients faced significant morbidity because of surgical complications and long-term immunosuppression.[53]

In 1992, Lindstedt and colleagues published a report of five children treated with nitisinone for HT.[48] All these patients experienced an almost miraculous improvement in their biochemical parameters and clinical condition. These dramatic results spurred additional research into nitisinone, revealing dramatic increases in the two- and four-year survival rates (88% and 88%, respectively, for children presenting when less than two months old, and 94% and 94%, respectively, for those presenting when less than six months old).[42] The improvements in survival are thought to be due to the drug's beneficial effects on the main complications of HT, as outlined next.

Effects on liver complications

Hepatocellular dysfunction, including acute and chronic failure, cirrhosis, and HCC, are the most significant complications of HT. Since the report of Lindstedt and colleagues in 1992, multiple studies have shown that nitisinone therapy results in a rapid improvement in LFTs, a reduction in the risk of acute liver failure (75%), an improvement of cirrhosis, and a drastic reduction in the need for liver transplantation, which was once the mainstay of therapy.[10,52] Today, liver transplantation is reserved for patients unresponsive to nitisinone treatment, or who have changes suggestive of HCC. The effect of nitisinone on the development of HCC is not as clear, however.

In the majority of patients treated with nitisinone, the AFP normalizes within six months to one year.[45,54] Despite this reduction and its implications, cases of HCC have been reported with nitisinone treatment.[55] In 1998, Holme and Lindstedt reported 2 patients of 101 who developed HCC after starting nitisinone within the first two years of life.[10] Santra and Baumman speculate that malignant transformation may have already occurred at the microscopic level prior to nitisinone treatment, and they cite cases of HCC diagnosed in patients before initiating, and years after taking, nitisinone.[45] Their impression is further supported by a report that abnormal gene expression, present in liver cells of knockout mice with HT, does not normalize after treatment with nitisinone.[56] Although patients on nitisinone may remain at risk for HCC, the degree of risk appears to be lower than that for patients treated with dietary treatment alone.[57] In fact, King and colleagues estimate that fewer than 5% of children placed on nitisinone before the age of two develop HCC.[4]

Effects on renal tubular dysfunction

Proximal tubular dysfunction (PTD), a well-known complication of HT affecting most patients, can cause nephrocalcinosis (16–33%) or rickets.[58] There has been some consensus that liver transplantation improves renal dysfunction, but outcomes have varied.[58] The beneficial effects of nitisinone on the liver have been well studied, but little is known about its effect on renal tubular dysfunction. In a long-term study by Masurel-Paulet and colleagues, 36 of 45 patients had evidence of tubulopathy at diagnosis, with 18 showing evidence of rickets. After long-term nitisinone treatment, 13 showed persistent signs of tubulopathy, without clinical consequences, and the symptoms of rickets resolved in all 18.[52] In 2008, Santra and colleagues described 21 children (median age 17 weeks), all of whom had biochemical evidence of renal tubular dysfunction, with four children showing radiological evidence of rickets. Within one year of nitisinone therapy and a tyrosine restricted diet, all 21 showed normalization of the biochemical parameters, and there was a complete clinical and biochemical response in the four children with rickets. The biochemical parameters remained normal even after 10 years of follow-up.[58]

Effects on neurologic complications

The painful porphyria-like neurologic crises characteristic of HT are unpredictable and dangerous complications that can be life-threatening. With dietary restriction as one of the mainstays of treatment prior to nitisinone, the reported incidence of these crises ranged from 7 to 20% per year.[6] The crises caused significant morbidity and were associated with a 10% mortality rate in some cohorts.[8] Nitisinone suppresses formation of SA, relieving the inhibition of gamma ALA dehydratase and consequently reducing formation of 5-ALA, thought to be responsible for the crises. Once feared complications of the disorder, neurological crises have been practically eliminated by sustained nitisinone therapy; in fact, interruption of therapy appears to be a risk factor for the occurrence of neurological crises.[59]

Effects on growth and development

Poor growth and development is a common complication of HT because of the effects of chronic liver and renal disease; dietary restriction of amino acids may exacerbate the problem. Current data indicate that correction of growth failure typically occurs within months of therapy.[3]

Effects on cardiomyopathy

Cardiomyopathy is a less-recognized complication of HT, and its mechanism is not known. The effect of dietary restriction, transplantation, or nitisinone on cardiomyopathy has not been studied extensively, probably because the cardiomyopathy is often subclinical and is easily missed. In 2006 Arora and colleagues published a study of 20 children with both the acute and chronic forms of HT; 30% (6 of 20) of the patients had some evidence of cardiomyopathy, with interventricular hypertrophy being the most common pattern. The authors found a significantly lower rate of myocardial hypertrophy in patients receiving nitisinone.[9] Another report described a newborn with severe obstructive cardiomyopathy as the presenting sign of HT.[60] Echocardiography showed both interventricular hypertrophy and left ventricular outflow tract obstruction. The child was treated with a beta-blocker and nitisinone. Within two weeks, the left ventricular outflow tract obstruction resolved; this improvement was considered to be due to the hemodynamic effects of beta blockade. The myocardial hypertrophy almost completely resolved in four months and, according to the investigators, was attributable to nitisinone and not beta blockade, because beta-blockers do not reverse hypertrophy.

Effects on tyrosine levels

Tyrosine levels can rise significantly in patients receiving nitisinone, and may respond in a dose-dependent manner. Rats fed a single dose of nitisinone (0.5 mg/kg) showed marked elevations of tyrosine in the plasma (2.5 mM), and in the aqueous humor (3.5 mM).[43] Nevertheless, elevations of plasma tyrosine are not always associated with the development of corneal toxicity in humans. (See "Side effects and toxicity" section.)

For AKU, nitisinone treatment remains investigational, and there is no other effective medical treatment. Complications, such as joint destruction and cardiac valvular disease, are managed initially with conservative medical treatments and then surgically in advanced disease.[28] Attempts at therapy with a tyrosine- and phenylalanine-restricted diet, intended to reduce the formation of HGA, and with vitamin C therapy, aimed at enhancing HGA degradation, are not efficacious.[28]

The first human trial investigating the effect of nitisinone in AKU involved two female patients in their fifties who took nitisinone for approximately 10 days, without dietary tyrosine or phenylalanine restriction.[28] One woman received 0.7 mg for seven days and then 2.8 mg for three days. Her urinary HGA excretion fell from 2.9 g/d to 0.13 g/d. The other patient's urinary HGA fell from 6.4 g/d to

1.7 g/d after nine days of treatment with nitisinone (0.7 mg/d). In both patients, the baseline plasma tyrosine concentrations were approximately 1.1 mg/dl (60 μmol/L), and they rose to approximately 12.8 mg/dl (700 μmol/L) in the first patient, and 23.6 mg/dl (1,300 μmol/L) in the second patient. No side effects were noted.

In 2005, Suwannarat and colleagues published a study of nine patients with nitisinone-treated AKU.[49] The treatment regimen included incremental dosing starting at 0.35 milligrams twice daily for one week, increasing to 1.05 milligrams twice daily, and then a low-protein diet during the final week. All nine patients had elevated urinary HGA at baseline, averaging 4.0 ± 1.8 (standard deviation [SD]) grams per day, and normal plasma tyrosine levels, averaging 68 ± 18 (SD) μmol/L. After initiation of nitisinone, urinary HGA levels fell rapidly within the first week of treatment on the starting dose, and continued to decline rapidly for another week, thereafter stabilizing at about 220 mg/d (a 94% reduction). The plasma tyrosine levels also rose rapidly during the first two and a half weeks of treatment, with seven of the patients on the higher dose having a mean tyrosine level of 760 μmol/L. The low-protein diet reduced the mean plasma tyrosine level of the five remaining patients from 755 to 603 μmol/L. Six of the seven patients who received nitisinone for more than seven days reported a decrease in their joint pain. No corneal toxicity was noted.

FUTURE DEVELOPMENTS

For HT, consideration might be given to liberalizing dietary restrictions and allowing plasma tyrosine levels to increase, based on AKU studies showing low toxicity associated with high plasma tyrosine concentrations. It will be interesting to determine whether nitisinone therapy can be stopped in patients who have undergone liver transplantation.

Abbreviations used in this chapter

HT	Hereditary tyrosinemia
AFP	α-Fetoprotein
FAH	Fumarylacetoacetate hydrolase
MAA	Maleylacetoacetate
FAA	Fumarylacetoacetate
SAA	succinylacetoacetate
SA	Succinylacetone
ALA	Aminolevulinic acid
AKU	Alkaptonuria
HGA	Homogentisic acid
HGD	Homogentisate 1,2-dioxygenase
HPPD	4-Hydroxyphenylpyruvate dioxygenase
HCC	Hepatocellular carcinoma
PTD	Proximal tubular dysfunction

A — Normal lysosome

Cystine

Lysine

B — Untreated cystinotic lysosome

Cystina

Lysine

C — Cysteamine-treated cystinotic lysosome

Cysteamine

Lysine

Mixed disulfide of cysteine and cysteamine

Cysteine

Plate 8–4: Mechanism of action of cysteamine in causing lysosomal cystine depletion. Reprinted with permission from Gahl WG, Thoene JG, Schneider JA. Cystinosis. *N Engl J Med.* 2002;347:111–121.

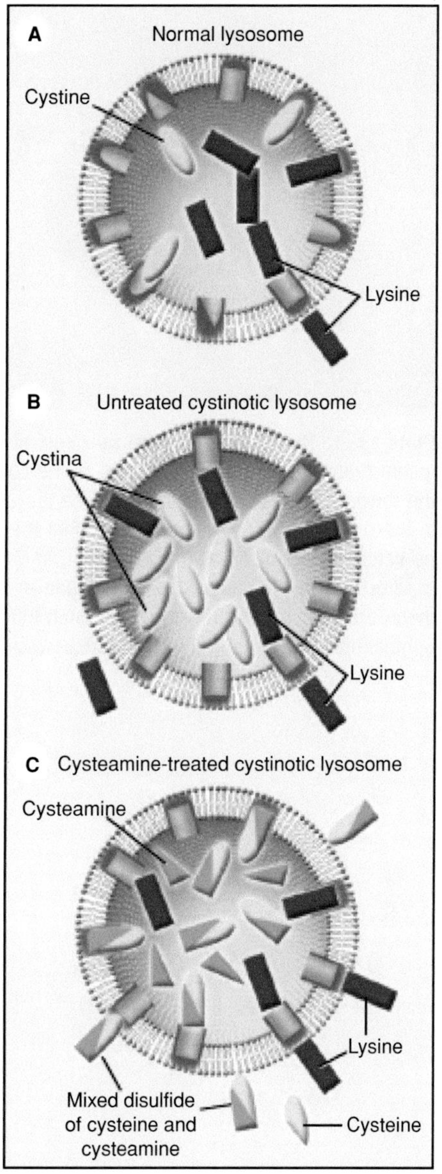

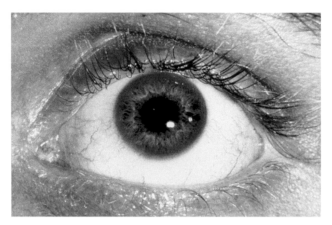

Plate 13–1: The KF ring, as seen by direct observation. These rings are brownish, sometimes greenish-brown, rings around the rim of the cornea. They begin in the upper pole, followed by the lower pole, then gradually complete the circle. They are the result of deposits of copper in these areas. It be emphasized that the presence of these partial or complete rings can be detected accurately, as in this patient, in only a minority of patients who really have them. In direct observation, errors may be made in seeing apparent rings when they are not really there (occasionally) and missing rings when they are there (often). A slit lamp examination by an ophthalmologist is required for accurate assessment of the presence or absence of KF rings.

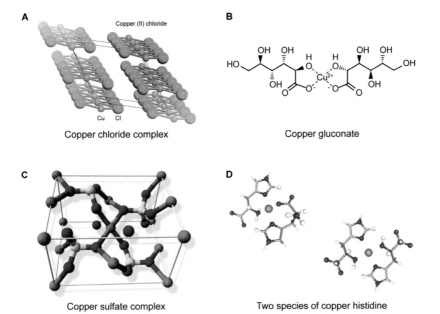

A Copper (II) chloride

Cu Cl

Copper chloride complex

B

Copper gluconate

C

Copper sulfate complex

D

Two species of copper histidine

Plate 14–1: Models illustrate the fundamental coordination chemistry of four small copper complexes used for treatment of acquired and inherited copper deficiency syndromes. The abundance of albumin in human serum (500 micromolar concentration) and its high affinity for copper imply that this protein may compete for copper atoms introduced as small complexes. (A) Cupric (2+) chloride. Copper atoms are pale red, chloride atoms are green, and coordination geometry is square planar. (B) In copper gluconate, four oxygen atoms coordinate a copper atom. (C) Copper sulfate complex. Sulfur atoms are yellow, oxygen atoms are red, and copper atoms are pale red. (D) Two species of copper histidine, based on density functional theory expected at physiological pH (7.3)[26] and modified to colorize nitrogen atoms (blue), oxygen atoms (red), and copper atoms (pale red).

A

Blood-brain barrier: Capillary endothelial cells

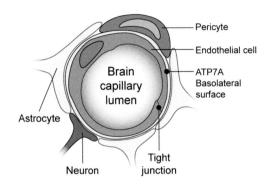

B

Blood-CSF barrier: Choroid plexus epithelium

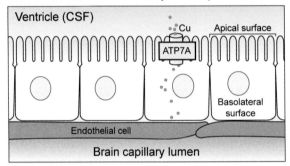

Plate 14–2: Paradigm of copper transport at the blood–brain barrier (A) and blood–CSF barrier (B). The usual basolateral membrane localization of ATP7A makes sense at the blood–brain barrier, however, apical localization in choroid plexus epithelial cells that comprise the blood–CSF barrier is proposed here. See text (Copper entry to the central nervous system) for further explanation.

For AKU patients, nitisinone might be efficacious even when given on a one-month-on-one-month-off basis. Furthermore, early treatment (e.g., in adolescence) may prevent all signs and symptoms of the disease, and this possibility should be investigated. All these pursuits await the results of the recently completed clinical trial of nitisinone in AKU (see http://clinicaltrials.gov/).

REFERENCES

1. Sakai K, Kitagawa T. An atypical case of tyrosinosis (1-para-hyroxyphenyllactic aciduria): I. Clinical and laboratory findings. *Jikei Med J.* 1957;2:1
2. Sakai K, Kitagawa T. An atypical case of tyrosinosis (1-para-hydroxyphenyllactic aciduria): II. A research on the metabolic block. *Jikei Med J.* 1957;2:11
3. Scott CR. The genetic tyrosinemias. *Am J Med Genet Part C.* 2006;142:121–126
4. King LS, Trahms C, Scott CR. Tyrosinemia type 1 in GeneReviews at GeneTests: Medical Genetics Information Resource [database online; updated October 2008]. Copyright, University of Washington, Seattle. 1997–2007. Available at: http://www.genetests.org
5. DeBraekeleer M, Larochelle J. Genetic epidemiology of hereditary tyrosinemia in Quebec and in Saguenay-Lac-St-Jean. *Am J Hum Genet.* 1990;47:302–307
6. Mitchell GA, Grompe M, Lambert M, Tanguay RM. Hypertyrosinemia. C. Scriver, A Beaudet, W. Sly, D. Valle, eds. *The Metabolic and Molecular Bases of Inherited Disease*, 8th edition, McGraw-Hill, 1777–1805, 2001
7. Mitchell G, Larochelle J, Lambert M, Michaud J, Grenier A, Ogier H, Gauthier M, Lacroix J, Vanasse M, Larbrisseau A, et al. Neurologic crises in hereditary tyrosinemia. *N Engl J Med.* 1990;322:432–437
8. van Spronsen FJ, Thomasse Y, Smit GPA, Leonard JV, Clayton PT, Fidler V, Berger R, Heymans HAS. Hereditary tyrosinemia type I: A new clinical classification with difference in prognosis on dietary treatment. *Hepatology.* 1994;20:1187–1191
9. Arora N, Stumper O, Wright J, Kelly DA, McKiernan PJ. Cardiomyopathy in tyrosinemia type I is common but usually benign. *J Inherit Metab Dis.* 2006;29:54–57
10. Holme E, Lindstedt S. Tyrosinaemia type I and NTBC (2-(2-nitro-4-trifluoro-methylbenzoyl)-1,3-cyclohexanedione). *J Inherit Metab Dis.* 1998;21:507–517
11. Sze YK, Dhawan A, Taylor RM, Bansal S, Mieli-Vergani G, Rela M, Heaton N. Pediatric liver transplantation for metabolic liver disease: Experience at King's College Hospital. *Transplantation.* 2009;87:87–93
12. Kayler LK, Rasmussen CS, Dykstra DM, Punch JD, Rudich SM, Magee JC, Maraschio MA, Arenas JD, Campbell DA, Merion RM. Liver transplantation in children with metabolic disorders in the United States. *Am J Transplant.* 2003;3:334–339
13. Mohan N, McKiernan P, Preece MA, Green A, Buckels J, Mayer AD, Kelly DA. Indications and outcome of liver transplantation in tyrosinaemia type 1. *Eur J Pediatr.* 1999;158(Suppl 2):S49–S54
14. Allard P, Grenier A, Korson MS, Zytkovicz TH. Newborn screening for hepatorenal tyrosinemia by tandem mass spectrometry: Analysis of succinylacetone extracted from dried blood spots. *Clin Biochem.* 2004;37:1010–1015
15. Turgeon C, Magera MJ, Allard P, Tortorelli S, Gavrilov D, Oglesbee D, Raymond K, Rinaldo P, Matern D. Combined newborn screening for succinylacetone, amino acids, and acylcarnitine in dried blood spots. *Clin Chem.* 2008;54:657–664
16. Lindblad B, Lindstedt S, Steen G. On the enzymic defects in hereditary tyrosinemia. *Proc Natl Acad Sci USA.* 1977;74:4641–4645
17. Grompe M. The pathophysiology and treatment of hereditary tyrosinemia type 1. *Semin Liver Dis.* 2001;21:563–571
18. Jorquera R, Tanguay RM. The mutagenicity of the tyrosine metabolite, fumarylacetoacetate, is enhanced by glutathione depletion. *Biochem Biophys Res Commun.* 1997;232:42–48

19. Phaneuf D, Labelle Y, Berube D, Arden K, Cavenee W, Gagne R, Tanguay RM. Cloning and expression of the cDNA encoding human fumarylacetoacetate hydrolase, the enzyme deficient in hereditary tyrosinemia: Assignment of the gene to chromosome 15. *Am J Hum Genet*. 1991;48:525–535

20. The Human Gene Mutation Database at the Institute of Medical Genetics in Cardiff. Available at: http://www.hgmd.cf.ac.uk/ac/index.php

21. Poudrier J, St-Louis M, Lettre F, Gibson K, Prevost C, Larochelle J, Tanguay RM. Frequency of the IVS12+5G→A splice mutation of the fumarylacetoacetate hydrolase gene in carriers of hereditary tyrosinemia in the French Canadian population of Saguenay-Lac-St.-Jean. *Prenat Diagn*. 1996;16:59–64

22. Arranz J, Pinol F, Kozak L, Perez-Cerda C, Cormand B, Ugarte M, Riudor E. Splicing mutations, mainly IVS6–1(G4T), account for 70% of fumarylacetoacetate hydrolase (FAH) gene alterations, including 7 novel mutations, in a survey of 29 tyrosinemia type I patients. *Hum Mutat*. 2002;20:180–188

23. Elpeleg ON, Shaag A, Holme E, Zughayar G, Ronen S, Fisher D, Hurvitz H. Mutation analysis of the FAH gene in Israeli patients with tyrosinemia type I. *Hum Mutat*. 2002;19(1):80–81

24. St-Louis M, Leclerc B, Laine J, Salo MK, Holmberg C, Tanguay RM. Identification of a stop mutation in five Finnish patients suffering from hereditary tyrosinemia type I. *Hum Mol Genet*. 1994;3:69–72

25. Poudrier J, Lettre F, Scriver CR, Larochelle J, Tanguay RM. Different clinical forms of hereditary tyrosinemia (type I) in patients with identical genotypes. *Mol Genet Metab*. 1998;64:119–125

26. Kvittingen EA, Rootwelt H, Berger R, Brandtzaeg P. Self-induced correction of the genetic defect in tyrosinaemia type I. *J Clin Invest*. 1994;94:1657–1661

27. Rootwelt H, Brodtkorb E, Kvittingen EA. Identification of a frequent pseudodeficiency mutation in the fumarylacetoacetase gene, with implications for diagnosis of tyrosinemia type 1. *Am J Hum Genet*. 1994;55:1122–1127

28. Phornphutkul C, Introne WJ, Perry MB, Bernardini I, Murphey M, Fitzpatrick DL, Anderson PD, Huizing M, Anikster Y, Gerber LH, Gahl WA. Natural history of alkaptonuria. *N Engl J Med*. 2002;347:2111–2121

29. Goicoechea de Jorge E, Lorda I, Gallardo ME, Perez B, Perez de Ferran C, Mendoza H, Rodriguez de Cordoba S. Alkaptonuria in the Dominican Republic: Identification of the founder AKU mutation and further evidence of mutation hot spots in the HGO gene. *J Med Genet*. 2002;39:e40

30. Srsen S, Cisaric F, Pasztor L, Harmecko L. Alkaptonuria in the Trencin district of Czechoslovakia. *Am J Med Genet*. 1978;2:159–166

31. Perry MB, Suwannarat P, Furst GP, Gahl WA, Gerber LH. Musculoskeletal findings and disability in alkaptonuria. *J Rheumatol*. 2006;33:2280–2285

32. De Haas V, Carbasius Weber EC, de Klerk JBC, Bakker HD, Smit GPA, Huijbers WAR, Duran M, Poll-The BT. The success of dietary protein restriction in alkaptonuria patients is age-dependent. *J Inherit Metab Dis*. 1998;21:791–798

33. Wolff JA, Barshop B, Nyhan WL, Leslie J, Seegmiller JE, Gruber H, Garst M, Winter S, Michals K, Matalon R. Effects of ascorbic acid in alkaptonuria: Alterations in benzoquinone acetic acid and an ontogenic effect in infancy. *Pediatr Res*. 1989;26:140–144

34. Spencer JMF, Maxime CL, Gibbons H, Sharp RJ, Carr AJ, Athanasou NA. Arthroplasty for ochronotic arthritis. *Acta Orthop Scand*. 2004;75:355–358

35. Introne WJ, Phornphutkul C, Bernardini I, McLaughlin K, Fitzpatrick D, Gahl WA. Exacerbation of the ochronosis of alkaptonuria due to renal insufficiency and improvement after renal transplantation. *Mol Genet Metab*. 2002;77:136–142

36. Kobak AC, Oder G, Kobak S, Argin M, Inal V. Ochronotic arthropathy: Disappearance of alkaptonuria after liver transplantation for hepatitis B-related cirrhosis. *J Clin Rheumatol*. 2005;11:323–325

37. Fernandez-Canon JM, Granadino B, Beltran-Valero de Bernabe D, Renedo M, Fernandez-Ruiz E, Penalva MA, Rodriguez de Cordoba S. The molecular basis of alkaptonuria. *Nature.* 1996;14:19–24

38. Titus GP, Mueller HA, Burgner J, Rodriguez de Cordoba S, Penalva MA, Timm DE. Crystal structure of human homogentisate dioxygenase. *Nat Struct Biol.* 2000;7:542–546.

39. Kayser MA, Introne W, Gahl WA. Alkaptonuria. Valle, Beaudet, Vogelstein, Kinzler, Antonarakis, Ballabio, Scriver, Childs, and Sly, eds. *The Online Metabolic & Molecular Bases of Inherited Disease.* Updated November 2007. Available at: http://www.ommbid.com/

40. Hall MG, Wilks MF, Provan WM, Eksborg S, Lumholtz B. Pharmacokinetics and pharmacodynamics of NTBC (2-(2-nitro-4-fluoromethylbenzoyl)-1,3-cyclohexanedione) and mesotrione, inhibitors of 4-hydroxyphenyl pyruvate dioxygenase (HPPD) following a single dose to healthy male volunteers. *Br J Clin Pharmacol.* 2001;52:169–177

41. Lock EA, Ellis MK, Gaskin P, Robinson M, Auton TR, Provan WM, Smith LL, Prisbylla MP, Mutter LC, Lee DL. From toxicological problem to therapeutic use: The discovery of the mode of action of 2-(2-nitro-4-trifluoromethylbenzoyl)-1,3-cyclohexanedione (NTBC), its toxicology and development as a drug. *J Inherit Metab Dis.* 1998;21:498–506

42. Swedish Orphan International AB. Orfadin package insert.

43. Lock EA, Gaskin P, Ellis MK, Provan WM, Robinson M, Smith LL, Prisbylla MP, Mutter LC. Tissue distribution of 2-(2-nitro-4-trifluoromethylbenzoyl) cyclohexane-1–3-dione (NTBC): Effect on enzymes involved in tyrosine catabolism and relevance to ocular toxicity in the rat. *Toxicol Appl Pharmacol.* 1996;141:439–447

44. Szczeciński P, Lamparska D, Gryff-Keller A, Gradowska W. Identification of 2-[2-nitro-4-(trifluoromethyl)benzoyl]-cyclohexane-1,3-dione metabolites in urine of patients suffering from tyrosinemia type I with the use of 1H and 19F NMR spectroscopy. *Acta Biochim Pol.* 2008;55:749–752

45. Santra S, Baumann U. Experience of nitisinone for the pharmacological treatment of hereditary tyrosinaemia type 1. *Expert Opin Pharmacother.* 2008;9:1229–1236

46. Kavana M, Moran GR. Interaction of (4-hydroxyphenyl)pyruvate dioxygenase with the specific inhibitor 2-[2-nitro-4-(trifluoromethyl)benzoyl]-1,3-cyclohexanedione. *Biochemistry.* 2003;42:10238–10245

47. Ellis MK, Whitfield AC, Gowans LA, Auton TR, Provan WM, Lock EA, Smith LL. Inhibition of 4-hydroxyphenylpyruvate dioxygenase by 2-(2-nitro-4-trifluoromethylbenzoyl)-cyclohexane-1,3-dione and 2-(2-chloro-4-methanesulfonylbenzoyl)-cyclohexane-1,3-dione. *Toxicol Appl Pharmacol.* 1995;133:12–19

48. Lindstedt S, Holme E, Lock EA, Hjalmarson O, Strandvik B. Treatment of hereditary tyrosinaemia type I by inhibition of 4-hydroxyphenylpyruvate dioxygenase. *Lancet.* 1992;340:813–817

49. Suwannarat P, O'Brien K, Perry MB, Sebring N, Bernardini I, Kaiser-Kupfer MI, Rubin BI, Tsilou E, Gerber LH, Gahl WA. Use of nitisinone in patients with alkaptonuria. *Metabolism.* 2005;54:719–728

50. Ahmad S, Teckman JH, Lueder GT. Corneal opacities associated with NTBC treatment. *Am J Ophthalmol.* 2002;134:266–268

51. Gissen P, Preece MA, Willshaw HA, McKiernan PJ. Ophthalmic follow-up of patients with tyrosinaemia type I on NTBC. *J Inherit Metab Dis.* 2003;26:13–16

52. Masurel-Paulet A, Poggi-Bach J, Rolland MO, Bernard O, Guffon N, Dobbelaere D, Sarles J, de Baulny HO, Touati G. NTBC treatment in tyrosinaemia type I: Long-term outcome in French patients. *J Inherit Metab Dis.* 2008;31:81–87

53. van Spronsen FJ, Berger R, Smit GP, de Klerk JB, Duran M, Bijleveld CM, van Faassen H, Slooff MJ, Heymans HS. Tyrosinaemia type I: Orthotopic liver transplantation as

the only definitive answer to a metabolic as well as an oncological problem. *J Inherit Metab Dis.* 1989;12(Suppl 2):339–342

54. Holme E, Lindstedt S. Nontransplant treatment of tyrosinemia. *Clin Liver Dis.* 2000;4:805–814

55. van Spronsen FJ, Bijleveld CM, van Maldegem BT, Wijburg FA. Hepatocellular carcinoma in hereditary tyrosinemia type I despite 2-(2 nitro-4-3 trifluoro-methylbenzoyl)-1,3-cyclohexanedione treatment. *J Pediatr Gastroenterol Nutr.* 2005;40:90–93

56. Luijerink MC, Jacobs SM, van Beurden EA, Koornneef LP, Klomp LW, Berger R, Van Den Berg IE. Extensive changes in liver gene expression induced by hereditary tyrosinemia type I are not normalized by treatment with 2-(2-nitro-4-trifluoromethylbenzoyl)-1,3-cyclohexanedione (NTBC). *J Hepatol.* 2003;39:901–909

57. Koelink CJ, van Hasselt P, Van Der Ploeg A, Van Den Heuvel-Eibrink MM, Wijburg FA, Bijleveld CM, van Spronsen FJ. Tyrosinemia type I treated by NTBC: How does AFP predict liver cancer? *Mol Genet Metab.* 2006;89:310–315

58. Santra S, Preece MA, Hulton SA, McKiernan PJ. Renal tubular function in children with tyrosinaemia type I treated with nitisinone. *J Inherit Metab Dis.* 2008;31:399–402

59. Schlump JU, Perot C, Ketteler K, Schiff M, Mayatepek E, Wendel U, Spiekerkoetter U. Severe neurological crisis in a patient with hereditary tyrosinaemia type I after interruption of NTBC treatment. *J Inherit Metab Dis.* 2008 [Epub ahead of print]

60. André N, Roquelaure B, Jubin V, Ovaert C. Successful treatment of severe cardiomyopathy with NTBC in a child with tyrosinaemia type I. *J Inherit Metab Dis.* 2005;28:103–106

10 Alternative waste nitrogen disposal agents for urea cycle disorders

Gregory M. Enns

NATURAL HISTORY OF UREA CYCLE DISORDERS

Urea cycle disorders (UCDs) are inborn errors of metabolism characterized by episodic, life-threatening hyperammonemia secondary to partial or complete inactivity of enzymes responsible for eliminating nitrogenous waste. The urea cycle was initially elucidated by Krebs and Henseleit in 1932.[1] In 1958, argininosuccinic acid lyase deficiency became the first enzymatic defect of the urea cycle to be identified, and reports of all others, except N-acetylglutamate synthetase (NAGS) deficiency, followed in the 1960s.[2] Ornithine transcarbamylase (OTC) deficiency is the most common UCD, followed by argininosuccinate synthetase (AS) deficiency (citrullinemia), carbamoyl phosphate synthetase (CPS) deficiency, and argininosuccinate lyase (AL) deficiency. NAGS deficiency was first described in 1981 and has been documented in only a few patients.[3] Estimates of overall incidence of UCDs in the United States have ranged from approximately 1 in 25,000 to 1 in 8,200 births.[4,5]

Historically, mortality and morbidity have been high, with survivors commonly showing devastating neurological sequelae.[2] UCDs are the most common cause of neonatal hyperammonemia and typically present with symptoms of poor feeding, lethargy, hypotonia, irritability, seizures, respiratory distress, grunting, and hyperventilation. Other disorders common in neonates, such as sepsis, cardiac failure, and intracranial hemorrhage, are also in the differential diagnosis because similar clinical findings may occur in these conditions. Therefore, in all neonates presenting with nonspecific symptoms of distress, a plasma ammonium level should be obtained. If the level of ammonium is elevated, diagnostic evaluations and treatment should be started immediately.

Although presentation in the neonatal period has been well-documented, patients who have a partial enzyme deficiency typically manifest after the neonatal period. UCDs may strike at any age. Indeed, approximately two thirds of cases initially present after the neonatal period.[5] Clinical features may be subtle in such late-onset cases, leading to delays in diagnosis. In addition to acutely altered mental status, later-onset patients may have episodic ataxia, psychiatric and behavioral symptoms, psychomotor delay, and gastrointestinal complaints, such as loss of appetite and episodic emesis.[6]

Many survivors of the initial hyperammonemic episode undergo recurrent attacks of hyperammonemia requiring hospitalization. Such episodes are typically preceded by an illness, especially a viral syndrome. Other events that contribute to hyperammonemic episodes include dietary or medication noncompliance and major life events, such as surgery, gastrointestinal bleeding, accidents, school stress, or parturition. Catabolic stress from viral illnesses appears to be a more significant risk factor than is increased intake of dietary nitrogen for causing hyperammonemia.[5,7]

A study of 260 UCD patients showed that onset of symptoms in the neonatal period results in the worst outcome (35% survival approximately 11 years after the start of the study period), and patients who presented initially in late infancy have the best outcome (87% survival; Figure 10–1). Percent survival to the final follow-up time point was highest for patients with AS deficiency (78%), followed by girls with OTC deficiency (74%), and CPS-I deficiency (61%).[5] Boys with OTC deficiency have the lowest survival rate over time (53%), as well as the lowest survival rate following hyperammonemic crises (71%).[5,8]

Although alternative pathway therapy and other therapies, especially hemodialysis, for UCDs has led to improved patient survival, cognitive impairment remains a common finding, especially in patients who have neonatal-onset disease.[9]

PATHOPHYSIOLOGY

Ammonia is present in all body fluids and exists mainly as ammonium ion at physiologic pH. Hyperammonemia is defined as a blood ammonia concentration greater than approximately 100 μmol/L in neonates or 50 μmol/L in children

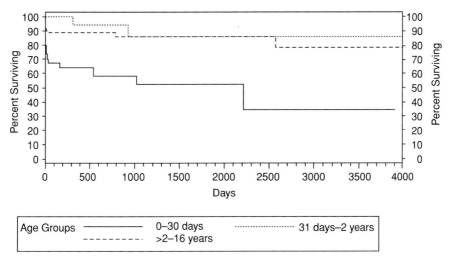

Figure 10–1: Kaplan–Meier survival by age at first episode of hyperammonemia. Survival time was calculated as the amount of time between the discharge date of the last episode and the admission date from the first episode. Only 35% of patients who presented with the first hyperammonemic episode during the neonatal period were still alive at the final follow-up time point (approximately 11 years after the start of the study period).[5] Reproduced with permission from *Acta Paediatrica*.

and adults (precise cutoffs vary depending on individual laboratory normative ranges). A five- to tenfold increase in blood ammonium levels is usually toxic to the nervous system.[10] Acute hyperammonemia causes astrocyte swelling and global cerebral edema, which affects brain white matter selectively. Changes involving the deep insular and perirolandic sulci may be reversible.[11] In cases of severe hyperammonemia, however, permanent changes occur. Neuropathological findings in patients who have neonatal-onset proximal UCDs consist of gross cerebral atrophy, ventriculomegaly, delayed myelination, the appearance of Alzheimer type II astrocytes, ulegyria, and spongiform degeneration of the cortex, gray–white matter junction, and deep gray nuclei, including the basal ganglia and thalamus.[11]

Hyperammonemia also causes increased cerebral cortical glutamine content, activation of astrocytic glutamine synthetase, and astrocyte swelling. Ammonia diffuses freely across the blood–brain barrier and is rapidly incorporated into glutamine via glutamine synthetase. Glutamine synthetase, a cytosolic enzyme primarily localized to the astrocyte in the brain, catalyzes the following reaction:

$$NH_3 + \text{L-Glutamate} + ATP \rightarrow \text{L-Glutamine} + ADP + P_i.$$

This reaction, therefore, represents a short-term means of buffering excess plasma ammonium. In theory, glutamine also may be an organic osmolyte that increases intracellular osmolarity. Such an increase in osmolarity would lead to increased cellular volume, as water enters the astrocyte, and subsequent cytotoxic cerebral edema.[9,12]

Although the "glutamine hypothesis" has been a leading explanation for the development of cerebral edema, other research has focused on glutamine-independent mechanisms to explain the pathogenesis of hyperammonemic encephalopathy. In particular, the role of impaired brain oxidative metabolism in causing cerebral dysfunction associated with hyperammonemia is an area of active investigation. Acute hyperammonemia causes a decrease in brain metabolic rate and high-energy phosphate concentration and increased production of toxic reactive oxygen species (ROS) by brain mitochondria.[13] Glutamine also enters mitochondria through a histidine-sensitive carrier. This process is potentiated by ammonia. Phosphate-activated glutaminase is located in the inner mitochondrial membrane and cleaves glutamine into glutamate and ammonia. Because of this localized production of ammonia, intramitochondrial ammonia levels have the potential to become high, leading to induction of mitochondrial permeability transition (MPT), increased oxidative and nitrosative stress, and astroglial dysfunction. The production of ROS and reactive nitrogen species and the induction of MPT have been hypothesized to initiate a cascade of events that includes activation of mitogen-activated protein kinases (MAPKs) and resultant failure of astrocytes to regulate their intracellular volume.[14]

In addition, ammonium ions have a multitude of effects on mammalian neurotransmitters, including systems involving cholinergic, serotonergic, and glutamatergic neurotransmission. The increased seizure predisposition in some UCD patients may be explained, in part, by increased brain concentrations of the excitatory amino acid neurotransmitters glutamate and aspartate. Increased levels of these amino acids are present in the sparse-fur (spf) mouse, a model of OTC deficiency.[15] Tryptophan, a precursor of serotonin, and quinolinic acid, an N-methyl-D-aspartate (NMDA) receptor agonist known to produce selective striatal cell loss, are similarly increased in spf mice and in rats following portacaval anastomosis. Ammonia also inhibits high-affinity transport of glutamate in astrocytes. This inhibition results in increased extracellular concentration of glutamate.[16] These biochemical and pathological findings suggest that NMDA-mediated excitotoxic brain injury may be occurring in UCD patients.[17] Ammonium ions also depress postsynaptic α-amino-3-hydroxy-5-methyl-4-isoxazolepropionic acid (AMPA) receptor–mediated currents.[16] AMPA receptors mediate fast synaptic transmission and are involved with learning and memory.

Chronic hyperammonemia activates the L-system carrier, which results in a loss of NMDA receptor densities and increased uptake of tryptophan into the brain.[16] Serotoninergic symptoms, such as anorexia, altered sleep patterns, and disorders of motor coordination, may be related to the increased brain turnover of serotonin observed in hyperammonemic states.[11] The adaptive changes in NMDA receptors that occur in chronic hyperammonemia result in a decrease in excitatory neurotransmission and impaired production of nitric oxide and cyclic guanosine monophosphate (cGMP). Decreased cGMP production may inhibit long-term potentiation (LTP) in the hippocampus. Because LTP is a long-lasting

Table 10–1. Molecular genetics of the UCDs

Disorder	Cellular compartment	Gene	Chromosomal location	Molecular characteristics
NAGS deficiency	Mitochondrial matrix	NAGS	17q21.31	7 exons, spans ~5 Kb, ORF* ~1.6 Kb, 534 amino acids
CPS deficiency	Mitochondrial matrix	CPS1	2q35	38 exons, spans ~201 Kb, ORF ~5.8 Kb, 1,500 amino acids
OTC deficiency	Mitochondrial matrix	OTC	Xp21.1	10 exons, spans ~94 Kb, ORF ~1.7 Kb, 354 amino acids
AS deficiency (citrullinemia)	Cytosol	ASS1	9q34.1	15 exons, spans ~57 Kb, ORF ~1.9 Kb, 412 amino acids
AL deficiency	Cytosol	ASL	7cen-q11.2	16 exons, spans ~79 Kb, ORF ~1.9 Kb, 464 amino acids
Arginase deficiency	Cytosol	ARG	6q23	8 exons, spans ~37 Kb, ORF ~1.4 Kb, 322 amino acids

* ORF: open reading frame.
Note: Molecular characteristics of the UCDs are shown. Data were obtained from the National Center for Biotechnology Information (NCBI) Web sites (www.ncbi.nlm.nih.gov/IEB/Research/Acembly/index.html [Ace View]; www.ncbi.nlm.nih.gov/nuccore [Entrez Nucleotide]; www.ncbi.nlm.nig.gov/omim [OMIM]).

enhancement of synaptic transmission efficacy, considered to be the basis for some forms of learning and memory, this effect of hyperammonemia may be related to the abnormal cognitive function observed in patients who have UCDs.[18] Abnormal axonal growth, accompanied by decreased creatine and phosphocreatine levels (creatine is essential for axonal elongation) and alteration of brain cytoskeletal elements, are also observed in hyperammonemia. Glial fibrillary acidic protein (GFAP) is an important astrocytic protein involved in a multitude of cellular functions. GFAP is reduced, and microtubule-associated protein-2 (MAP-2) and neurofilament protein (NF-M) exhibit decreased phosphorylation, possibly through abnormal MAPK function caused by hyperammonemia.[19] Although the precise interrelationship between these proposed pathogenetic mechanisms is unclear, it is reasonable to suspect that these processes play at least some role in the mental impairment observed in UCD patients.

INHERITANCE

Urea cycle defects, with the exception of OTC deficiency, are inherited as autosomal recessive traits. OTC deficiency is X-linked and, therefore, typically manifests more severely in males. Approximately fifteen percent of females with OTC deficiency display symptoms, such as protein intolerance, cyclical vomiting, behavioral and neurologic abnormalities, and even hyperammonemic coma, and are termed "manifesting heterozygotes." The severity of symptoms in such females is related to random X-inactivation and allelic heterogeneity, as well as to degree of environmental stress. Further details regarding the molecular genetics of the UCDs are provided in Table 10–1.

EARLY EFFORTS AT HYPERAMMONEMIA THERAPY

A number of different therapies aimed at removing accumulated ammonia in cases of hyperammonemic encephalopathy have been attempted, including lactulose (reduces the production or absorption of the end products of bacterial nitrogen metabolism in the colon), exchange transfusion, peritoneal dialysis (PD), hemodialysis, and supplementation with nitrogen-free analogues of essential amino acids. Although children treated with α-keto amino acid analogues showed some clinical improvement, such as improved seizure control attention span and weight gain, death in infancy was still common. Exchange transfusions are ineffective in managing hyperammonemia. PD has shown variable efficacy in treating hyperammonemia but, in general, is far inferior to hemodialysis. The early use of these treatments prolonged survival in some cases, but overall efficacy has been disappointing.[20]

ALTERNATIVE PATHWAY MEDICATIONS

In 1914, Lewis demonstrated that sodium benzoate could divert urea nitrogen to hippurate (HIP) nitrogen in two normal subjects. After ingestion of sodium benzoate, blood urea nitrogen and ammonia levels fell and urine HIP excretion rose markedly, with little change in total urine nitrogen excretion.[21] Shiple and Sherwin later showed that oral administration of phenylacetate results in substitution of phenylacetylglutamine (PAGN) nitrogen for urea nitrogen in urine. Coadministration of benzoate and phenylacetate resulted in as much as 60% of urine nitrogen being excreted as HIP and PAGN.[22] Subsequently, the enzymes responsible for these reactions (acyl-coenzyme A [CoA]:glycine and acyl-CoA glutamine N-acyltransferases) were identified and localized to both kidney and liver in humans and primates. Synthesis of HIP (from conjugation of glycine with benzoate) and PAGN (from conjugation of glutamine with phenylacetate) requires adenosine triphosphate (ATP) and CoA. Pharmacogenetic factors partly determine the activity of enzymes responsible for formation of HIP and PAGN and, therefore, play a role in determining the individual rate of nitrogen removal.[23]

MECHANISM OF ACTION

In 1979, Brusilow and colleagues suggested that the use of endogenous biosynthetic pathways of non-urea waste nitrogen excretion could substitute for defective urea synthesis in patients who have UCDs. By promoting the synthesis of non-urea nitrogen-containing metabolites (the excretion rates of which are high or may be augmented), in theory, total body nitrogen load could be decreased despite abnormal urea cycle function.[24] The two classes of alternative pathway metabolites are (1) urea cycle intermediates (citrulline and argininosuccinate) and (2) amino acid acylation products (HIP and PAGN).

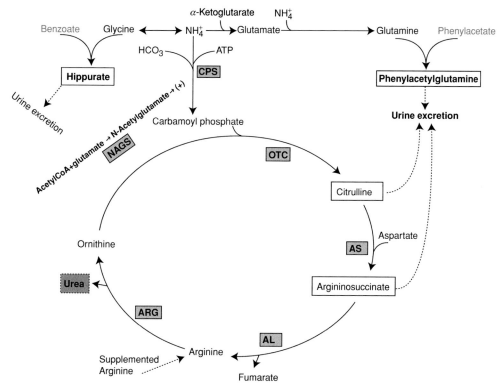

Figure 10–2: The urea cycle and alternative pathway therapy. Nitrogen flux through the urea cycle may be decreased by excretion of HIP and PAGN, molecules which contain one and two waste nitrogen atoms, respectively. In addition, citrulline (which contains one waste nitrogen atom) or argininosuccinate (which contains two waste nitrogen atoms) can serve as a vehicle of waste nitrogen excretion, depending on the location within the urea cycle of the deficient enzyme. For example, in AL deficiency, there is a block in argininosuccinate conversion to arginine. Supplementing AL deficiency patients with arginine increases production of argininosuccinate, which is then excreted in the urine along with its waste nitrogen. ARG: arginase. Reproduced with permission from *NeoReviews*, Vol. 7, page e490, Copyright © 2006 by the AAP.

Urea cycle intermediates

In AL deficiency, argininosuccinate accumulates and is excreted in the urine. Because argininosuccinate contains two waste nitrogen atoms, production of this metabolite can be exploited to excrete waste nitrogen in AL deficiency, provided that an adequate amount of ornithine is present to supply the necessary carbon skeletons for argininosuccinate biosynthesis. By administering pharmacologic doses of arginine, ornithine is synthesized by the action of arginase. Citrulline and argininosuccinate are then produced in turn by the sequential action of OTC and AS. In AL deficiency, argininosuccinate cannot be further metabolized and is excreted in the urine, along with waste nitrogen (Figure 10–2).[4]

Similarly, as long as sufficient arginine is supplied, citrulline can serve as a vehicle for waste nitrogen excretion in AS deficiency (citrullinemia; Figure 10–2). When compared to argininosuccinate, however, citrulline has two major

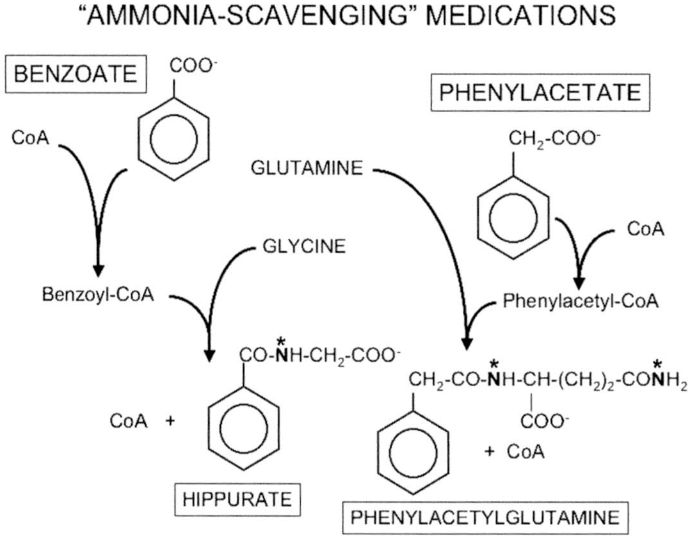

"AMMONIA-SCAVENGING" MEDICATIONS

Figure 10–3: Mechanism of nitrogen scavenging by sodium benzoate and sodium phenylacetate: HIP and PAGN are formed by conjugation of benzoate with glycine and phenylacetate with glutamine, respectively. These reactions are performed by specific liver and kidney N-acyltransferases. HIP contains one waste nitrogen atom, and phenylacetylglutamine contains two waste nitrogen atoms. Both HIP and PAGN are excreted in the urine, effectively decreasing nitrogen flux through the urea cycle. *Nitrogen atoms excreted. Reproduced with permission from *NeoReviews*, Vol. 7, Page e490, Copyright © 2006 by the AAP.

disadvantages: (1) It contains only one waste nitrogen atom, and (2) a high percentage of filtered citrulline is reabsorbed, so urine excretion is relatively poor.[4,23]

Amino acylation products

Because of high renal clearance (five times the glomerular filtration rate), HIP is easily excreted by the kidneys. HIP biosynthesis, by conjugation of benzoate with glycine, is accomplished by the action of mitochondrial matrix enzymes (benzoyl thiokinase and a glycine-specific N-acyltransferase; Figure 10–3). Similarly, PAGN is formed by sequential action of phenylacetyl thiokinase and a glutamine-specific N-acyltransferase. Because phenylacetate has the ability to conjugate glutamine, forming PAGN (a compound that contains two waste nitrogen atoms), its nitrogen-scavenging ability was hypothesized to be twice as effective as benzoate (which contains one nitrogen atom).[24]

Brusilow and colleagues suggested using combined therapy with sodium phenylacetate and sodium benzoate (Ammonul; Ucyclyd Pharma, Inc., Scottsdale, AZ) along with intravenous arginine HCl for treating hyperammonemic coma. Ammonul, a combination of sodium phenylacetate (10%) and sodium benzoate (10%), is an intravenously administered drug used as adjunctive therapy for the treatment of acute hyperammonemia and associated encephalopathy in patients with UCDs (Table 10–2).[24] The concomitant use of Ammonul with protein restriction, high caloric nutrition, arginine HCl, adequate hydration, and

Table 10–2. Acute management of patients with UCDs

Administration	Components of infusion solution			Dosage provided		
	Ammonul	Arginine HCl injection, 10%	Dextrose injection, 10%	Sodium phenylacetate	Sodium benzoate	Arginine HCl injection, 10%
Patients weighing 0–20 kg						
AL deficiency						
Loading dose: over 90–120 min.	2.5 mL/kg	6.0 mL/kg	25 mL/kg	250 mg/kg	250 mg/kg	600 mg/kg
Maintenance dose: over 24 h	2.5 mL/kg	6.0 mL/kg	25 mL/kg	250 mg/kg	250 mg/kg	600 mg/kg
AS deficiency						
Loading dose: over 90–120 min	2.5 mL/kg	6.0 mL/kg	25 mL/kg	250 mg/kg	250 mg/kg	600 mg/kg
Maintenance dose: over 24 h	2.5 mL/kg	6.0 mL/kg	25 mL/kg	250 mg/kg	250 mg/kg	600 mg/kg
CPS deficiency						
Loading dose: over 90–120 min	2.5 mL/kg	2.0 mL/kg	25 mL/kg	250 mg/kg	250 mg/kg	200 mg/kg
Maintenance dose: over 24 h	2.5 mL/kg	2.0 mL/kg	25 mL/kg	250 mg/kg	250 mg/kg	200 mg/kg
OTC deficiency						
Loading dose: over 90–120 min	2.5 mL/kg	2.0 mL/kg	25 mL/kg	250 mg/kg	250 mg/kg	200 mg/kg
Maintenance dose: over 24 h	2.5 mL/kg	2.0 mL/kg	25 mL/kg	250 mg/kg	250 mg/kg	200 mg/kg
Patients weighing >20 kg						
AL deficiency						
Loading dose: over 90–120 min	55 mL/m^2	6.0 mL/kg	25 mL/kg	5.5 g/m^2	5.5 g/m^2	600 mg/kg
Maintenance dose: over 24 h	55 mL/m^2	6.0 mL/kg	25 mL/kg	5.5 g/m^2	5.5 g/m^2	600 mg/kg
AS deficiency						
Loading dose: over 90–120 min	55 mL/m^2	6.0 mL/kg	25 mL/kg	5.5 g/m^2	5.5 g/m^2	600 mg/kg
Maintenance dose: over 24 h	55 mL/m^2	6.0 mL/kg	25 mL/kg	5.5 g/m^2	5.5 g/m^2	600 mg/kg
CPS deficiency						
Loading dose: over 90–120 min	55 mL/m^2	2.0 mL/kg	25 mL/kg	5.5 g/m^2	5.5 g/m^2	200 mg/kg
Maintenance dose: over 24 h	55 mL/m^2	2.0 mL/kg	25 mL/kg	5.5 g/m^2	5.5 g/m^2	200 mg/kg
OTC deficiency						
Loading dose: over 90–120 min	55 mL/m^2	2.0 mL/kg	25 mL/kg	5.5 g/m^2	5.5 g/m^2	200 mg/kg
Maintenance dose: over 24 h	55 mL/m^2	2.0 mL/kg	25 mL/kg	5.5 g/m^2	5.5 g/m^2	200 mg/kg

Note: Appropriate dosing of alternative pathway therapy medications for patients weighing up to 20 kg and greater than 20 kg is shown. Arginine HCl may be mixed directly with Ammonul or infused via a separate line. A central line is recommended for delivery of Ammonul and arginine HCl, because serious burns have resulted from extravasation from a peripheral catheter. The loading dose infusion should be given in 10% glucose at 25–35 mL/kg (or in 10% glucose at 400–600 mL/m^2 in older patients). Odansetron may be given (0.15 mg/kg) over the first 15 minutes of the priming infusion to decrease the risk of emesis.[4] Medical management of UCDs has the potential to decrease plasma ammonium levels; however, in cases associated with extreme hyperammonemia, a form of hemodialysis or hemofiltration is typically needed. Although institution of alternative pathway therapy and appropriate caloric support should be started without delay, the possibility of transferring the neonate to a specialist center with hemodialysis capacity should be explored concurrently if the initial point-of-care facility lacks appropriate resources to perform urgent dialysis.

Table 10–3. Chronic management of patients with UCDs

UCD		g/kg/d	g/m²/d
CPS or OTC deficiency	Sodium phenylbutyrate	0.45–0.60	9.9–13.0
	Citrulline or arginine (free base)	0.17	3.8
AS deficiency	Sodium phenylbutyrate	0.45–0.60	9.9–13.0
	Arginine (free base)	0.40–0.70	8.8–15.4
AL deficiency	Arginine (free base)	0.40–0.70	8.8–15.4

Note: Long-term care of UCD patients requires careful evaluation of nutritional status and provision of adequate protein (including essential amino acid formulas), calories, and essential vitamins and nutrients to promote growth, in addition to appropriate medications. The g/kg/d dosing is used for patients weighing up to 20 kg, and the g/m²/d dosing is used for older patients weighing more than 20 kg. Tablets or powder should be taken in equally divided amounts with each meal or feeding (i.e., three to six times daily). Patients should be followed by a center skilled in management of inborn errors of metabolism.

hemodialysis in acute hyperammonemia associated with altered mental status helps to increase waste nitrogen excretion through the formation of HIP and PAGN by the two different pathways discussed earlier in text (Figures 10–1 and 10–2). Hemodialysis is recommended in cases of severe hyperammonemia or if ammonium levels are not significantly reduced within four to eight hours after starting Ammonul.[4]

Sodium phenylbutyrate (Buphenyl; Ucyclyd Pharma, Inc.) is a prodrug of sodium phenylacetate that is used for chronic management of UCDs. Buphenyl, administered enterally in tablet or powder form, is used as adjunctive therapy, along with appropriate dietary management, for outpatient treatment of CPS, OTC, and AS deficiencies (Table 10–3).[4] A clinical trial has started to evaluate whether Buphenyl, in conjunction with decreased arginine dosing, will be beneficial in treating AL deficiency, especially with respect to liver function. Sodium benzoate in powder form is also sometimes used, either alone or in conjunction with Buphenyl, for chronic management of UCD patients.

Pharmacokinetics of Ammonul

Both phenylacetate and benzoate demonstrate saturable, nonlinear elimination, with a decrease in clearance with increased dose. Therefore, following established treatment protocol dosing guidelines is important to avoid an overdose. A second bolus infusion is not recommended if plasma ammonium levels do not drop significantly after the initial bolus.[4] Brusilow and colleagues studied the pharmacokinetics of intravenous sodium phenylacetate and sodium benzoate in two children (five months old and one year old) with CPS deficiency. The peak levels of phenylacetate and benzoate occurred at the same time (approximately two to three hours following dosing), and the benzoate level decreased faster. Phenylacetate levels were initially higher than benzoate levels and remained so throughout the period of study. HIP reached a peak earlier than PAGN but PAGN levels remained high for a longer period when compared to HIP in both patients. Urinary HIP nitrogen (18–57% of waste nitrogen) and urinary PAGN nitrogen (15–53% of waste nitrogen) combined accounted for approximately 60% of "effective" urinary waste nitrogen.[25]

There are no published pharmacokinetic studies on Ammonul performed exclusively in neonates. Green and colleagues, however, monitored the disposition of intravenous sodium benzoate alone in hyperammonemic newborn infants ($n = 4$) following administration of 460 mg/kg/d in four divided doses. An eightfold range in serum benzoate concentrations between treated neonates was noted. The elimination half-life of benzoate was 2.8 ± 3.1 hours. The total plasma clearance of benzoate was 1.00 ± 0.61 mg/kg/min, the majority being attributed to glycine conjugation in three of four neonates. The excreted total of benzoate and HIP was 84% ($\pm31\%$) of the administered benzoate. One neonate with reduced renal clearance excreted only 12% of benzoate as HIP. In this case, PD was the major route of benzoate clearance.[26] Intravenous infusions of benzoate and phenylacetate (given on different days) were administered to five children with lysinuric protein intolerance who were clinically stable during the period of study. Plasma benzoate levels peaked at 6.0 mmol/L (range 5.2–7.0 mmol/L) two hours after the start of the infusion (2.0 mmol/kg over 90 minutes) and decreased linearly with a mean half-life of 273 minutes. Plasma HIP levels peaked 120 minutes after the start of the infusion at 0.24 mmol/L (range 0.14–0.40 mmol/Lm) and remained stable for three hours. Less than 2% of the administered dose of benzoate appeared unchanged in the urine. Plasma phenylacetate levels also peaked at 120 minutes and decreased similarly to benzoate ($t_{1/2} = 253$ minutes), although peak levels were lower (4.8 mmol/L, range 3.7–6.1 mmol/L). Plasma PAGN levels peaked at 270 minutes with a mean concentration of 0.48 mmol/L (range 0.22–1.06 mmol/L). Forty percent (range 15–110%) of infused phenylacetate was excreted as PAGN in 24 hours.[27]

Both sodium phenylacetate and sodium benzoate are low-molecular-weight molecules with poor protein binding. Hemodialysis and hemofiltration result in significant dialytic and convective clearances of Ammonul, respectively, although therapeutic plasma levels of Ammonul may still be obtained despite high extracorporeal clearance.[28]

DOSAGE

Infants and young children (weighing up to 20 kg) with CPS deficiency, OTC deficiency, or AS deficiency should be treated with Ammonol at a load of 250 mg/kg intravenously over a period of 90–120 minutes. Older children and adults (weighing more than 20 kg) should be treated with Ammonul at 5.5 g/m^2 as an intravenous load over a period of 90–120 minutes (Table 10–2). After the loading dose, maintenance infusions of the same dose over 24 hours may be continued until the patient is no longer hyperammonemic and oral therapy can be tolerated.[4,8] Specific guidelines for administering Ammonul are not provided for treatment of AL deficiency or arginase deficiency. AL deficiency may respond to intravenous arginine HCl alone (although other interventions, including Ammonul use and hemodialysis, are needed in some cases), and arginase deficiency has only rarely been associated with significant hyperammonemia. Loading and maintenance infusions should contain arginine HCl (210 mg/kg for patients with OTC or CPS deficiency or 630 mg/kg for patients with AS or AL deficiency). Ammonul is diluted in sterile 10% dextrose in both loading and maintenance infusions. Ten percent arginine HCl can be mixed in the same dextrose solution as Ammonul. Because of the saturable pharmacokinetics of phenylacetate, no more than one loading dose of Ammonul is recommended regardless of the initial level of plasma ammonium. The maintenance infusion can be continued until plasma ammonium levels are within normal limits.[4] Ammonul should be administered through a central line because extravasation may cause irritation, burns, and necrosis.

Appropriate nutrition, temporary protein restriction, and adequate hydration must also be used in conjunction with Ammonul and arginine HCl to maximize clearance of plasma ammonium. Hemodialysis and/or continuous hemofiltration should be started without delay if alternative pathway therapy and other interventions do not result in adequate control of plasma ammonium levels. Central access is critical to provide high-dextrose fluids and fat emulsion (Intralipid), with the goal of administering approximately 100–120 kcal/kg/d to neonates. An insulin drip is often needed to control hyperglycemia and promote anabolism.[29] In older patients and adults, a nutritional regimen providing 80 kcal/kg/d is a reasonable initial goal.[7] Protein should be withdrawn immediately and then slowly reintroduced after 24–48 hours.[29]

SIDE EFFECTS

Because of the difficulty in distinguishing symptoms related to hyperammonemia from symptoms caused by a reaction to medication, side effects are similarly difficult to attribute directly to alternative pathway therapy. Oral benzoate therapy has been associated with nausea and vomiting, but overall toxicity appears to be low as long as standard dosing guidelines are followed.[30] The use of benzyl alcohol as a bacteriostatic agent in neonatal intensive care units has resulted in severe metabolic acidosis, lethargy progressing to coma, seizures, and death. Benzoate and HIP, breakdown products of benzyl alcohol, were identified in the urine of these neonates.[31] A theoretical concern related to benzoate use in neonates is its potential ability to displace bilirubin from high-affinity albumin binding sites. There are no known cases of significant hyperbilirubinemia or kernicterus attributable to benzoate use, however.

No side effects, other than an unpleasant odor, were reported in normal human subjects and two patients with urea cycle defects receiving between 1 and 10 grams of phenylacetate.[32] Buphenyl use is associated with body odor caused by the metabolite phenylacetate, and patients have reported an aversion to the medication because of its bad taste. Abdominal discomfort and gastritis may also occur.

The most common adverse reaction reported to be associated with Ammonul is vomiting, occurring in approximately 9% of patients.[33] In a study of healthy adults, MacArthur and colleagues reported nausea, vomiting, and somnolence following administration of Ammonul in doses used to treat hyperammonemia.[34] In a report documenting responses to Ammonul in 299 UCD patients, adverse events were reported in a little more than 50% of treated patients. Most adverse events were likely related to the underlying primary disease or patient clinical status and were reported during treatment for hyperammonemia. Metabolic (hypokalemia, hyperammonemia, hyperglycemia, acidosis), nervous system (seizures, cerebral edema, mental impairment), and respiratory system abnormalities (respiratory distress or failure, hyperventilation) were reported most frequently and occurred in 22%, 18%, and 14% of patients, respectively.[8]

The most significant side effects and toxicity related to Ammonul use have occurred in cases of inadvertent overdose. Continuous intravenous infusion rates that result in plasma phenylacetate levels that saturate the capacity of conversion of phenylacetate to PAGN result in rapid phenylacetate accumulation and subsequent toxicity. Three patients (two to six years old) who were given inappropriately high doses of intravenous Ammonul (915 mg/kg over 12 hours, 1,750 mg/kg over 18 hours, and 750 mg/kg over 10 hours) had plasma benzoate and phenylacetate levels of approximately 10 mmol/L four hours after infusion and developed altered mental status, Kussmaul breathing, metabolic acidosis, cerebral edema, and hypotension. Two of the three patients died; one survived after hemodialysis.[35] Other signs of intoxication with Ammonul include hypernatremia, hyperosmolarity, and cardiovascular collapse.[4] Clearly written medical prescriptions and cross-checking of drug dosage are important safeguards.

U.S. FOOD AND DRUG ADMINISTRATION STATUS

Ammonul received U.S. Food and Drug Administration (FDA) new drug approval on February 17, 2005. Data collected over approximately 25 years of clinical investigation by a multitude of investigators throughout the country was used as a basis for the FDA decision. Ammonul is labeled a Category C drug, so it is not known whether Ammonul can cause harm to the fetus when administered to a pregnant woman or if reproduction capacity can be affected. Therefore, Ammonul use in pregnancy is recommended only if the medication is clearly needed. Caution should also be exercised if Ammonul is administered to pregnant women because it is unknown whether excretion in breast milk occurs. Buphenyl received FDA new drug approval on April 30, 1996 and is also a Category C drug.

RESULTS OF THERAPY

Treatment with Ammonul results in decreased plasma ammonium levels and improved neurological status in most cases, although, if severe hyperammonemia

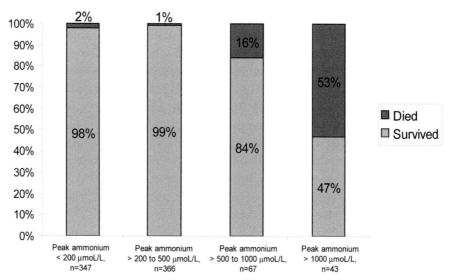

Figure 10–4: Hyperammonemic episodes survived according to peak ammonium levels. Patient survival of hyperammonemic episodes depends on peak plasma ammonium level, with significantly improved survival for patients who experience hyperammonemic episodes with a peak plasma ammonium level of up to 500 μM ($p < 0.001$). Neonates with a peak plasma ammonium level greater than 1,000 μM are least likely to survive a hyperammonemic episode (survival, 38%; $p < 0.001$).[8] From Enns et al. Survival after Treatment with Phenylacetate and Benzoate for Urea Cycle Disorder, *The New England Journal of Medicine*, F2. 2007, Massachusetts Medical Society. All rights reserved.

is present, alternative pathway therapy may be insufficient to have any appreciable effect. Early reports of alternative pathway therapy use in relatively small cohorts documented improved survival compared to that in historical controls.[23,25,26,36] A large study reported the outcome of 299 UCD patients who were treated with Ammonul. Patients sustained 1,181 episodes of hyperammonemia over a 25-year period with an episode survival rate of 96% (neonates: 73%; patients older than 30 days: 98%) and overall patient survival of 84%, a clear improvement when compared to historical data. Survival was also related to the peak plasma ammonium level and patient age. Nearly all episodes in which the ammonium level did not rise above 500 μmol/L resulted in survival, with survival decreasing as ammonium levels increased (Figure 10–4).[8] Because patients were primarily treated by metabolic centers with experience in caring for acute hyperammonemia caused by UCDs, the high survival rate in this study may in part reflect the expertise available at treating institutions. The improved outcome following use of alternative pathway medication is also apparent when comparison is made to outcome data detailed in a European report of 217 UCD patients who did not receive alternative pathway therapy for acute management of hyperammonemia. Only 16% of patients with neonatal-onset disease survived overall, and patient survival in late-onset disease was 72%.[6]

Although alternative pathway therapy in conjunction with other therapies, especially hemodialysis, has led to improved UCD patient survival, cognitive impairment remains a common finding, especially in patients who have neonatal-onset disease. The age at which the first symptom is noted, however, is not necessarily predictive of outcome in individual cases, because patients who have neonatal-onset disease may still have a normal long-term outcome. A study of 26 children who survived neonatal hyperammonemia was discouraging with respect to neurological outcome; the overwhelming majority (79%) had one or more developmental disabilities at 12–74 months of age. IQ correlated with the depth of coma, but not the peak plasma ammonium level over a range of 351–1,800 μmol/L.[33]

Other studies have found a correlation between the peak plasma ammonium level and cognitive outcome, although Ammonul was not used in these reports. When the concentration of plasma ammonium exceeded 350 μmol/L at the time of the first episode of hyperammonemia, patients either died or had severe neurological deficits in a Japanese study of 108 UCD patients.[37] In a European questionnaire study, no surviving UCD patients with an initial plasma ammonium level greater than 300 μmol/L or a peak plasma ammonium level greater than 480 μmol/L had normal psychomotor development.[38]

Neonatal-onset OTC deficiency is particularly devastating with respect to neurological outcome. Prospective neonatal therapy following prenatal diagnosis by deoxyribonucleic acid (DNA) or biochemical analysis, however, decreases the risk of neonatal hyperammonemia. Infants at risk for hyperammonemia caused by UCDs based on family history may be treated with Ammonul prospectively to prevent hyperammonemic coma. If such proactive therapy is instituted, neonates have a more favorable outcome compared to patients who are rescued from hyperammonemic coma. The brief period of prospective treatment while confirmatory diagnostic studies are pending does not appear to have any adverse effect on the growth and development of those infants who turn out to be unaffected.[36]

The use of Ammonul to treat other conditions that can cause neonatal hyperammonemia, such as organic acidemias, fatty acid oxidation disorders, and transient hyperammonemia of the newborn, has not been studied in detail. These conditions may be difficult to distinguish from UCDs on initial presentation in some instances. Clinicians have used Ammonul to treat non-UCD conditions, such as organic acidemias or transient hyperammonemia of the newborn, with variable efficacy.

FUTURE DEVELOPMENTS

The National Institutes of Health has sponsored the formation of a Rare Disease Clinical Research Center network for UCDs. This establishment of a network of specialized centers with expertise in providing state-of-the-art treatment for metabolic disorders has the potential to improve neurologic outcomes. A multicenter longitudinal study has been initiated and has already provided new information about the natural history of these disorders.[39] The prospective treatment of children at risk for hyperammonemic coma and other therapeutic modalities, especially liver transplantation, also play significant roles in the management of patients with UCDs and may improve outcome. Although hepatocyte transplantation is a promising new approach for the treatment of liver-based metabolic disorders, only limited success has been reported to date.[40] Gene therapy also holds promise for the treatment of these disorders, but significant technical hurdles need to be overcome, as is clear following the fatal occurrence of systemic inflammatory response syndrome in an OTC patient following adenoviral gene transfer.[41] Until the aforementioned technologies can be developed for wider application, liver transplantation is currently the only definitive therapy for these patients.

A new oral medication is being developed for hyperammonemia control and is currently in clinical trials. Glycerol phenylbutyrate [glyceryl tri-(4-phenylbutyrate)] is an investigational agent that is a prodrug of sodium phenylbutyrate (currently marketed as Buphenyl). Like sodium phenylbutyrate, glycerol phenylbutyrate is metabolized in the liver to phenylacetate, which in turn conjugates to glutamine and forms PAGN. Glycerol phenylbutyrate is a triglyceride containing three molecules of 4-phenylbutyric acid joined via ester linkage to glycerol. Glycerol phenylbutyrate is an organic liquid (oil) with little odor or taste that delivers the same amount of phenylbutyrate in a compact form (e.g., ~17.4 milliliters of glycerol phenylbutyrate [a little more than one teaspoon three times daily] delivers the same amount of phenylbutyric acid as do 40 tablets of sodium phenylbutyrate). Pharmacological data from Cynomolgus monkeys, which have the capacity to metabolize phenylacetate to form PAGN, suggest that glycerol phenylbutyrate acts as a slow-release product which may be converted to PAGN more efficiently than sodium phenylbutyrate.[42] Ten adult UCD subjects were switched to glycerol phenylbutyrate from sodium phenylbutyrate. Compared to treatment with sodium phenylbutyrate, glycerol phenylbutyrate treatment resulted in approximately 30% lower plasma ammonium values (as assessed by time-normalized area under the curve, findings not statistically significant), similar plasma PAGN and amino acid levels, and similar urinary excretion of PAGN. Somewhat fewer adverse events were reported during the glycerol phenylbutyrate period of this trial (21 adverse events in seven subjects during sodium phenylbutyrate treatment compared to 15 adverse events in five subjects during glycerol phenylbutyrate treatment), and the only two hyperammonemic events during this study occurred in subjects on sodium phenylbutyrate.[43] Given the difficulties facing urea cycle patients with respect to daily pill burden and the noxious taste of sodium phenylbutyrate, glycerol phenylbutyrate has the potential to improve compliance and chronic plasma ammonium control if the promise of the initial small trial results is confirmed in larger-scale studies.

REFERENCES

1. Krebs HA, Henseleit K. Untersuchungen über die harnstoffbildung im tierkorper. *Hoppe-Seyler's Z Physiol Chem.* 1932;210:325–332
2. Shih VE. Hereditary urea-cycle disorders. S. Grisolia, R. Báguena, F. Mayor, eds. *The Urea Cycle*, John Wiley, New York, 367–414, 1976

3. Morizono H, Caldovic L, Shi D, Tuchman M. Mammalian N-acetylglutamate synthase. *Mol Genet Metab.* 2004;81(Suppl 1):S4–S11
4. Brusilow SW, Maestri NE. Urea cycle disorders: Diagnosis, pathophysiology, and therapy. *Adv Pediatr.* 1996;43:127–170
5. Summar ML, Dobbelaere D, Brusilow S, Lee B. Diagnosis, symptoms, frequency and mortality of 260 patients with urea cycle disorders from a 21-year, multicentre study of acute hyperammonaemic episodes. *Acta Paediatr.* 2008;97(10):1420–1425
6. Nassogne MC, Heron B, Touati G, Rabier D, Saudubray JM. Urea cycle defects: Management and outcome. *J Inherit Metab Dis.* 2005;28(3):407–414
7. Summar ML, Barr F, Dawling S, Smith W, Lee B, Singh RH, Rhead WJ, Sniderman King L, Christman BW. Unmasked adult-onset urea cycle disorders in the critical care setting. *Crit Care Clin.* 2005;21:S1–S8
8. Enns GM, Berry SA, Berry GT, Rhead WJ, Brusilow SW, Hamosh A. Survival after treatment with phenylacetate and benzoate for urea-cycle disorders. *N Engl J Med.* 2007;356(22):2282–2292
9. Enns GM. Neurologic damage and neurocognitive dysfunction in urea cycle disorders. *Semin Pediatr Neurol.* 2008;15(3):132–139
10. Colombo JP, Peheim E, Kretschmer R, Dauwalder H, Sidiropoulos D. Plasma ammonia concentrations in newborns and children. *Clin Chim Acta.* 1984;138(3):283–291
11. Gropman AL, Summar M, Leonard JV. Neurological implications of urea cycle disorders. *J Inherit Metab Dis.* 2007;30(6):865–879
12. Brusilow SW. Hyperammonemic encephalopathy. *Medicine* (Baltimore). 2002;81(3):240–249
13. Norenberg MD, Jayakumar AR, Rama Rao KV, Panickar KS. New concepts in the mechanism of ammonia-induced astrocyte swelling. *Metab Brain Dis.* 2007;22(3–4):219–234
14. Albrecht J, Norenberg MD. Glutamine: A Trojan horse in ammonia neurotoxicity. *Hepatology.* 2006;44(4):788–794
15. Ratnakumari L, Qureshi IA, Butterworth RF. Regional amino acid neurotransmitter changes in brains of spf/Y mice with congenital ornithine transcarbamylase deficiency. *Metab Brain Dis.* 1994;9(1):43–51
16. Butterworth RF. Glutamate transporter and receptor function in disorders of ammonia metabolism. *Ment Retard Dev Disabil Res Rev.* 2001;7(4):276–279
17. Robinson MB, Hopkins K, Batshaw ML, McLaughlin BA, Heyes MP, Oster-Granite ML. Evidence of excitotoxicity in the brain of the ornithine carbamoyltransferase deficient sparse fur mouse. *Brain Res Dev Brain Res.* 1995;90(1–2):35–44
18. Monfort P, Munoz MD, Felipo V. Molecular mechanisms of the alterations in NMDA receptor-dependent long-term potentiation in hyperammonemia. *Metab Brain Dis.* 2005;20(4):265–274
19. Bachmann C, Braissant O, Villard AM, Boulat O, Henry H. Ammonia toxicity to the brain and creatine. *Mol Genet Metab.* 2004;81(Suppl 1):S52–S57
20. Niemi AK, Enns GM. Sodium phenylacetate and sodium benzoate in the treatment of neonatal hyperammonemia. *NeoReviews.* 2006;7(9):e486–e495
21. Lewis HB. Studies in the synthesis of hippuric acid in the animal organism. *J Biol Chem.* 1914;18:225
22. Shiple GJ, Sherwin CP. Synthesis of amino acids in animal organisms I. Synthesis of glycocoll and glutamine in the human organism. *J Am Chem Soc.* 1922;44(3):618–624
23. Batshaw ML, MacArthur RB, Tuchman M. Alternative pathway therapy for urea cycle disorders: Twenty years later. *J Pediatr.* 2001;138(1 Suppl):S46–S54; discussion S54–S55
24. Brusilow SW, Valle DL, Batshaw M. New pathways of nitrogen excretion in inborn errors of urea synthesis. *Lancet.* 1979;2(8140):452–454
25. Brusilow SW, Danney M, Waber LJ, Batshaw M, Burton B, Levitsky L, Roth K, McKeethren C, Ward J. Treatment of episodic hyperammonemia in children with inborn errors of urea synthesis. *N Engl J Med.* 1984;310(25):1630–1634
26. Green TP, Marchessault RP, Freese DK. Disposition of sodium benzoate in newborn infants with hyperammonemia. *J Pediatr.* 1983;102(5):785–790

27. Simell O, Sipila I, Rajantie J, Valle DL, Brusilow SW. Waste nitrogen excretion via amino acid acylation: Benzoate and phenylacetate in lysinuric protein intolerance. *Pediatr Res*. 1986;20(11):1117–1121

28. Bunchman TE, Barletta GM, Winters JW, Gardner JJ, Crumb TL, McBryde KD. Phenylacetate and benzoate clearance in a hyperammonemic infant on sequential hemodialysis and hemofiltration. *Pediatr Nephrol*. 2007;22(7):1062–1065

29. Singh RH, Rhead WJ, Smith W, Lee B, King LS, Summar M. Nutritional management of urea cycle disorders. *Crit Care Clin*. 2005;21(4 Suppl):S27–S35

30. Batshaw ML, Brusilow SW. Evidence of lack of toxicity of sodium phenylacetate and sodium benzoate in treating urea cycle enzymopathies. *J Inherit Metab Dis*. 1981;4(4):231

31. Gershanik J, Boecler B, Ensley H, McCloskey S, George W. The gasping syndrome and benzyl alcohol poisoning. *N Engl J Med*. 1982;307(22):1384–1388

32. Thibault A, Samid D, Cooper MR, Figg WD, Tompkins AC, Patronas N, Headlee DJ, Kohler DR, Venzon DJ, Myers CE. Phase I study of phenylacetate administered twice daily to patients with cancer. *Cancer*. 1995;75(12):2932–2938

33. Batshaw ML, Brusilow S, Waber L, Blom W, Brubakk AM, Burton BK, Cann HM, Kerr D, Mamunes P, Matalon R, Myerberg D, Schafer IA. Treatment of inborn errors of urea synthesis: Activation of alternative pathways of waste nitrogen synthesis and excretion. *N Engl J Med*. 1982;306(23):1387–1392

34. MacArthur RB, Altincatal A, Tuchman M. Pharmacokinetics of sodium phenylacetate and sodium benzoate following intravenous administration as both a bolus and continuous infusion to healthy adult volunteers. *Mol Genet Metab*. 2004;81(Suppl 1):S67–S73

35. Praphanphoj V, Boyadjiev SA, Waber LJ, Brusilow SW, Geraghty MT. Three cases of intravenous sodium benzoate and sodium phenylacetate toxicity occurring in the treatment of acute hyperammonaemia. *J Inherit Metab Dis*. 2000;23(2):129–136

36. Maestri NE, Hauser ER, Bartholomew D, Brusilow SW. Prospective treatment of urea cycle disorders. *J Pediatr*. 1991;119(6):923–928

37. Uchino T, Endo F, Matsuda I. Neurodevelopmental outcome of long-term therapy of urea cycle disorders in Japan. *J Inherit Metab Dis*. 1998;21(Suppl 1):151–159

38. Bachmann C. Outcome and survival of 88 patients with urea cycle disorders: A retrospective evaluation. *Eur J Pediatr*. 2003;162(6):410–416

39. Tuchman M, Lee B, Lichter-Konecki U, Summar ML, Yudkoff M, Cederbaum SD, Derr DS, Dias GA, Seashore MR, Lee H-S, McCarter RJ, Jeffrey P, Krischer JP, Batshaw ML. Cross-sectional multicenter study of patients with urea cycle disorders in the United States. *Mol Genet Metab*. 2008;94:397–402

40. Enns GM, Millan MT. Cell-based therapies for metabolic liver disease. *Mol Genet Metab*. 2008;95(1–2):3–10

41. Raper SE, Chirmule N, Lee FS, Wivel NA, Bagg A, Gao GP, Wilson JM, Batshaw ML. Fatal systemic inflammatory response syndrome in a ornithine transcarbamylase deficient patient following adenoviral gene transfer. *Mol Genet Metab*. 2003;80(1–2):148–158

42. John BA, Taylor LM, Johnson S, Lees MJ, Johns P, Gargosky S, Dickinson K. The disposition of HPN-100, a novel pharmaceutical under development for potential treatment of hyperammonemia, in Cynomolgus monkeys. Presented at American College of Medical Genetics Annual Meeting 2009; Abstract 66.

43. Lee B, Mian A, Shchelochkov O, Martinez T, Mokhtarani M, Scharschmidt B, et al. Phase 2 study of a novel ammonia scavenging agent in adults with urea cycle disorders. Presented at American College of Medical Genetics Annual Meeting 2009; Abstract 17.

11 PDMP-based glucosylceramide synthesis inhibitors for Gaucher and Fabry diseases

James A. Shayman

INTRODUCTION

Sphingolipids are enigmatic compounds that have been the object of study for more than 100 years. By definition, a sphingolipid is any compound that contains a long-chain (sphingoid) base. These compounds were originally studied because of their observed tendency to accumulate in rare monogenic disorders resulting in lysosomal storage diseases. These disorders include, but are not limited to,

Gaucher disease, Fabry disease, Tay–Sachs disease, and GM1 gangliosidosis. In recent years, scientists have focused on the normal biological functions of sphingolipids. Sphingolipids have been discovered to be important molecules serving a diverse range of biological functions, including circulating ligands, receptors, and second messengers. Investigators have also asked what role, if any, these compounds might play in more common diseases, including cancer and diabetes. These studies have produced a number of compelling findings and suggest that targeting sphingolipid-metabolizing enzymes may provide targets for novel therapeutics in these disorders.

With a rising interest in sphingolipid biology, a number of small molecules were identified that act as inhibitors of important sphingolipid-metabolizing enzymes. These compounds not only have served as important reagents for probing the biology of sphingolipids, but also have been the focus of clinical development of the treatment of sphingolipid-associated diseases. D-*threo*-1-phenyl-2-decanoyl-3-morpholino-propanol (PDMP) was one of the first small molecule inhibitors of sphingolipid metabolism to be identified. PDMP inhibits the activity of glucosylceramide, the first dedicated step in the formation of more than 80% of mammalian glycosphingolipids. A class of related homologues has been developed based on a core pharmacophore. These compounds not only have achieved widespread use among biochemists and cell biologists probing sphingolipid biology, they have also entered clinical trials for the treatment of Gaucher disease. In this chapter the development, characterization, and biological activities of the PDMP family of inhibitors are reviewed and contrasted with other small molecules for the treatment of Gaucher and Fabry disease.

LYSOSOMAL STORAGE DISORDERS

The seminal discovery and characterization of the lysosome by de Duve and colleagues occurred only 54 years ago.[1] These organelles referred to by them as "a new group of particles with lytic properties" were quickly associated with a group of diseases termed "lysosomal storage disorders." Currently, there are more than 40 lysosomal storage disorders associated with inherited enzyme deficiencies, with the absence of activators of the catalytic enzymes, or with a loss in transporter activity. Of these 40 known disorders, 10 are associated with the accumulation of sphingolipids, and seven of these are characterized by the lysosomal accumulation of glycosphingolipids.[2]

Recent publications on the lysosomal proteome indicate that there are more than 90 lysosomal proteins of which 75 are well characterized with regard to their biochemical and biological function.[3] Thus approximately two thirds of the characterized lysosomal proteins are associated with distinct storage disorders. It is interesting that the loss of function is not restricted to soluble hydrolytic enzymes directly involved in the catabolism of substrates but also includes membrane-bound proteins. There appears to be no a priori means of determining which lysosomal proteins would be associated with observed disease and which might be incompatible with survival. Thus for those gene products not associated with recognized diseases, it remains to be established whether a loss of function is lethal or whether an associated disease has yet to be described.

Gaucher and Fabry diseases

Gaucher type I and Fabry disease represent the prototypic sphingolipid storage disorders. Gaucher disease is the most common lysosomal storage disorder with an incidence of 1 in 40,0000 to 1 in 60,0000. Gaucher disease is an autosomal recessive disease that arises from a deficiency in β-glucocerebrosidase.[4] A deficiency in this enzyme results in the accumulation of glucosylceramide in macrophages of the spleen, liver, bone marrow, and lung. Clinical manifestations include massive hepatosplenomegaly, pulmonary disease, and debilitating bone deformities associated with necrosis and lytic lesions. Patients suffer from significant anemia and thrombocytopenia. Type II and type III Gaucher disease are distinguished from type I by the presence of central nervous system involvement.[5] Fortunately, these variants occur less frequently. Importantly, type I Gaucher patients retain some residual β-glucocerebrosidase activity. All three variants are due to mutations of the GBA gene located at chromosome 1q21.

Fabry disease is an X-linked sphingolipid storage disease arising from a loss of activity of α-galactosidase A. The loss of this enzyme activity results in the accumulation of glycosphingolipids with terminal gal-α-1,4-gal residues, primarily globotriaosylceramide (Gb3).[6] Because Gb3 is predominately localized to the vascular endothelium, vascular complications (including stroke) are prominent clinical expressions of the disease. Affected males also suffer from major complications that include renal failure and cardiac disease, the latter due to infiltration of the myocardium with glycolipid and left ventricular hypertrophy. Less clinically significant symptoms include anhidrosis, angiokeratomas, and corneal opacities. Although X-linked, heterozygous females may have significant clinical disease. The incidence is less frequent than Gaucher disease with 1 in 40,000 to 1 in 120,000 affected individuals. The gene encoding α-galactosidase A is located on the long arm of the X chromosome. The encoded protein is heavily glycosylated. Both nonsense and missense mutations have been described. Approximately 40% of affected males have no detectable enzyme activity.[7]

STRATEGIES FOR THE TREATMENT OF LYSOSOMAL STORAGE DISEASES

The primary approaches to the treatment of lysosomal storage disorders have focused on the replacement or substitution of the absent or defective catabolic enzyme. The most successful and accepted means of "enzyme replacement" has been through the direct administration of recombinant enzyme to patients with inherited deficiencies. The principle behind enzyme replacement therapy is based on the seminal observations of Kornfeld and Kornfeld[8] and Stahl,[9] who discovered and characterized the role of mannose-terminated proteins in lysosomal trafficking and cellular uptake, respectively. Brady and his colleagues proved the therapeutic utility of this approach by demonstrating the ability of puri-fied, mannose-terminated β-glucocerebrosidase to reverse the phenotype of type I Gaucher disease.[10] There are currently six lysosomal storage disorders for which recombinant enzyme replacement is now approved. These disorders include imiglucerase for type I Gaucher disease, α-galactosidase A for Fabry disease, laronidase for mucopolysaccharidosis type I, arylsulfatase B for mucopolysac-charidosis type VI, alglucosidase α for infantile Pompe disease, and idursulfase for Hunter disease. Although enzyme replacement therapies have been acknowl-edged to have a high degree of clinical success, their application remains limited. First, they do not cross the blood–brain barrier, thus the central nervous sys-tem complications of the lysosomal storage disorders have not been amenable to recombinant protein therapy. Second, because patients receiving these pro-teins often carry null mutations, it is not uncommon for an immune response to develop to repeated administration. This not only results in potentially harmful allergic reactions but can be associated with a loss of efficacy of the drug. Third, the cost of recombinant enzyme therapy remains inordinately high. Indeed, these biologics represent among the most expensive drugs that are FDA-approved, in some cases costing hundreds of thousands of dollars per year. The economic and social costs, in addition to the ethical challenges raised by the use of these agents, have received a significant amount of attention in the lay press in recent years. These concerns have led to the realization that alternative forms of treatment would be desirable.

Several other experimental yet promising alternatives have been studied: They include gene therapy,[11] bone marrow transplantation,[12] and, more recently, chemical chaperones.[13] These alternatives are similar to enzyme replacement to the extent that they are based on the strategic goal of increasing the activity of the defective lysosomal hydrolase. In the examples of gene therapy and bone marrow transplantation, the desired outcome is the formation of new normal enzyme. With chemical chaperone therapy, the therapeutic goal is to protect a misfolded protein from premature degradation, permitting the protein to traffic to its site of action, viz. the lysosome. When within the lysosome, the chemical chaperone dissociates from the misfolded protein. The excess substrate present is then degraded by the chaperoned, albeit defective protein.

Synthesis inhibition therapy

In contrast to those therapies that seek to normalize the catabolic function of a lysosomal enzyme, synthesis inhibition provides a unique alternative to the treatment of glycosphingolipidoses. This strategy was first proposed in 1972 by Norman Radin and his colleagues.[14,15] They subsequently initiated a search for a small molecule inhibitor of glucosylceramide synthase (ceramide:UDP-glucose glucosyltransferase [EC 2.4.1.80]), the first glycosylation step for the synthesis of more than 80% of mammalian glycosphingolipids. According to this hypothe-sis, the inhibition of glucosylceramide formation would directly lower the levels of the cerebroside in Gaucher disease and indirectly result in the lowering of

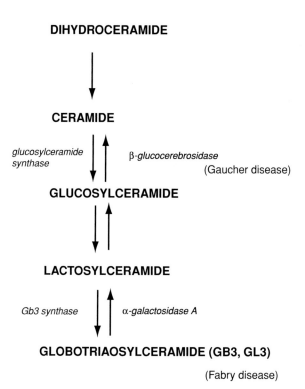

DIHYDROCERAMIDE

CERAMIDE

glucosylceramide synthase   β-*glucocerebrosidase*
(Gaucher disease)

GLUCOSYLCERAMIDE

LACTOSYLCERAMIDE

Gb3 synthase   α-*galactosidase A*

GLOBOTRIAOSYLCERAMIDE (GB3, GL3)

(Fabry disease)

Figure 11–1: Pathways for simple glycosphingolipid synthesis. Glucosylceramide and Gb3 accumulate in Gaucher and Fabry diseases due to loss of glycosidase activities associated with β-glucocerebrosidase and α-galactosidase A, respectively.

more highly glycosylated glycosphingolipids in other sphingolipidoses, such as Fabry disease and Tay–Sachs disease (Figure 11–1). Because the levels of accumulated sphingolipid represent a balance between synthesis and degradation, this approach would be particularly promising for those conditions in which residual enzyme activity were present (e.g., type I Gaucher disease). Patients who might be less likely to benefit would be those with null mutations in which there would be no alternative pathway for glycolipid degradation. Although this strategy has been focused on the development of inhibitors of glucosylceramide synthase, in principle it could also be applied to other anabolic enzymes in the glycosphingolipid synthesis pathways. For example, an inhibitor of GalTIV, the glycosyltransferase responsible for the creation of gal-α-1,4-gal linkages such as those found on globotriaosylceramide, could provide a more specific inhibitor for use in Fabry disease.

DISCOVERY AND DESIGN OF PDMP-BASED GLUCOSYLCERAMIDE SYNTHASE INHIBITORS

In 1980 the first glucosylceramide synthase inhibitor was reported. DL-2-Decanoylamino-3-morpholinopropiophenone-1 was identified based on its

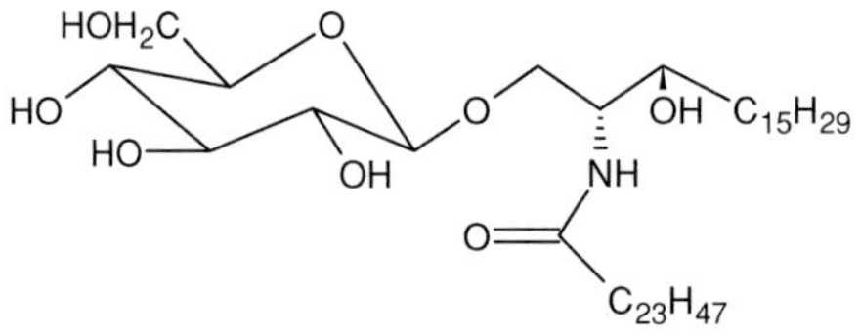

GLUCOSYLCERAMIDE

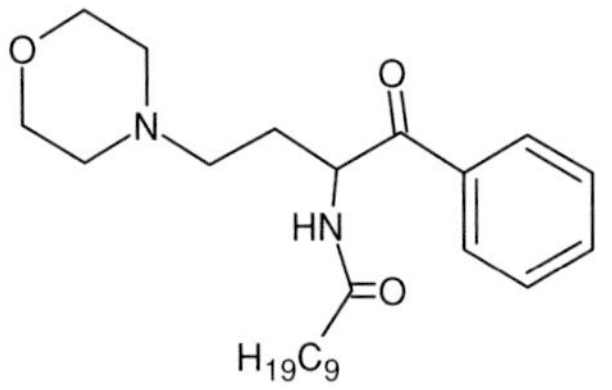

DL-2-DECANOYLAMINO-3-MORPHOLINO-
PROPIOPHENONE

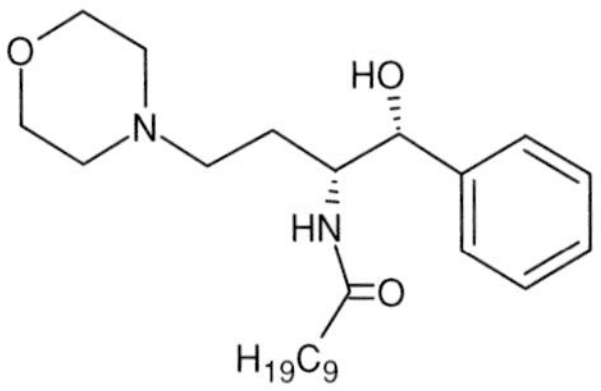

D-*threo*-1-PHENYL-2-DECANOYLAMINO
-3-MORPHOLINO-PROPANOL

Figure 11–2: Chemical structures of glucosyl-ceramide, DL-2-decanoylamino-3-morpholino-propiophenone, and D-*threo*-1-phenyl-2-deca-noylamino-3-morpholino-propanol (PDMP). Of note is the structural homology between the cerebroside and the first-generation glucosylcer-amide synthase inhibitors.

structural similarity to both gluco-sylceramide and chloramphenicol. This compound completely and irreversibly inhibited the enzyme at approximately 300 micromolar, probably because of its covalent bind-ing at the catalytic site, and was there-fore a suicide substrate inhibitor.[16] By reduction of the ketone, a new com-pound, 1-phenyl-2-decanoylamino-3-morpholino-propanol (PDMP), was produced. This compound not only was more potent in inhibiting gluco-sylceramide, but, more importantly, it acted reversibly (Figure 11–2).

Following the reduction of the pro-piophenone two chiral centers were formed, and thus PDMP consisted of four distinct enantiomers. The resolu-tion of the enantiomers by thin layer chromatography and ultimately crys-tallization revealed that only the D-*threo*-PDMP was an inhibitor of gluco-sylceramide synthase. The IC$_{50}$ of the D-*threo* enantiomer was 20 micromo-lar. The enantioselectivity of PDMP was surprising in that ceramide dis-plays a different stereochemistry, viz. a D-*erythro* structure. This observed enantioselectivity, however, is preserved throughout the entire family of PDMP-related homologues.

PDMP consists of three functional groups that include an aromatic ring, fatty acid in amide linkage, and cyclic amine. Empiric substitutions of both the fatty acyl group and the cyclic amine were initially made in an attempt to identify structural homologues of PDMP that might exhibit greater inhibitory activity. A strong correlation was established between fatty acid chain length and activity, with a peak activity observed for a C16 fatty acyl group.[17] A series of compounds was also generated substituting various amines for the morpholino group. We observed that a cyclic amine was absolutely required for the preservation of activ-ity and that a pyrrolidino substitution displayed significantly enhanced activity. Based on these studies, a second generation compound was identified: D-*threo*-1-phenyl-2-palmitoylamino-3-pyrrolidino-propanol (P4) (Figure 11–3).[18]

Whereas the improved activity of P4 was encouraging, the IC$_{50}$ of one micro-molar remained in a range that was deemed unsuitable for potential therapeutic

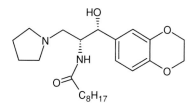

D-*threo*-1-phenyl-2-palmitoylamino
-3-pyrrolidinopropanol

D-*threo*-1-4'-hydroxyphenyl-2-palmitoylamino-
3-pyrrolidinopropanol

D-*threo*-1-(3',4')ethylenedioxyphenyl-2-
palmitoylamino-3-pyrrolidinopropanol

D-*threo*-1-(3',4')ethylenedioxyphenyl-2-
octanoylamino-3-pyrrolidinopropanol
(Genz-112638)

Figure 11–3: Chemical structures of the fatty acyl- and phenyl-substituted PDMP homologues. These structures preserved the pharmacophore that was observed to be required for the retention of inhibitory activity against glucosylceramide synthase.

use. We therefore focused on substitutions of the aromatic function to identify more active homologues. Instead of shotgun substitutions of the phenyl group, Hansch analysis was applied to identify substitutions that, based on partitioning and electronic parameters, would predictably display higher activities.[19] Two promising leads were identified. These included the 4'-hydroxyphenyl- and ethylenedioxyphenyl-substituted homologues. Both D-*threo*-4'-hydroxyphenyl-P4 and D-*threo*-ethylenedioxyphenyl-P4 displayed markedly enhanced inhibitory activities with IC$_{50}$ values of less than 100 nanomolar against soluble enzyme. When these compounds were evaluated in intact cells, the IC$_{50}$ values were approximately 10 nanomolar, reflecting the tendency of these lipophilic compounds to concentrate within cells.

SPECIFICITY OF GLUCOSYLCERAMIDE SYNTHASE INHIBITION BY PDMP HOMOLOGUES

PDMP, P4, and ethylenedioxyphenyl-P4 have been widely used as probes for the study of the biochemistry and cellular biology of glycosphingolipids. More than 250 studies have been reported since 1989 using these inhibitors in a wide range of models. An important consideration for the use of these inhibitors (or other metabolic inhibitors, for that matter) is their specificity. Because ceramide is a substrate for glucosylceramide formation, we assumed that significant inhibition of glucosylceramide synthase would result in the accumulation of this lipid with subsequent shunting toward other ceramide-related metabolites. These metabolites might include sphingomyelin, galactosylceramide, sphingosine, sphingosine-1-phosphate, and ceramide-1-phosphate. Indeed, in an early study we observed that a time- and concentration-dependent increase in ceramide was observed in MDCK cells treated with PDMP. At high concentrations cells underwent apoptosis, consistent with a potential role for ceramide in the signaling of programmed cell death. At lower concentrations, the cells underwent cell cycle arrest. These observations suggested that the PDMP compounds might have a role in the treatment of cellular proliferative disorders, such as cancer, but raised concerns that the toxicity would preclude their use for treating sphingolipidoses.

This concern was dispelled when subsequent studies revealed that it was possible to dissociate inhibition of glucosylceramide synthesis from ceramide accumulation. The first demonstration of this dissociation arose when stereospecific deoxyceramides such as D-*threo*-1-morpholino-1-deoxyceramide and D-*threo*-1-pyrrolidino-1-deoxyceramide were synthesized and studied.[20] These compounds demonstrated moderate activity as inhibitors of glucosylceramide synthase but were not associated with any increase in ceramide levels. The second demonstration of this dissociation was based on studies of cellular growth with the use of the 4′-hydroxyphenyl- and ethylenedioxyphenyl-P4 homologues.[19] These compounds potently blocked glucosylceramide formation at low nanomolar concentrations but only increased ceramide content and inhibited cell growth at low micromolar concentration. The third demonstration of the dissociation between glucosylceramide synthesis and ceramide accumulation resulted from studies of the four enantiomers of the 4′-hydroxyphenyl- and ethylenedioxyphenyl-P4 homologues. Whereas the D-*threo* enantiomers were uniformly active against glucosylceramide synthase, all four enantiomers elevated ceramide levels at comparable, albeit higher, concentrations. The results of these studies suggested that the PDMP compounds were elevating ceramide levels through a second site of action.

PDMP is a cationic amphiphilic drug that inhibits lysosomal phospholipase A2

A search was undertaken for a second site of action of the PDMP enantiomers. An important clue was the observation that fluorescently tagged PDMP localized in part to the lysosome and that chronic treatment of cultured cells with PDMP resulted in the accumulation of lysosomal lipids akin to what is observed in drug-induced phospholipidosis. An empiric study of known ceramide-using enzymes, including sphingomyelin synthase, ceramidase, galactosylceramide synthase, and ceramide kinase, failed to demonstrate either activation or inhibition of the respective enzymes. By use of radiolabeled *N*-acetylsphingosine, however, it was observed that PDMP inhibited the formation of a novel metabolite, 1-*O*-acylceramide.[21]

This enzyme activity was characterized as an acidic phospholipase A2 with ceramide transacylase activity. The enzyme was purified from calf brain, sequenced, and subsequently cloned.[22] The target was identified as a novel acidic, lysosomally localized phospholipase A2. Lysosomal phospholipase A2 was found to contain a catalytic domain that was highly homologous to lecithin cholesterol acyltransferase and was a member of the αβ-hydrolase fold family of proteins. The expressed protein was observed to be inhibited by PDMP as well as by other cationic amphiphilic drugs, including amiodarone.[23] Recently, we have reported that the basis for the inhibition is the disruption of an electrostatic charge interaction between the lysosomal phospholipase A2 and anionic phospholipids within membranes.[24] Transgenic mice lacking normal lysosomal phospholipase A2 expression have been created, and they display a phenotype associated with early foam cell formation in the lung and surfactant lipid accumulation.[25]

Other activities of PDMP and related compounds

Two additional activities of PDMP have been observed. Basu and colleagues have reported that PDMP blocks the activity of ceramide glycanase at high concentrations.[26] Inokuchi and coworkers have observed that the L-*threo* enantiomer of PDMP stimulates glycosphingolipid synthesis. His group has pursued this observation in demonstrating that L-*threo*-PDMP may mitigate brain injury from cerebral ischemia.[27]

IN VITRO AND IN VIVO PROOF-OF-CONCEPT STUDIES

With the identification and characterization of glucosylceramide synthase inhibitors with high specificity and nanomolar inhibitory activity, we sought to test whether these compounds could demonstrate promising pharmacodynamic effects with regard to glycosphingolipid reduction in suitable models of sphingolipidoses. Although a β-glucocerebrosidase knockout mouse had been generated, these mice died a few days postpartum because of a water-permeability defect in their skin and thus were unsuitable for testing the new compounds. By contrast, an α-galactosidase A knockout mouse had been created and characterized. Male mice lacking the glycosidase activity were phenotypically normal at birth and exhibited an age-dependent increase in Gb3 levels in their kidneys, livers, hearts, and arteries. Three models of vasculopathy have also been identified in these mice: oxidant-induced thrombosis,[28] accelerated atherogenesis when bred on an apolipoprotein E–null background,[29] and impaired vascular reactivity.[30]

Epstein–Barr virus–transformed lymphoblasts from patients with Fabry disease were first studied. D-*threo*-ethylenedioxy-P4 and D-*threo*-4′-hydroxy-P4 potently lowered both glucosylceramide and Gb3 levels in the lymphoblasts.[31] Ten nanomolar of either inhibitor lowered Gb3 levels 80%. By contrast, N-butyl-deoxynojirimycin (miglustat), even at concentrations as high as 10 micromolar, only minimally decreased glucosylceramide and Gb3. Both total cell levels and cell surface levels of Gb3 as measured by B subunit Shiga toxin binding were significantly lowered by the PDMP homologues.

Based on these findings we were encouraged to undertake a more extensive in vivo study in the α-galactosidase A knockout mouse.[32] The pharmacodynamic response of C57BL/6 mice was first studied following intraperitoneal injections of D-*threo*-ethylenedioxy-P4. A concentration-dependent reduction of glucosylceramide was observed in the kidneys, spleens, and livers of the mice treated every 12 hours for three days. An 80% reduction in glucosylceramide was observed in all three organs with inhibitor at 10 mg/kg. Remarkably, a single injection at 10 mg/kg resulted in an 80% reduction of glucosylceramide by 24 hours in the kidney and a 55% reduction in the liver of these mice. These results were consistent with a high basal level of turnover of the cerebroside.

α-Galactosidase A–null mice were next treated with D-*threo*-ethylenedioxy-P4. No changes in either body weight or organ weights were observed in mice treated for up to 60 days with the drug. Highly significant dose- and time-dependent effects of the drug were observed in mice treated for up to eight weeks with intraperitoneal injections. Significant reductions in Gb3 were observed in the kidneys, livers, and hearts of the treated mice. By contrast, age-dependent increases in Gb3 were observed in the vehicle-treated control groups. The improvement in renal Gb3 levels correlated with a marked reduction of lysosomal lipid bodies as observed by electron microscopy.

Surprisingly, despite the fact that the mice are completely deficient in α-galactosidase A activity and that there are no known alternative pathways for Gb3 degradation, the Gb3 levels in the kidneys of the treated mice were lower than those observed in the eight-week-old mice prior to the initiation of treatment. These findings suggest that there must be an alternative means for the clearance of Gb3 from the kidney. We speculate that the lysosomal contents can be extruded into the urinary space. This hypothesis is supported by the observation that lysosomal enzymes are readily detected in the urine.

DEVELOPMENT OF A PDMP HOMOLOGUE FOR CLINICAL TRIALS

Based on the proof-of-principle studies with D-*threo*-ethylenedioxyphenyl-P4, the University of Michigan and Genzyme Corporation entered into a license agreement for the clinical development of the PDMP homologues as oral agents for the treatment of lysosomal storage disorders. Although the specificity and potency of D-*threo*-ethylenedioxyphenyl-P4 made the compound a reasonable candidate for clinical trials, initial studies on the pharmacokinetics of this palmitoyl derivative indicated that it was unsuitable for clinical development. Specifically, the high lipophilicity of the compound resulted in a highly prolonged half-life. Additionally, the potency of the compound was sufficiently high that the plasma levels were at the limit of detection. A substitution of the 16-carbon palmitoyl group with an eight-carbon octanoyl group resulted in a homologue that retained sufficiently potent inhibitory activity (IC_{50}: 115 nanomolar in whole-cell homogenates; 14–79 nanomolar in cultured cells), but with a significantly shorter half-life (one to two hours). A formulation using the L-tartrate salt was also observed to demonstrate excellent oral bioavailability as opposed to the free base (55% bioavailability in rats). This homologue was assigned the name Genz-112638 for further development (Figure 11–3).

Concurrent with the identification of Genz-112638 as the lead clinical compound for clinical development, a knock-in mouse that more closely resembled type I Gaucher disease was reported.[33] The D409V/null mouse retains a low level of β-glucocerebrosidase activity. These mice survive postnatally and develop an age-dependent accumulation of glucosylceramide in association with the development of Gaucher cells in their spleens. The treatment of 10-week-old mice with orally delivered drug resulted in the prevention of glucosylceramide accumulation in the liver, spleen, and lungs of the Gaucher mice in association with the absence of Gaucher cells in these organs. When seven-month-old mice were similarly treated, cerebroside accumulation and foamy macrophage numbers were similarly reduced. Thus the C8 and C16 ethylenedioxyphenyl homologues were effective in preventing the accumulation of glycosphingolipids in models of Gaucher and Fabry disease.[34]

Preinvestigational new drug enabling studies

Prior to the submission of an investigational new drug (IND) application and the initiation of clinical trials, a series of enabling studies were conducted to assess drug toxicity, chemical stability, and pharmacokinetics. For most measures of toxicity, including genotoxicity, toxicity of the central nervous and respiratory systems, gastrointestinal motility, and hepatic function, no significant effects were observed at drug concentrations near the median effective dose (ED_{50}). The inhibition of hERG ($K_V11.1$, voltage-gated potassium channel) in an in vitro assay, however, suggested that QT prolongation might represent a potentially significant toxicity. Upon further study, however, the effect of the drug was observed to not result from potassium channel inhibition, it was instead a sodium channel effect as manifest by a decrease in the action potential duration. Although QT prolongation was observed in in vivo dog studies at high dosing levels, it was determined that the safety margin for use in humans would be 30-fold based on allometric scaling, which was performed by comparing the pharmacokinetic results in mouse, rat, and dog to estimate the appropriate dosing in humans. Based on observed ED_{50} values for these animals, it was estimated that an effective dose in humans would be 0.6 mg/kg.

Phase I studies

Following the approval of an IND application submitted in December 2003, Phase I studies were initiated with the primary goal of assessing the safety, tolerability, and pharmacokinetics of Genz-112638 in healthy volunteers. A single-dose Phase

Ia trial was conducted in 99 male volunteers. Thirteen cohorts received a single oral dose of drug or placebo with a dose escalation ranging from 0.01 to 30 mg/kg. The drug was well tolerated, and only mild gastrointestinal side effects were observed at higher doses.

In a Phase Ib study, 36 male and female volunteers received twice-a-day administration of Genz-112638 for 13 days. The participants received placebo or drug at 50, 200, or 350 milligrams orally twice a day, corresponding to 0.5–1.0, 2–4, or 3.5–7 mg/kg. Again, the drug was well tolerated. This study established that a dose of 1.6 mg/kg produced a mean maximum (peak) concentration (C_{max}) of 7 ng/mL.

The pharmacodynamic response to the drug was measured as a change in plasma glucosylceramide concentrations. A time- and dose-dependent decrease in plasma glucosylceramide level was observed. By 13 days a 40% decline in glucosylceramide concentrations was observed in subjects receiving 50 milligrams orally twice a day; a 90% decline was observed in subjects receiving 350 milligrams orally twice a day. Thus, in healthy volunteers, the drug displayed no significant toxicity and potently lowered plasma cerebroside levels.

Phase II studies

Based on the promising results of the Phase I data, an open label, Phase II trial was initiated in July 2006 to assess the efficacy, safety, and pharmacokinetics of Genz-112638 in patients with type I Gaucher disease from sites in Israel, Russia, North America, and South America. The study duration was 52 weeks, and subjects received either 50 or 100 milligrams orally twice a day. Hemoglobin, platelet counts, and spleen volume were identified as the primary endpoints. By design, a positive response to treatment was defined as a clinically meaningful response in two of three endpoints, an increase in hemoglobin of greater than or equal to 0.5 g/dL an increase in platelet counts of greater than or equal to 15%, and a reduction of spleen volume of greater than or equal to 15%.

The inclusion criteria included a diagnosis of type I Gaucher disease by enzyme assay, age of 18–65 years, weight of 50–120 kilograms, use of contraceptives, and a negative pregnancy test for female participants. In addition, subjects were to have a spleen volume at baseline greater than 10 times normal. Finally, subjects were to either be thrombocytopenic (45,000–100,000 per cubic millimeter) or anemic with a hemoglobin of 8.0–10.0 g/dL for female subjects and 8.0–11.0 g/dL for male subjects.

Exclusion criteria included splenectomy, hemoglobin less than 8.0 g/dL, platelet count less than 45,000, anemia due to causes other than Gaucher disease, transfusion dependence, pregnancy, or other significant medical problems. Subjects were not to have received enzyme replacement therapy or miglustat within 12 months of enrollment. Patients could not be pregnant. Finally, patients were not to have had other complications of Gaucher disease, including pulmonary complications, neurologic complications, bone infarction, osteonecrosis, lytic lesions of the bone or liver, or bleeding varices.

Twenty-six patients were enrolled in the study and 22 patients completed 52 weeks of therapy. Of the four patients who dropped out, two discontinued on Day 1 following their first dose of Genz-112638 when they were observed to have a short run of nonsustained ventricular tachycardia. Follow-up evaluation indicated the presence of baseline arrhythmias in these subjects, and thus this complication was not believed to be the result of a single dose of drug. Two additional patients discontinued when they became pregnant. Of the 22 patients who completed the study, 20 have opted to continue therapy on the extension arm of the study. One patient did not continue because of pregnancy, and one patient did not continue when a lytic bone lesion was observed at the end of the study.

Two primary biomarkers were followed to assess the pharmacodynamic response to the drug. Chitotriosidase, a well-established biomarker of Gaucher disease,[35] activity followed a time-dependent decrease when measured every 90 days. The mean decrement in activity was 51%. Plasma glucosylceramide levels, markedly elevated at the initiation of the study, were normalized within three months of treatment and fell from a mean of 12 μg/mL to 2.1 μg/mL.

The primary endpoints of spleen-size reduction and improvement in thrombocytopenia and anemia were met by six months of treatment. By 12 months of treatment, even greater improvements were seen. A mean reduction in spleen size of 39%, a mean increase in platelet count of 40%, and a mean increase in hemoglobin of 1.6 g/dL were observed. These responses are comparable to those observed for enzyme replacement where spleen size is reportedly decreased 36% and hemoglobin increased 2.1 g/dL.[36] It should be noted, however, that these agents were not directly compared in this study. Nevertheless, based on these highly promising results, a Phase III, randomized, controlled study of type I Gaucher patients naïve to therapy was initiated in June 2009.

Recently, the preliminary results from the Phase II extension trial were reported. Twenty patients elected to continue on Genz-112638. Further improvements in spleen and liver volumes and hemoglobin and platelet counts were observed (Table 11–1). Chitotriosidase activities decreased further, and plasma glucosylceramide levels remained within the normal range. Finally, the number of adverse effects remained low and were minor.

ALTERNATIVE SMALL MOLECULAR ENTITIES FOR GAUCHER DISEASE

In addition to the PDMP-based glucosylceramide synthase inhibitors, two other classes of chemical entities have been identified as treatment options for type I Gaucher disease. Miglustat was originally developed as an α-glucosidase inhibitor and potential antiviral agent.[37] Platt and coworkers reported that this agent had mid-micromolar inhibitory activity against glucosylceramide synthase.[38] This compound inhibits a variety of other enzymes, including α-glucosidase I and II and β-glucocerebrosidase. Although preclinical studies reported activity in

Table 11–1. Comparison of clinical data for the treatment of Gaucher type I patients with miglustat and Genz-112638

	Miglustat				Genz-112638		
Months of treatment	6	12	24	36	6	12	18
Number of subjects	23	22	14	13	22	22	20
Spleen volume (% change)	−15	−19	−14.5	−17.5	−25	−39	−47
Liver volume (% change)	−7	−12	−14.5	−17.5	NR*	−17	−20
Hemoglobin (g/dL)	+0.03	+0.26	+0.9	+0.95	+1.0	+1.6	+1.84
Platelets	$+3.7 \times 10^9$	$+8.3 \times 10^9$	$+13.6 \times 10^9$	$+22.2 \times 10^9$	+19%	+40%	$+39.7 \times 10^9$
Chitotriosidase (% change)	−0.9	−16.4	−21.9	−32	−25	−51	NR

Note: The miglustat data are from the initial study (OGT918–001) and extension study (OGT918–001X) as reported.[39,40] Twenty-eight patients were enrolled in the initial miglustat trial, and 23 patients completed 12 months of therapy. Seven of the 28 patients had undergone splenectomy, which was not an exclusion criterion for the miglustat trial. The Genz-112638 data are derived from the Genzyme Analyst Day report and the American Society of Hematology 2009 meeting abstract and had not been peer-reviewed at the time this chapter was written.

* NR: not reported.

models of GM2 gangliosidoses,[41] the compound was noted to have a number of nonspecific effects, including lymphoid atrophy and weight loss.[42] Nevertheless, this agent was developed as a clinical alternative to enzyme replacement therapy. Because of a significant degree of toxicity that includes peripheral neuropathy, potential memory loss, and diarrhea associated with weight loss, the drug was approved for type I Gaucher disease patients in whom enzyme replacement is not an option. These untoward effects have led to a high dropout rate among patients treated with miglustat.

This agent has received limited acceptance, and some investigators have questioned whether the modest clinical response to this agent is based on its effects as a glycolipid synthesis inhibitor. This skepticism is based on several observations. First, some (but not all) investigators have identified miglustat as a chemical chaperone.[43] Miglustat binds to and has been cocrystallized with β-glucocerebrosidase.[44] Because miglustat induces lymphoid atrophy in normal mice, it has been suggested that the clinical responses, most notably a decrease in spleen size, may be independent of its effects on glucosylceramide levels.[45] The in vitro effects of miglustat on glucosylceramide reduction are observed at the mid to high micromolar range whereas the clinically attained plasma and spinal fluid levels are in the low micromolar range. Miglustat is ineffective in blocking the accumulation of Gb3 in the α-galactosidase A mouse, an unexpected result for an inhibitor of glucosylceramide synthase.[46] Finally, miglustat homologues, most notably isofagamine, are potent chemical chaperones of the β-glucocerebrosidase.[47] Notably, miglustat did not lower plasma glucosylceramide levels in type I Gaucher disease patients in a statistically significant manner.[40]

Even though the mechanism of action remains a subject of debate, a comparison of its clinical efficacy compared to Genz-112638 can be made (Table 11–1). Based on the Phase II data, it appears that the 12-month response to Genz-112638 exceeded the response to miglustat observed at 36 months of treatment.

A potential advantage of miglustat over Genz-112638 is its distribution across the blood–brain barrier. Pharmacokinetic studies with radiolabeled Genz-112638 failed to demonstrate any significant accumulation in the central nervous system. Although this result may be a distinct advantage for the avoidance of potential side effects resulting from the inhibition of brain glycolipid synthesis, this property renders the drug ineffective in the treatment of sphingolipidoses such as Tay–Sachs, Sandhoff disease, and GM1 gangliosidosis. Two randomized controlled studies on the use of miglustat for type III Gaucher disease and late-onset Tay–Sachs disease failed, however, to demonstrate any clinical benefit.[48,49]

Pharmacological chaperones have been explored as an alternative way to treat Gaucher disease. To date, most of the described chaperones are glucose-based azasugars, including miglustat and N-nonyl-deoxynojirimycin. Isofagomine is an azasugar lacking an alkylated side chain and is currently in Phase II trials for Gaucher disease. These compounds stabilize β-glucocerebrosidase activity through a mechanism believed to be due to the stabilization of the substrate binding pocket. Three loops surrounding this pocket that include residues 311–319, 342–354, and 393–396 are believed to be involved.[44] Recently, two novel carbohydrate inhibitory molecules have been identified.[50] 1-Deoxygalacto-nojirimycin has been identified as a chemical chaperone for α-galactosidase A and is being pursued as a therapeutic for Fabry disease.[51]

The efficacy of pharmacological chaperones is highly dependent on the presence and nature of the mutation of the target enzyme. Sixty percent of patients with Fabry disease have missense mutations of α-galactosidase A. More than 500 distinct mutations have been identified. Approximately 40% of Fabry disease patients have a null mutation and thus would not be candidates for chaperone therapy. Type I Gaucher disease patients typically retain 5–20% of their residual β-glucocerebrosidase activity. Ninety percent of these patients carry one of four alleles (N370S, F213I, L444P, or G202R) with N370S accounting for 75% of patients. Thus, type I Gaucher disease would appear to be a more suitable target for this strategy.

COMBINATION THERAPY WITH PDMP-BASED INHIBITORS

Enzyme replacement therapy, pharmacological chaperones, and gene therapy share one common feature. These strategies are designed to increase the activity of the defective glycosidase in Gaucher or Fabry disease. Synthesis inhibition therapy is distinct in that it targets the production of the accumulating glycosphingolipid. Predictably, glucosylceramide synthase inhibitors would act additively or synergistically with these other therapeutic alternatives. Some manifestations of Gaucher disease, such as bone and pulmonary involvement, have been less responsive to enzyme replacement, and significant renal involvement in Fabry disease does not appear to benefit from enzyme replacement alone. Combination therapy involving enzyme replacement with Genz-112638 in these settings should be explored in the future.

CONCLUSIONS

More than 35 years have passed since Norman Radin first proposed the strategy of synthesis inhibition for the treatment of sphingolipidoses. The identification of PDMP as a lead inhibitor of glucosylceramide synthase and the subsequent identification of structural homologues that were more potent and selective in their inhibition of the cerebroside synthase paved the way for proof-of-concept studies and, more recently, Phase I and Phase II clinical studies for type I Gaucher disease. The high bioavailability, low toxicity, and potential for synergistic interactions with either enzyme replacement therapy or chemical chaperones suggest that the C8 ethylenedioxyphenyl homologue of PDMP may represent a significant advance in the therapeutics of this disorder and potentially of Fabry disease.

It remains a matter of debate whether the mechanism of action of miglustat is as a weak glucosylceramide synthase inhibitor or as a chemical chaperone for β-glucocerebrosidase. The markedly superior clinical response of the type I Gaucher patients to C8-ethylenedioxyphenyl-P4 and the comparatively lower toxicity profile suggest, however, that the PDMP homologue is a significantly more promising oral therapeutic. Given the lower costs of production of small molecules compared to recombinant enzyme, this agent also is anticipated to provide significant cost savings for the Gaucher patient population.

A significant amount of future work is required to fully exploit the potential clinical benefits of the PDMP class of drugs. Because C8-ethylenedioxyphenyl-P4 does not distribute into the central nervous system, a group of sphingolipi-doses (including Tay–Sachs, GM1 gangliosidosis, and Sandhoff disease) are not amenable to treatment. Designing homologues with the physical characteristics that would promote distribution across the blood–brain barrier is an obvious opportunity for future work.

The additional work, albeit preliminary, indicating that glucosylceramide synthase inhibition may be a suitable target for other, more common diseases, including diabetes, viral illness, and cancer, provides a large range of promising opportunities for future investigation as well. These studies remind us that glycosphingolipids play an important role in normal cell biology and as mediators of disease outside of the conventional, but historically important, area of lysosomal storage disorders. Clearly, we are only at the dawn of an exciting era in sphingolipid research.

REFERENCES

1. de Duve C, Wattiaux R. Functions of lysosomes. *Annu Rev Physiol.* 1966;28:435–492
2. Futerman AH, van Meer G. The cell biology of lysosomal storage disorders. *Nat Rev Mol Cell Biol.* 2004;5:554–565
3. Lubke T, Lobel P, Sleat DE. Proteomics of the lysosome. *Biochim Biophys Acta.* 2009;1793:625–635
4. Brady RO. Sphingolipidoses. *Annu Rev Biochem.* 1978;47:687–713
5. Grabowski GA, Horowitz M. Gaucher's disease: Molecular, genetic and enzymological aspects. *Baillieres Clin Haematol.* 1997;10:635–656
6. Shayman JA, Killen PD. Fabry disease. D.B. Mount, M.R. Pollaks, eds. *Molecular and Genetic Basis of Renal Disease.* Philadelphia, Saunders Elsevier, 195–199, 2008
7. Branton MH, Schiffmann R, Sabnis SG, Murray GJ, Quirk JM, Altarescu G, Goldfarb L, Brady RO, Balow JE, Austin HA III, Kopp JB. Natural history of Fabry renal disease: Influence of alpha-galactosidase A activity and genetic mutations on clinical course. *Medicine (Baltimore).* 2002;81:122–138
8. Kornfeld R, Kornfeld S. Assembly of asparagine-linked oligosaccharides. *Annu Rev Biochem.* 1985;54:631–664
9. Stahl PD. The mannose receptor and other macrophage lectins. *Curr Opin Immunol.* 1992;4:49–52
10. Brady RO, Pentchev PG, Gal AE, Hibbert SR, Dekaban AS. Replacement therapy for inherited enzyme deficiency. Use of purified glucocerebrosidase in Gaucher's disease. *N Engl J Med.* 1974;291:989–993
11. Cabrera-Salazar MA, Novelli E, Barranger JA. Gene therapy for the lysosomal storage disorders. *Curr Opin Mol Ther.* 2002;4:349–358

12. Krivit W, Peters C, Shapiro EG. Bone marrow transplantation as effective treatment of central nervous system disease in globoid cell leukodystrophy, metachromatic leukodystrophy, adrenoleukodystrophy, mannosidosis, fucosidosis, aspartylglucosaminuria, Hurler, Maroteaux-Lamy, and Sly syndromes, and Gaucher disease type III. *Curr Opin Neurol.* 1999;12:167–176

13. Yu Z, Sawkar AR, Kelly JW. Pharmacologic chaperoning as a strategy to treat Gaucher disease. *FEBS J.* 2007;274:4944–4950

14. Radin NS, Arora RC, Ullman MD, Brenkert AL, Austin J. A possible therapeutic approach to Krabbe's globoid leukodystrophy and the status of cerebroside synthesis in the disorder. *Res Commun Chem Pathol Pharmacol.* 1972;3:637–644

15. Radin NS. Treatment of Gaucher disease with an enzyme inhibitor. *Glycoconj J.* 1996;13:153–157

16. Vunnam RR, Radin NS. Analogs of ceramide that inhibit glucocerebroside synthetase in mouse brain. *Chem Phys Lipids.* 1908;26:265–278

17. Abe A, Inokuchi J, Jimbo M, Shimeno H, Nagamatsu A, Shayman JA, Shukla GS, Radin NS. Improved inhibitors of glucosylceramide synthase. *J Biochem.* 1992;111:191–196

18. Abe A, Radin NS, Shayman JA, Wotring LL, Zipkin RE, Sivakumar R, Ruggieri JM, Carson KG, Ganem B. Structural and stereochemical studies of potent inhibitors of glucosylceramide synthase and tumor cell growth. *J Lipid Res.* 1995;36:611–621

19. Lee L, Abe A, Shayman JA. Improved inhibitors of glucosylceramide synthase. *J Biol Chem.* 1999;274:14662–14669

20. Shayman JA, Lee L, Abe A, Shu L. Inhibitors of glucosylceramide synthase. *Methods Enzymol.* 2000;311:373–387

21. Abe A, Shayman JA, Radin NS. A novel enzyme that catalyzes the esterification of N-acetylsphingosine. Metabolism of C2-ceramides. *J Biol Chem.* 1996;271:14383–14389

22. Abe A, Shayman JA. Purification and characterization of 1-O-acylceramide synthase, a novel phospholipase A2 with transacylase activity. *J Biol Chem.* 1998;273:8467–8474

23. Abe A, Hiraoka M, Shayman JA. A role for lysosomal phospholipase A2 in drug induced phospholipidosis. *Drug Metab Lett.* 2007;1:49–53

24. Abe A, Shayman JA. The role of negatively charged lipids in lysosomal phospholipase A2 function. *J Lipid Res.* 2009;50:2027–2035

25. Hiraoka M, Abe A, Lu Y, Yang K, Han X, Gross RW, Shayman JA. Lysosomal phospholipase A2 and phospholipidosis. *Mol Cell Biol.* 2006;26:6139–6148

26. Basu M, Kelly P, O'Donnell P, Miguel M, Bradley M, Sonnino S, Banerjee S, Basu S. Ceramide glycanase activities in human cancer cells. *Biosci Rep.* 1999;19:449–460

27. Inokuchi J, Mizutani A, Jimbo M, Usuki S, Yamagishi K, Mochizuki H, Muramoto K, Kobayashi K, Kuroda Y, Iwasaki K, Ohgami Y, Fujiwara M. A synthetic ceramide analog (L-PDMP) up-regulates neuronal function. *Ann N Y Acad Sci.* 1998;845:219–224

28. Eitzman DT, Bodary PF, Shen Y, Khairallah CG, Wild SR, Abe A, Shaffer-Hartman J, Shayman JA. Fabry disease in mice is associated with age-dependent susceptibility to vascular thrombosis. *J Am Soc Nephrol.* 2003;14:298–302

29. Bodary PF, Shen Y, Vargas FB, Bi X, Ostenso KA, Gu S, Shayman JA, Eitzman DT. Alpha-galactosidase A deficiency accelerates atherosclerosis in mice with apolipoprotein E deficiency. *Circulation.* 2005;111:629–632

30. Park JL, Whitesall SE, D'Alecy LG, Shu L, Shayman JA. Vascular dysfunction in the alpha-galactosidase A-knockout mouse is an endothelial cell-, plasma membrane-based defect. *Clin Exp Pharmacol Physiol.* 2008;35:1156–1163

31. Abe A, Arend LJ, Lee L, Lingwood C, Brady RO, Shayman JA. Glycosphingolipid depletion in Fabry disease lymphoblasts with potent inhibitors of glucosylceramide synthase. *Kidney Int.* 2000;57:446–454

32. Abe A, Gregory S, Lee L, Killen PD, Brady RO, Kulkarni A, Shayman JA. Reduction of globotriaosylceramide in Fabry disease mice by substrate deprivation. *J Clin Invest.* 2000;105:1563–1571

33. Xu YH, Quinn B, Witte D, Grabowski GA. Viable mouse models of acid beta-glucosidase deficiency: The defect in Gaucher disease. *Am J Pathol.* 2003;163:2093–2101

34. McEachern KA, Fung J, Komarnitsky S, Siegel CS, Chuang WL, Hutto E, Shayman JA, Grabowski GA, Aerts JM, Cheng SH, Copeland DP, Marshall J. A specific and potent inhibitor of glucosylceramide synthase for substrate inhibition therapy of Gaucher disease. *Mol Genet Metab.* 2007;91:259–267

35. Hollak CE, van Weely S, van Oers MH, Aerts JM. Marked elevation of plasma chitotriosidase activity. A novel hallmark of Gaucher disease. *J Clin Invest.* 1994;93:1288–1292

36. Weinreb NJ, Barranger JA, Charrow J, Grabowski GA, Mankin HJ, Mistry P. Guidance on the use of miglustat for treating patients with type 1 Gaucher disease. *Am J Hematol.* 2005;80:223–229

37. Ratner L, vander Heyden N, Dedera D. Inhibition of HIV and SIV infectivity by blockade of alpha-glucosidase activity. *Virology.* 1991;181:180–192

38. Platt FM, Neises GR, Dwek RA, Butters TD. N-butyldeoxynojirimycin is a novel inhibitor of glycolipid biosynthesis. *J Biol Chem.* 1994;269:8362–8365

39. Cox T, Lachmann R, Hollak C, Aerts J, van Weely S, Hrebicek M, Platt F, Butters T, Dwek R, Moyses C, Gow I, Elstein D, Zimran A. Novel oral treatment of Gaucher's disease with N-butyldeoxynojirimycin (OGT 918) to decrease substrate biosynthesis. *Lancet.* 2000;355:1481–1485

40. Elstein D, Hollak C, Aerts JM, van Weely S, Maas M, Cox TM, Lachmann RH, Hrebicek M, Platt FM, Butters TD, Dwek RA, Zimran A. Sustained therapeutic effects of oral miglustat (Zavesca, N-butyldeoxynojirimycin, OGT 918) in type I Gaucher disease. *J Inherit Metab Dis.* 2004;27:757–766

41. Platt FM, Neises GR, Reinkensmeier G, Townsend MJ, Perry VH, Proia RL, Winchester B, Dwek RA, Butters TD. Prevention of lysosomal storage in Tay-Sachs mice treated with N-butyldeoxynojirimycin. *Science.* 1997;276:428–431

42. Platt FM, Reinkensmeier G, Dwek RA, Butters TD. Extensive glycosphingolipid depletion in the liver and lymphoid organs of mice treated with N-butyldeoxynojirimycin. *J Biol Chem.* 1997;272:19365–19372

43. Sanchez-Olle G, Duque J, Egido-Gabas M, Casas J, Lluch M, Chabas A, Grinberg D, Vilageliu L. Promising results of the chaperone effect caused by imino sugars and aminocyclitol derivatives on mutant glucocerebrosidases causing Gaucher disease. *Blood Cells Mol Dis.* 2009;42:159–166

44. Brumshtein B, Greenblatt HM, Butters TD, Shaaltiel Y, Aviezer D, Silman I, Futerman AH, Sussman JL. Crystal structures of complexes of N-butyl- and N-nonyl-deoxynojirimycin bound to acid beta-glucosidase: Insights into the mechanism of chemical chaperone action in Gaucher disease. *J Biol Chem.* 2007;282:29052–29058

45. Mistry PK. Treatment of Gaucher's disease with OGT 918. *Lancet.* 2000;356:676–677

46. Heare T, Alp NJ, Priestman DA, Kulkarni AB, Qasba P, Butters TD, Dwek RA, Clarke K, Channon KM, Platt FM. Severe endothelial dysfunction in the aorta of a mouse model of Fabry disease; partial prevention by N-butyldeoxynojirimycin treatment. *J Inherit Metab Dis.* 2007;30:79–87

47. Sawkar AR, Cheng WC, Beutler E, Wong CH, Balch WE, Kelly JW. Chemical chaperones increase the cellular activity of N370S beta-glucosidase: A therapeutic strategy for Gaucher disease. *Proc Natl Acad Sci USA.* 2002;99:15428–15433

48. Shapiro BE, Pastores GM, Gianutsos J, Luzy C, Kolodny EH. Miglustat in late-onset Tay-Sachs disease: A 12-month, randomized, controlled clinical study with 24 months of extended treatment. *Genet Med.* 2009;11:425–433

49. Schiffmann R, Fitzgibbon EJ, Harris C, DeVile C, Davies EH, Abel L, van Schaik IN, Benko W, Timmons M, Ries M, Vellodi A. Randomized, controlled trial of miglustat in Gaucher's disease type 3. *Ann Neurol.* 2008;64:514–522

50. Tropak MB, Kornhaber GJ, Rigat BA, Maegawa GH, Buttner JD, Blanchard JE, Murphy C, Tuske SJ, Coales SJ, Hamuro Y, Brown ED, Mahuran DJ. Identification of

pharmacological chaperones for Gaucher disease and characterization of their effects on beta-glucocerebrosidase by hydrogen/deuterium exchange mass spectrometry. *Chembiochem.* 2008;9:2650–2662

51. Fan JQ, Ishii S, Asano N, Suzuki Y. Accelerated transport and maturation of lysosomal alpha-galactosidase A in Fabry lymphoblasts by an enzyme inhibitor. *Nat Med.* 1999;5:112–115

12 Betaine treatment for the homocystinurias

Amy Lawson-Yuen and Harvey L. Levy

INTRODUCTION

The methionine metabolic pathway is one of the most interesting and complex pathways in biochemical genetics. At least 11 inborn errors of metabolism involve this pathway. In many of these disorders betaine has a major role in therapy. The methionine pathway is in reality a cycle in which methionine loses a methyl group (transmethylation) and then regains a methyl group (remethylation). Figure 12–1 depicts this pathway, indicating the key enzymes and disorders associated with these enzymes. Because an increase of homocysteine occurs in a number of these disorders and seems to be toxic, a major goal of therapy is to reduce the level of homocysteine. In the remethylation disorders, decreased methionine may be the major pathogenic factor; therefore, increasing the level of methionine may be critical. For both of these goals, betaine, a methyl donor that activates an alternative remethylation path (Figure 12–1), is a key therapeutic agent. The following description of the disorders in the methionine pathway will feature those associated with hyperhomocysteinemia and will be divided into two groups: homocystinuria, the disorder of transsulfuration, and the several disorders of remethylation.

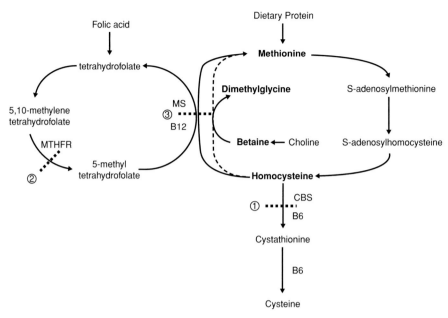

Figure 12–1: The methionine cycle. Enzyme or transport defects as follows lead to elevated homocysteine: (1) CBS deficiency; (2) MTHFR deficiency; and (3) the five cobalamin C-G defects.

DISORDER OF TRANSSULFURATION

Homocystinuria was first described in 1962.[1,2] It is caused by a deficiency of cystathionine ß-synthase (CBS), a B6-dependent enzyme responsible for the transsulfuration of homocysteine to cystathionine (Figure 12–1). More than 140 homocystinuria-causing mutations have been identified in the CBS gene. The mutations are mostly private and include a wide range of changes, including missense and nonsense mutations, deletions, insertions, and splice site changes. The majority of these mutations interfere with the CBS active core. The most frequent mutations are p. Ile278Thr, causing the usually milder pyridoxine-responsive form of homocystinuria, and p. Gly307Ser, causing severe pyridoxine-nonresponsive homocystinuria. Deficient activity of CBS results in an accumulation of homocysteine and, via enhanced remethylation, an increased concentration of methionine. The clinical features of homocystinuria include ectopia lentis, mental retardation, osteoporosis with a marfanoid habitus, thromboembolism, and, on occasion, psychiatric manifestations.

The pathogenesis of homocystinuria seems to primarily center around the increased concentration of homocysteine. Homocysteine interferes with disulfide bonds that are important to protein secondary structure. This interference results in ectopia lentis by disruption of the disulfide bonds in cysteine-rich fibrillin, a protein in the zonular fibers that connects the optic lens to the ciliary body.[3] The changes in fibrillin are analogous to the cause of ectopia lentis in Marfan syndrome, which is due to a genetic defect in fibrillin-1.[4] The disulfide bonds in the calcium binding epidermal growth factor (cbEGF)-like domain fragments from fibrillin-1 may be the key disulfides involved.[5] The marfanoid skeletal abnormalities are a consequence of disruption of collagen cross-linking by the increased homocysteine. The exact mechanisms for the thromboembolism and mental retardation in homocystinuria are unexplained but almost certainly are related to the increase in homocysteine.

Presymptomatic therapy can prevent most or all of the clinical complications of homocystinuria. For this reason, homocystinuria has been included in newborn screening.[6] The screening indicator of the disorder is an increase in methionine. It seems, however, that some affected infants do not have an increased level of methionine during the first days of life when the blood specimen for screening is collected.[6,7] A normal methionine level in newborn screening may particularly apply to infants with pyridoxine-responsive homocystinuria in whom there may be a later increase in methionine and usually a milder clinical course. Thus, homocystinuria may be found later in life in previously undetected individuals because of clinical complications, notably thromboembolic events.[8]

Treatment includes a methionine-restricted diet, vitamin B6 (pyridoxine; especially in patients with the pyridoxine-responsive form of homocystinuria), folic acid and vitamin B12 to enhance remethylation, and betaine. The role of betaine in the therapy of homocystinuria is described in the section "Betaine."

DISORDERS OF REMETHYLATION

There are six inborn errors of remethylation, all of which produce increased homocysteine. Unlike homocystinuria, however, methionine in these disorders is decreased rather than increased. Five errors are due to defects in cobalamin (B12) metabolism or in the relationship between cobalamin and methionine synthase (cobalamin C-G disorders), and one (methyltetrahydrofolate reductase deficiency) is due to a defect in folate metabolism. The most frequent of the remethylation disorders, cblC disorder, limits the conversion of precursor cobalamin to its coenzymatically active derivatives, deoxyadenosylcobalamin (AdoCbl) and methylcobalamin (MeCbl), and results in both hyperhomocysteinemia and methylmalonic aciduria. Patients with cblC disorder are at risk for developmental delay, pigmentary retinopathy with resulting poor vision or blindness, and megaloblastic anemia. Recently, the gene responsible for the conversion of precursor cobalamin to its coenzymatic forms, designated MMACHC, and mutations in the gene responsible for cblC disorder, have been reported.[9,10] The function of the MMACHC gene product has not yet been specified but seems to possibly be a lysosomal transport protein.[9] Treatment for cblC disorder includes megadoses of B12 (hydroxycobalamin), usually 1 mg/d intramuscularly but perhaps even as much as 30 mg/d intramuscularly,[11] and betaine (see section "Betaine"). A low-methionine diet has also been used in an attempt to control the accumulation of homocysteine, but it may be counterproductive because it also can accentuate the hypomethioninemia, a potentially critical pathophysiological factor.[12,13] See also Chapter 6.

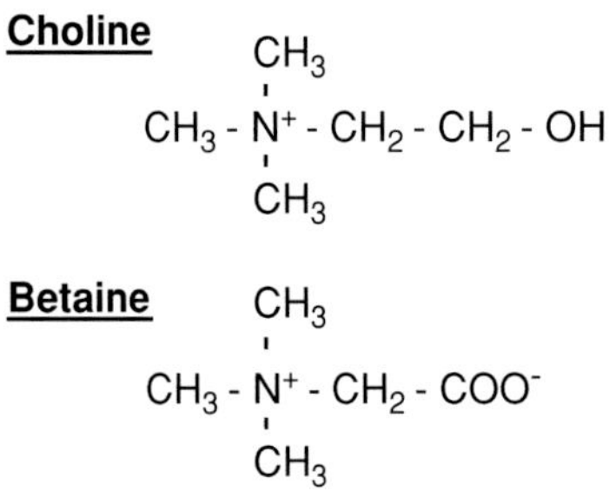

Choline

$$CH_3$$
$$|$$
$$CH_3 - N^+ - CH_2 - CH_2 - OH$$
$$|$$
$$CH_3$$

Betaine

$$CH_3$$
$$|$$
$$CH_3 - N^+ - CH_2 - COO^-$$
$$|$$
$$CH_3$$

Figure 12–2: Structures of choline and betaine.

The other disorder of remethylation in which betaine has been used effectively is methylenetetrahydrofolate reductase (MTHFR) deficiency. MTHFR converts 5, 10-methylenetetrahydrofolate to 5-methyltetrahydrofolate, the donor of the methyl group required for the conversion of homocysteine to methionine (Figure 12–1). Deficient MTHFR activity, therefore, results in hyperhomocysteinemia and hypomethioninemia.

BETAINE

Betaine (N, N, N-trimethylglycine) (Figure 12–2) as a substrate for betaine-homocysteine methyltransferase is a potent alternative methyl donor for the remethylation of methionine (Figure 12–1). As such, it is used in the therapy of homocystinuria as well as the remethylation disorders. Its chemical structure is similar to that of choline (Figure 12–2). The molecular weight of betaine is 117.

Homocystinuria

The principle for the use of betaine in treating homocystinuria is to reduce the concentration of homocysteine. Although betaine also accentuates the hypermethioninemia in homocystinuria, this is usually inconsequential in that increased methionine seems to be benign except when extraordinarily elevated (see "Side effects").

The concept of using a supplementary methyl donor to reduce the concentration of homocysteine in homocystinuria was introduced by Perry and colleagues in 1968.[14] They used choline, the precursor of betaine. Three years later, Komrower and Sardharwalla reported the use of betaine with excellent biochemical benefit in two patients with homocystinuria.[15] Subsequently, a number of studies have reported biochemical benefit from betaine therapy in homocystinuria.[16,17]

Clinical evidence of benefit in homocystinuria has so far been limited to the prevention of vascular events. The evidence for this benefit is impressive, however. Wilcken and Wilcken showed that, among 15 Australian pyridoxine-nonresponsive homocystinuria patients who had had at least one vascular event before being treated with betaine, none had another event while on betaine.[18] This experience has been supported by subsequent reports.[19,20] With regard to osteoporosis, a small and relatively short crossover study indicated that betaine did not improve vertebral body density.[21] Obviously, much further study will be required before it can be determined whether betaine is effective in reducing the impact of the full range of complications in homocystinuria. These studies will be difficult to interpret because of potential confounding by early and continuous dietary therapy. Nevertheless, should it be shown that, when patients become noncompliant with diet, betaine therapy alone over the long term improves or retards the development of osteoporosis, as well as improves cognitive and emotional functioning, betaine would assume an even more substantial role than at present in the treatment of homocystinuria.

Remethylation disorders

In these disorders betaine assumes a twofold role, to increase the level of methionine and to decrease the level of homocysteine. In fact, the former role may be more important than the latter. The benefit of betaine by increasing the methionine level in MTHFR deficiency was suggested in a girl reported by Wendel and Bremer[22] but has recently been dramatically illustrated in a patient of Strauss and colleagues.[12] This patient was identified at birth by a targeted analysis for a frequent MTHFR mutation present in the Amish population of central Pennsylvania. She was treated only with betaine and aspirin beginning at 16 days of age. Her increased plasma homocysteine level was reduced but remained far greater than normal, whereas the plasma methionine and S-adenosylmethionine levels markedly increased. Moreover, the calculated brain uptake of methionine increased threefold on betaine. Unlike other Amish children in whom MTHFR deficiency was not identified until after irreversible brain damage occurred, this girl remained clinically normal and maintained a fully developed and appropriately myelinated brain by magnetic resonance imaging (MRI).

Betaine therapy has been employed in other disorders of remethylation, notably in cblC disorder, to decrease the level of homocyst(e)ine and increase methionine.[23,24] It may be especially important in increasing the level of methionine and preventing subacute combined degeneration (SCD) of the spinal cord. We have reported the neuropathological findings in a boy who died from cblC disorder. Despite lifelong therapy with megadoses of vitamin B12 (hydroxycobalamin), his spinal cord had striking changes of SCD, identical to the characteristic changes in vitamin B12 deficiency pernicious anemia.[13] Because SCD of the spinal cord in monkeys and pigs rendered hypomethioninemic by inhibition of methionine synthase is prevented by methionine dietary supplementation,[25,26] we suggested that a deficiency of central nervous system methionine may be the central cause of the SCD in cblC disorder as well as in other disorders of remethylation. If so, large doses of betaine may be protective in cblC disorder as seems to be the case in MTHFR deficiency.[12]

Dosage

In adolescents and adults, betaine (Cystadane; Chronimed Pharmacy, Minnetonka, MN) is administered orally in a dose of 6–12 grams divided into two to three doses daily, depending on the response in reducing the level of homocysteine. In patients younger than three years, betaine is started at a dose of

100 mg/kg/d and can be increased weekly by 50 mg/kg until the desired decrease in homocysteine or, in remethylation defects, increase in methionine levels is achieved. It is supplied as an anhydrous powder. One level 1.7–cubic centimeter scoop contains one gram of betaine and can be mixed into four to six ounces of water or juice or can be mixed with food.

Pharmacokinetic studies have been performed on a limited number of healthy volunteers and patients with classic homocystinuria.[27] Absorption and distribution are rapid after oral ingestion. Elimination is predominately by metabolism with only a minor amount eliminated by renal clearance. Pharmacological studies do not suggest any benefit to dosing more frequently than twice daily.[28]

Side effects

Betaine is generally well-tolerated and appears to be safe. As betaine works to lower homocysteine levels, methionine levels may rise. The hypermethioninemia appears to be benign and is tolerated well by most patients. Case reports suggest, however, that extremely high levels of methionine may result in cerebral edema in rare individuals.

The first report of this toxicity described a 10-year-old girl who began betaine in a dose of 6 g/d (200 mg/kg/d) as adjunctive therapy for homocystinuria.[29] Methionine levels increased to more than 3,000 μmol/L (normal range 14–54 μmol/L). She developed headache, vomiting, visual changes, and evidence of brain edema on head computed tomography (CT) and MRI. At this point, betaine was discontinued, methionine was restricted, and vitamins B6, B12, and folate were supplemented. The neurological symptoms and the MRI abnormalities completely resolved.

The second report described a five-year-old boy with homocystinuria only minimally responsive to pyridoxine and folic acid.[30] Betaine was given at a dose of 3 g/d with dietary restriction of protein and methionine. Subsequently, the patient developed headaches, emesis, papilledema, and increased pressure on lumbar puncture. The symptoms worsened when the betaine dose was increased to three grams twice daily. His serum methionine level increased to 1,190 μmol/L with a cerebrospinal fluid (CSF) methionine level of 235 μmol/L (normal CSF methionine: 1–5 μmol/L). CT scan showed diffuse brain swelling. Discontinuation of betaine resulted in the serum methionine levels decreasing to near normal (43–111 μmol/L) and resolution of the symptoms.

A third report described a boy with isolated hypermethioninemia due to methionine adenosyltransferase (MAT) I/III deficiency who had been treated with betaine because of an initial diagnosis of homocystinuria.[31] The plasma methionine level increased to 1,560 μmol/L and MRI disclosed T1 and T2 prolongation in subcortical regions and in the brainstem. These MRI findings were subsequently interpreted as consistent with cerebral edema.[32] Betaine was discontinued, his plasma methionine levels decreased, and the MRI findings largely normalized.

These cases indicate that caution should be employed in the use of betaine, especially when treating homocystinuria. Metabolic monitoring of all patients receiving betaine must include the measurement of plasma methionine. Clinical attention must be paid to headache, vomiting, change in mental status, or any new neurological symptoms. Should any of these signs appear in association with an increased level of methionine, especially if the plasma methionine concentration is greater than 1,000 μmol/L, betaine should immediately be discontinued. Most patients receiving betaine, however, have had an elevated methionine level, even an extremely high level, and remained stable with no new neurological symptoms, so if the patient remains well with only an elevated methionine level, betaine can safely be continued.

U.S. Food and Drug Administration status

Betaine (betaine anhydrous powder) is available as an orphan product known as Cystadane. It was approved by the U.S. Food and Drug Administration on October 20, 1996.

It is listed as a category C drug and betaine should be used in pregnancy only if the benefits outweigh the risks. It is not known if betaine is excreted in breast milk. Pregnancy and offspring outcome in maternal homocystinuria are usually normal, but there may be a risk of maternal thromboembolic events and spontaneous abortion, thus treatments that lessen the risk of thrombosis in pregnancy may be beneficial.[33] Vilaseca and colleagues reported two successful pregnancies in a woman with pyridoxine-nonresponsive homocystinuria.[34] She was treated with betaine in a dose of a 6 g/d, cystine, increased pyridoxine, folate, and acetylsalicylic acid. The patient had one early spontaneous abortion between the two successful pregnancies. Both of the children are reported to have normal development and are attending regular school. Pierre and colleagues reported successful treatment of a 19-year-old pregnant woman with poorly controlled pyridoxine-nonresponsive homocystinuria by betaine at a dose of 150 mg/kg combined with a low protein diet, anticoagulation, and close monitoring.[35] The pregnancy was successful, and she delivered the infant at term.

FUTURE DEVELOPMENTS

Betaine therapy has been used in a study of Angelman syndrome. The rationale has been to increase the ratio of S-adenosylmethionine to S-adenosylhomocysteine, thereby enhancing methylation. The data from this study are currently being examined. Betaine has also been used to lower the homocysteine level in mild hyperhomocysteinemia that seems to increase the risk of vascular disease. At present, the benefit of betaine in this context is unproven. It is conceivable that, in the future, we will see other potential benefits from betaine therapy.

REFERENCES

1. Carson NA, Neill DW. Metabolic abnormalities detected in a survey of mentally backward individuals in Northern Ireland. *Arch Dis Child*. 1962;37:505–513

2. Gerritsen T, Vaughn JG, Waisman HA. The identification of homocysteine in the urine. *Biochem Biophys Res Commun*. 1962;9:493–496

3. Mudd SH, Levy HL, Kraus JP. Disorders of transsulfuration. C.R. Scriver, A.L. Beaudet, W.S. Sly, D. Valle, eds. *The Metabolic and Molecular Bases of Inherited Disease*, New York, McGraw-Hill, 2007–2056, 2001

4. Hubmacher D, Tiedemann K, Bartels R, Brinckmann J, Vollbrandt T, Bätge B, Notbohm H, Reinhardt DP. Modification of the structure and function of fibrillin-1 by homocysteine suggests a potential pathogenetic mechanism in homocystinuria. *J Biol Chem*. 2005;280(41):34946–34955

5. Hutchinson S, Aplin RT, Webb H, Kettle S, Timmermans J, Boers GH, Handford PA. Molecular effects of homocysteine on cbEGF domain structure: Insights into the pathogenesis of homocystinuria. *J Mol Biol*. 2005;346(3):833–844

6. Peterschmitt MJ, Simmons JR, Levy HL. Reduction of false-negative results in screening of newborns for homocystinuria. *N Engl J Med*. 1999;341:1572–1576

7. Wagstaff J, Korson M, Kraus JP, Levy HL. Severe folate deficiency and pancytopenia in a nutritionally-deprived infant with homocystinuria caused by cystathionine beta-synthase deficiency. *J Pediatr*. 1991;118:569–572

8. Scovby F, Gaustadnes M, Mudd SH. A revisit to the natural history of homocystinuria due to cystathionine B-synthase deficiency. *Molec Genet Metab*. 2010;99:1–3

9. Lerner-Ellis JP, Tirone JC, Pawelek PD, Dore C, Atkinson JL, Watkins D, Morel CF, Fujiwara TM, Moras E, Hosack AR, Dunbar GV, Antonicka H, Forgetta V, Dobson CM, Leclerc D, Gravel RA, Shoubridge EA, Coulton JW, Lepage P, Rommens JM, Morgan K, Rosenblatt DS. Identification of the gene responsible for methylmalonic aciduria and homocystinuria, cblC type. *Nat Genet*. 2006;38:93–100

10. Lerner-Ellis JP, Anastasio N, Liu J, Coelho D, Suormala T, Stucki M, Loewy AD, Gurd S, Grundberg E, Morel CF, Watkins D, Baumgartner MR, Pastinen T, Rosenblatt DS, Fowler B. Spectrum of mutations in MMACHC, allelic expression, and evidence for genotype-phenotype correlations. *Hum Mutat*. 2009;30:1–10

11. Carrillo-Carrasco N, Sloan J, Valle D, Hamosh A, Venditti CP.. Hydroxocobalamin dose escalation improves metabolic control in cblC. *J Inherit Metab Dis*. 2009;32:728–731

12. Strauss KA, Morton DH, Puffenberger EG, Hendrickson C, Robinson DL, Wagner C, Stabler SP, Allen RH, Chwatko G, Jakubowski H, Niculescu MD, Mudd SH. Prevention of brain disease from severe 10-methylenetetrahydrofolate reductase deficiency. *Molec Genet Metab*. 2007;91:165–175

13. Smith SE, Kinney HC, Swoboda KJ, Levy HL. Subacute combined degeneration of the spinal cord in cblC disorder despite treatment with B12. *Mol Genet Metab*. 2006;88:138–145

14. Perry TL, Hansen S, Love DL, Crawford LE, Tischler B. Treatment of homocystinuria with a low-methionine diet, supplementary cystine, and a methyl donor. *Lancet*. 1968;2:474–478

15. Komrower GM, Sardharwalla IB. The dietary treatment of homocystinuria. N.A. Carson, D.N. Raine, eds. *Inherited Disorders of Sulfur Metabolism*. Churchill Livingstone, Edinburgh, 254–263, 1971

16. Smolin LA, Benevenga NJ, Berlow S. The use of betaine for the treatment of homocystinuria. *J Pediatr*. 1981;99:467–472

17. Wilcken DE, Wilcken B, Dudman NP, Tyrrell PA. Homocystinuria – the effects of betaine in the treatment of patients not responsive to pyridoxine. *N Engl J Med*. 1983;309:448–453

18. Wilcken DE, Wilcken B. The natural history of vascular disease in homocystinuria and the effects of treatment. *J Inherit Metab Dis*. 1997;20:295–300

19. Walter JH, Wraith JE, White FJ, Bridge C, Till J. Strategies for the treatment of cystathionine beta-synthase deficiency: The experience of the Willink Biochemical Genetics Unit over the past 30 years. *Eur J Pediatr*. 1998;157(Suppl 2):S71–S76

20. Yap S, Boers GH, Wilcken B, Wilcken DE, Brenton DP, Lee PJ, Walter JH, Howard PM, Naughten ER. Vascular outcome in patients with homocystinuria due to cystathionine

beta-synthase deficiency treated chronically: A multicenter observational study. *Arterioscler Thromb Vasc Biol.* 2001;21:2080–2085

21. Gahl WA, Bernardini I, Chen S, Kurtz D, Horvath K. The effect of oral betaine on vertebral body bone density in pyridoxine-nonresponsive homocystinuria. *J Inherit Metab Dis.* 1988;11:291–298

22. Wendel U, Bremer U. Betaine in the treatment of homocystinuria due to 5, 10-methylenetetrahydrofolate reductase deficiency. *Eur J Pediatr.* 1984;142:147–150

23. Rosenblatt DS, Aspler AL, Shevell MI, Pletcher BA, Fenton WA, Seashore MR. Clinical heterogeneity and prognosis in combined methylmalonic aciduria and homocystinuria (cblC). *J Inherit Metab Dis.* 1997;20:528–538

24. Bartholomew DW, Batshaw ML, Allen RH, Roe CR, Rosenblatt D, Valle DL, Francomano CA. Therapeutic approaches to cobalamin-C methylmalonic academia and homocystinuria. *J Pediatr.* 1988;112:32–39

25. Scott JM, Dinn JJ, Wilson P, Weir DG. Pathogenesis of subacute combined degeneration: A result of methyl group deficiency. *Lancet.* 1981;2:334–337

26. Weir DG, Keating S, Molloy A, McPartlin J, Kennedy S, Blanchflower J, Kennedy DG, Rice D, Scott JM. Methylation deficiency causes vitamin B12-associated neuropathy in the pig. *J Neurochem.* 1988;51(6):1949–1952

27. Schwahn BC, Hafner D, Hohlfeld T, Balkenhol N, Laryea MD, Wendel U. Pharmacokinetics of oral betaine in healthy subjects and patients with homocystinuria. *Br J Clin Pharmacol.* 2003;55(1):6–13

28. Matthews A, Johnson TN, Rostami-Hodjegan A, Chakrapani A, Wraith JE, Moat SJ, Bonham JR, Tucker GT. An indirect response model of homocysteine suppression by betaine: Optimising the dosage regimen of betaine in homocystinuria. *Br J Clin Pharmacol.* 2002;54(2):140–146

29. Yaghmai R, Kashani AH, Geraghty MT, Okoh J, Pomper M, Tangerman A, Wagner C, Stabler SP, Allen RH, Mudd SH, Braverman N. Progressive cerebral edema associated with high methionine levels and betaine therapy in a patient with cystathionine beta-synthase (CBS) deficiency. *Am J Med Genet.* 2002;108(1):57–63

30. Devlin, A.M., Hajipour L, Gholkar A, Fernandes H, Ramesh V, Morris AA. Cerebral edema associated with betaine treatment in classical homocystinuria. *J Pediatr.* 2004;144(4):545–548

31. Tada H, Takanashi J, Barkovich AJ, Yamamoto S, Kohno Y. Reversible white matter lesion in methionine adenosyltransferase I/III deficiency. *Am J Neuroradiol.* 2004;144:545–548

32. Braverman NE, Mudd SH, Barker PB, Pomper MG. Characteristic MR imaging changes in severe hypermethioninemic states. *Am J Neuroradiol.* 2005;26:2705–2706

33. Levy HL, Vargas JE, Waisbren SE, Kurczynski TW, Roeder ER, Schwartz RS, Rosengren S, Prasad C, Greenberg CR, Gilfix BM, MacGregor D, Shih VE, Bao L, Kraus JP. Reproductive fitness in maternal homocystinuria due to cystathionine beta-synthase deficiency. *J Inherit Metab Dis.* 2002;25(4):299–314

34. Vilaseca MA, Cuartero ML, Martinez de Salinas M, Lambruschini N, Pintó X, Urreizti R, Balcells S, Grinberg D. Two successful pregnancies in pyridoxine-nonresponsive homocystinuria. *J Inherit Metab Dis.* 2004;27(6):775–777

35. Pierre G, Gissen P, Chakrapani A, McDonald A, Preece M, Wright J. Successful treatment of pyridoxine-unresponsive homocystinuria with betaine in pregnancy. *J Inherit Metab Dis.* 2006;29(5):688–689

SECTION IV
METAL ION THERAPY

13 Zinc and tetrathiomolybdate for the treatment of Wilson disease

George J. Brewer

OVERVIEW OF WILSON DISEASE

Wilson disease is an autosomal recessive disease of copper accumulation and copper toxicity.[1–5] It is a rare disease, occurring in approximately 1 in 40,000 births in most populations. The disease can present as a liver disease, as a neurologic movement disorder, or with psychiatric symptoms. In Western countries, presentation is primarily in the second and third decades of life, with a peak at approximately 20 years of age.[6] In India and other Asian countries, presentation is usually in much younger people, as young as early childhood.[7]

The liver disease presentation can look like hepatitis and, if not diagnosed, can remit and relapse numerous times.[1–5] It can also present as a complication of chronic cirrhosis, perhaps with bleeding from esophageal or gastric varices, or with leukopenia or thrombocytopenia from hypersplenism. Occasionally it presents with liver failure and, if fulminant, may require immediate liver transplantation.

This work has been supported by grant FD-R-0021353-03 from the FDA's Orphan Products Office, and by the General Clinical Research Center of the University of Michigan Hospitals, supported by the National Institutes of Health (grant number MO1-RR000042), and Clinical and Translational Science Awards (grant number Ul1-RR024986).

The neurologic presentation is that of a movement disorder.[8–10] The full-blown syndrome includes tremor, dystonia, and incoordination, although the patient may have an isolated symptom, such as tremor, for a long period. Speech and swallowing problems are common, and the disease may progress to complete anarthria. Dystonia may progress, pulling limbs out of physiologic positions, causing abnormal posture and, eventually, an inability to walk or even get out of bed.

Approximately half of patients who eventually present neurologically have psychiatric problems such that they see a behavioral health care worker before neurologic symptoms develop.[11] Behavioral abnormalities are quite varied and may be present for up to several years before neurologic symptoms appear. Inability to focus on tasks is common, leading to failure in school and/or loss of a job. Emotional instability is also common and includes temper tantrums, depression, manic behavior, and sexual disinhibition. Development of these behavioral problems in a previously healthy young person often leads to a misdiagnosis of substance abuse.

Some patients may be diagnosed prior to clinical presentation, generally because of a family workup, because the disease is inherited as an autosomal recessive gene, and siblings have a 25% risk of being affected. Such patients are called presymptomatic. Because in general the genes appear to be close to fully penetrant, these patients are destined to become symptomatic and should be treated prophylactically.[12,13]

If untreated, the natural history of the liver form of the disease is one of progression to liver failure and death, in the absence of liver transplantation.[14] In the meantime, the patient may suffer and even die from the complications of the disease, such as bleeding from esophageal or gastric varices. In the progression to severe liver failure the patient may develop ascites and/or hepatic encephalopathy. If untreated, the natural history of the primary neurologic form of the disease is also progression to increasing disability, anarthria, dysphagia, being wheelchair or bed bound, and eventually death from intercurrent infection. In the meantime, the patient may suffer from aspiration as a result of dysphagia, leading to pulmonary disease. He or she may suffer from under- and/or malnutrition from dysphagia unless a gastrostomy and tube feeding are carried out. Patients may also have concomitant progression of hepatic and neurologic disease.

The pathophysiology of Wilson disease is due to accumulation and toxicity of copper.[6] The average diet contains approximately 1.0 milligrams of copper per day, which is in excess by approximately 0.25 milligrams. Healthy people excrete excess copper in the bile for loss in the stool. Wilson disease patients have mutations in one of the genes coding for a liver protein in the excretory pathway[15–17] and can not excrete excess copper in the bile.[18] The excess copper accumulates and is first stored in the liver. As the storage capacity of the liver is exceeded, liver damage begins, probably in early childhood in most patients. In addition, excess "free" copper begins to circulate in the blood and accumulate in other organs. The next most sensitive organ is the brain, particularly those parts of the brain that coordinate movement. Damage in these brain areas leads

Table 13–1. Usefulness of various tests for diagnosis of Wilson disease

Test	Difficulty	Usefulness
Serum Cp assay	Easy	Some: 80–90% of patients have low values, but 10–20% have intermediate to normal values; 20% of carriers have low to intermediate values. Infants up to six months old have low values.
24-hour urine copper assay	Fairly easy	Useful in symptomatic patients whose levels are always elevated. Results of half of the presymptomatic patients are normal. Obstructive liver disease can give false positive results.
Slit lamp examination for KF rings	Easy	Some: Diagnostic in neurologic/psychiatric patients; positive only part of the time in other patients
Hepatic copper assay from liver biopsy	Hard and invasive	Excellent: Closest to a "gold standard"; false negatives are rare, but can occur in obstructive liver disease
DNA mutation analysis	Requires a specialized laboratory	Only small from a practical standpoint; too many mutations for accurate testing of many affected patients
DNA haplotype analysis	Patients and family samples must be sent to a special laboratory.	Excellent for genotyping full siblings of an affected patient. Siblings can be accurately typed into affected, carrier, and clear.

to a neurologic movement disorder in approximately half of the patients. There is no information as to why these patients develop brain damage and the others do not.

In healthy people, approximately 90% of serum copper is covalently bound to the ceruloplasmin (Cp) molecule and is "safe" in the sense that it is not available to cause copper toxicity. The other 10% is more loosely bound to albumin and small molecules in the blood and is called "free." In Wilson disease, the Cp levels are usually low, but the free copper pool is greatly expanded, leading to copper toxicity. The mechanism of copper toxicity is generally considered to be oxidant damage.[6] Copper causes oxidant damage to proteins, lipids, deoxyribonucleic acid (DNA), membranes, and so forth.

Wilson disease is inherited as an autosomal recessive gene. The causative gene is ATP7b, which is located on chromosome 13 and codes for a protein in the biliary excretory pathway.[15-17] There are more than 300 causative mutations worldwide,[19] and, in most populations, no small set of mutations is common enough to allow DNA diagnosis in a large proportion (e.g., 95%) of the cases. Thus, DNA mutation analysis with current technology is not available as a primary diagnostic tool. The nature of various mutations has not clarified why some patients are primarily hepatic and some are primarily neurologic, so the answer to this question must be elsewhere, such as in modifying genes or environmental effects.

The usefulness of various tests for the diagnosis of Wilson disease is shown in Table 13–1. Table 13–2 shows diagnostic criteria for the different presentations

Table 13–2. Diagnostic criteria for different presentations of Wilson disease

Presentation	Diagnostic criteria	Comment
Neurologic	Positive KF rings and 24-h urine copper > 100 μg	These two tests are adequate for diagnosis.
Hepatic (with no or little obstructive component)	Liver copper > 200 μg/g dry weight, and 24-h urine copper > 100 μg	These two tests are diagnostic in the absence of obstructive disease.
Hepatic (with significant obstructive component)	Liver copper > 200 μg/g dry weight, 24-h urine copper > 100 μg, and serum Cp < 15 mg/dL	Low Cp adds to a positive diagnosis when an obstructive component is present.
None (presymptomatic patient)	Positive KF rings and 24-h urine copper > 100 μg or If KF rings are negative and/or if 24-h urine copper < 100 μg: Liver copper > 200 μg/g dry weight	These two tests are adequate for diagnosis. If either or both KF rings and urine copper are negative, a liver copper will be diagnostic.

of Wilson disease. The diagnosis of Wilson disease in the neurologic form of the disease is straightforward (Table 13–2).[4,6] More than 99% of these patients have Kayser–Fleischer (KF) rings – copper deposits at the rim of the cornea that can best be reliably detected by a slit lamp examination by an ophthalmologist (Figure 13–1). Thus, heavy use of this simple test in young patients with tremor, apparent Parkinson disease, dystonia, the sudden appearance of loss of focus or odd behaviors would lead to more rapid diagnosis in many patients who may go months or years before a proper diagnosis is made. A 24-hour urine copper value, always greater than 100 micrograms in symptomatic patients (normal: 20–50 micrograms), can be used for confirmation.[4,6] A liver biopsy need not be done, but if it is it will show a diagnostic liver copper greater than 200 μg/g dry weight (normal: 20–50 μg/g).

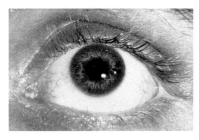

Figure 13–1: The KF ring, as seen by direct observation. These rings are brownish, sometimes greenish-brown, rings around the rim of the cornea. They begin in the upper pole, followed by the lower pole, then gradually complete the circle. They are the result of deposits of copper in these areas. It must be emphasized that the presence of these partial or complete rings can be detected accurately, as in this patient, in only a minority of patients who really have them. In direct observation, errors may be made in seeing apparent rings when they are not really there (occasionally) and missing rings when they are there (often). A slit lamp examination by an ophthalmologist is required for accurate assessment of the presence or absence of KF rings. *See color plate.*

The diagnosis of Wilson disease in the liver presentation is sometimes more difficult.[1-6] The KF rings are present in only approximately half of patients. Twenty-four-hour urine copper and liver copper are always elevated but can be elevated in other liver diseases, particularly those with a good deal of obstruction (Table 13–2). The serum Cp value can be useful because it is low in 90% of patients, but it is also low in

Table 13–3. Oral anticopper drugs used in Wilson disease

Drug	Mechanism of action	Usual dose regimen	Comment
Zinc	Induction of intestinal MT and blockade of copper absorption	50 mg 3 × /d, avoid food	Quite well tolerated with few side effects but slow acting
Trientine	Copper chelation and increased urinary excretion of copper	250 mg 4 × /d or 500 mg 2 × /d, avoid food	Causes neurologic worsening in about $1/4$ of neurologic patients; an cause several serious side effects
Penicillamine	Copper chelation and increased urinary excretion of copper	250 mg 4 × /d or 500 mg 2 × /d, avoid food	Causes neurologic worsening in about $1/2$ of neurologic patients; many and frequent serious side effects
TM	Complexes copper and protein, preventing copper absorption, and complexing toxic copper of the blood rendering it nontoxic	20 mg 3 × /d with meals, and 20 mg 3 × /d between meals for 2 weeks, then 10 mg 3 × /d with meals and 10 mg 3 × /d between meals for 14 weeks	Optimal therapy for the neurologic presentation because it prevents almost all neurologic worsening, but not yet commercially available

approximately 20% of gene carriers, who comprise approximately 1% of the population. Diagnostically elevated urine and liver copper, in the absence of serious obstructive liver disease, are generally enough to make the diagnosis, with a low Cp and/or the presence of KF rings helpful confirmation.

The diagnosis of the presymptomatic patient is straightforward if he or she has KF rings (approximately one third) and diagnostically elevated urine copper (approximately one half).[4,6] If the patient has normal urine copper by age 15 years, he or she is considered clear. If the urine copper falls between 50 and 100 μg/d, the patient will require a liver biopsy, which will be greater than 200 μg/g dry weight in affected presymptomatic patients (Table 13–2).

OVERVIEW OF THERAPEUTIC AGENTS

Many drugs are used to treat the hepatic, neurologic, and psychiatric manifestations of Wilson disease. There is nothing specific to Wilson disease with regard to the use of these drugs, so here we will focus only on agents designed to attack the basic cause of the disease, excess copper. These drugs are called anticopper drugs: Three are commercially available, and one is in development. They are listed, along with information about each, in Table 13–3. Our recommendations for which drug or drugs to use in various categories of Wilson disease patients are shown in Table 13–4.

Penicillamine

Penicillamine was developed by Walshe in 1956 and was the first orally effective anticopper agent for the treatment of Wilson disease.[20] It is a reductive chelator,

Table 13–4. Recommended therapies for various categories of Wilson disease

Category of patient	First-choice therapy	Second-choice therapy
Maintenance after initial therapy	Zinc	Trientine
Presymptomatic	Zinc	Trientine
Pregnant	Zinc	Trientine
Pediatric	Zinc	Trientine
Initial neurologic/psychiatric	TM	Zinc
Initial hepatic failure	Zinc and trientine	Zinc and penicillamine

which means that it reduces copper to Cu^+ from Cu^{++}, thus lowering its affinity for proteins and allowing chelation. Penicillamine mobilizes copper from body stores, primarily the liver stores, and flushes it through the bloodstream for excretion in the urine. It is effective at producing a large negative copper balance. For example, it is not unusual for urinary excretion of copper during early penicillamine therapy to reach 10 mg/d, which, with a 1.0-milligram intake, means a 9 milligram negative copper balance.

Penicillamine is effective for the treatment of the liver-disease patient and the presymptomatic patient. Generally, abnormal liver function tests (LFTs) will return to normal values within 6–12 months.[3] The dose is generally 1.0 g/d in two or four divided doses.[3] Each dose should be given at least one-half hour before meals or at least two hours after meals. Penicillamine has a long list of side effects, many of them serious.[6] Perhaps 20% of patients have an initial hypersensitivity reaction, which can be overcome with steroids or a drug holiday and restarted at a much lower dose. Other side effects of varying frequency and severity include proteinuria; bone-marrow depression; skin wrinkling and other dermatologic disorders; autoimmune effects, such as systemic lupus erythematosus or Goodpasture syndrome; arthralgias and arthritis; susceptibility to infections; possible aneurysms; and others.

Penicillamine therapy in terms of efficacy is often monitored by following 24-hour urine copper, but using the 24-hour urine copper value is problematic because the drug effect, and the remaining load of mobilizable body copper, both contribute to urine copper. A better way to monitor is to follow the free copper of the blood by simultaneously measuring serum copper and Cp, and subtracting the Cp copper from the serum copper.

I do not recommend penicillamine for the treatment of neurologically presenting Wilson disease because of the high risk (approximately 50%) of making the neurologic disease worse, with many of the patients who worsen never recovering (Table 13–3).[21]

Penicillamine is approved for the treatment of Wilson disease without specification as to the type or phase of the disease.

Trientine

Trientine was also developed by Walshe, in 1982,[22] and was approved for the treatment of Wilson disease patients intolerant of penicillamine. It is also a copper chelator that causes increased excretion of copper in the urine, although at a considerably lower level than penicillamine.

The dose of trientine and the prohibition against concomitant food intake are identical to those of penicillamine.[3] Although it is approved only for penicillamine-intolerant patients, it is increasingly seeing somewhat broader use. (See, e.g., our recommendations in Table 13–4). Some doctors use it for treating the pregnant Wilson disease patient, because penicillamine is teratogenic, and it seems to be effective and well tolerated in this use.[23] We use it in combination with zinc for the initial four- to six-month treatment of the liver-failure presentation (Table 13–4).[24] It is sometimes used as maintenance therapy, even though the patients are not penicillamine intolerant. The monitoring of trientine therapy for efficacy is identical to that of penicillamine therapy.

We do not recommend the use of trientine for the treatment of neurologically presenting patients because we have found that it makes these patients worse about one fourth of the time, and five of the six patients who worsened on trientine did very badly, three dying and two others never recovering (Table 13–3).[25]

The side effects of trientine therapy are similar to those of penicillamine in that they include proteinuria, bone-marrow depression, and autoimmune effects, but at a much lower frequency.

Zinc

Zinc was first used in a few Wilson disease patients by Schouwink, in The Netherlands, who published his work only in a thesis.[26] There was some follow-up work on zinc sulfate therapy by Hoogenraad and colleagues, also in The Netherlands,[27,28] but most of the development of zinc, leading to U.S. Food and Drug Administration (FDA) approval in 1997, was done by our group using zinc acetate.[13,24,29–45] Zinc is officially designated as an orphan drug.

Zinc acts by inducing metallothionein (MT) in the intestinal cell.[39] The MT has a high affinity for copper and binds food copper as well as copper from endogenous secretions, such as saliva and gastric juices. The MT copper complex is held in the intestinal cell, without transfer to the blood, until the cells slough, with an approximately six-day turnover time, causing the excretion of the copper in the stool. Thus, zinc produces an intestinal block of copper absorption. It takes approximately two weeks of zinc administration to fully induce intestinal MT.[39] Zinc produces a mild negative copper balance, up to approximately 1.5 mg/d, as a result of blocking absorption of both food and endogenously secreted copper.[30,37,41]

Zinc is approved for maintenance therapy of Wilson disease patients,[43] and this includes the treatment of the presymptomatic patient from the beginning,[13] the treatment of the pregnant patient,[45] and the treatment of pediatric patients in the maintenance phase (Table 13–4).[44] The adult dose is 50 milligrams three times per day, each dose separated from food and beverages other than water by at least one hour. It has been shown that the minimal dose to keep MT induced is 25 milligrams three times per day or 37.5 milligrams two times per day,[41] but the 50 milligrams three times per day dose is designed to produce a safety factor against poor compliance in this lifelong therapy. The recommended pediatric doses are 25 milligrams two times per day until age six, 25 milligrams three times per day until age 15 or until a body weight of 125 pounds is reached, and then the adult dose.[44,46]

The main side effect of zinc is gastric irritation (or sometimes nausea in approximately 10% of patients).[43] This side effect often wears off after a few doses. Often the offending dose is the one taken before breakfast. Taking the first dose halfway between breakfast and lunch often relieves this problem. In cases of continuing intolerance, offending doses can be taken together with a little protein, such as a piece of lunchmeat or cheese, because protein interferes the least with zinc penetration into the intestinal cell.

Monitoring of zinc therapy for efficacy[43] is much easier and more straightforward than is monitoring of penicillamine and trientine because zinc has no direct effect on urine copper excretion. Thus, the 24-hour urine copper is a direct reflection of the mobilizable body load of copper. The 24-hour urine copper should decrease during the first year of zinc therapy to 125 micrograms or less. It will remain fairly stable between 50 and 125 micrograms for years.[43] When it begins to get into the normal range (20–50 micrograms), the patient should be occasionally evaluated for overtreatment copper deficiency, the first indication of which would be anemia and/or leukopenia. A significant increase in urine copper level (e.g., more than 25% or so, confirmed by a second test) suggests poor compliance. Another excellent way to evaluate compliance is to measure zinc on the same 24-hour urine sample.[43] In well-complying patients, the 24-hour urine zinc level should be a least 2.0 milligrams (normal: 0.2–0.5 milligrams). With poor compliance, the urine zinc level will decrease well before the urine copper level increases. We recommend monitoring urine copper and zinc levels every 3–6 months in the beginning, reducing the monitoring to every 6–12 months in well-complying patients, but never less than annually.

Tetrathiomolybdate

Tetrathiomolybdate (TM) is not yet FDA-approved. It is being developed by our group for the initial treatment of the neurologic presentation of Wilson disease.[25,47-50] It is officially designated as an orphan product.

TM has a unique mode of action. It forms a tripartite complex with copper, protein, and itself (Tables 13–3 and 13–4).[51-54] If given with food, it uses food protein to form the complex with food and endogenously secreted copper. This copper is not absorbed, and this blockade of copper absorption puts the patient into an immediate negative copper balance.[47] If given between meals, it is well-absorbed and forms the complex with free copper of the blood, albumin, and itself. The copper in this complex is not available for cellular uptake. The complex builds up in the blood, reaching a stable level in a few days, when the metabolism of the complex by the liver equals the buildup of new complex.[47] The free copper in the blood is reduced to zero within two weeks or less.[47-50] Thus further copper toxicity, which is dependent on free copper, is stopped within two weeks or less.

The dose of TM that has been used in most of our studies is 120 mg/d, with 20 milligrams three times per day with meals and 20 milligrams three times per day between meals given for eight weeks.[25,47–50] With this dose, approximately 16% of Wilson disease patients develop significant elevations of transaminase enzymes, and approximately 12% develop anemia and/or leukopenia.[25] The first side effect seems to be due to shifting copper pools, because it has not been seen in TM-treated non-Wilson patients.[55–58] It is easily treatable with a drug holiday and/or halving the dose. It is transitory and does not involve abnormalities in other LFTs. The second side effects appears to be due to bone-marrow depletion of copper. It also responds to a drug holiday and/or halving the dose. A new dose regimen, presented in Table 13–3, and discussed in the "TM" subsection of the "Results of Therapy" section, is now recommended to reduce these two side effects.

It is important to monitor TM therapy weekly after approximately Week 3 for transaminase levels and blood counts, but there is no efficacy monitoring recommended other than frequent neurologic examinations.

RESULTS OF THERAPY

If patients with Wilson disease are not treated with an anticopper drug, they progress with liver disease and/or neurologic disease and die. There is one exception to this that we know about: Vegetarianism can halt the progression of the disease or prevent it from becoming symptomatic[59] because the copper from vegetables is not as well absorbed as the copper from meat, and this seems to offset the failure to excrete excess copper in the bile. Not enough vegetarians with Wilson disease have been studied to know that this approach is always effective, so we should not rely on it.

Patients with Wilson disease can be treated with the chelators, penicillamine and trientine. These are effective maintenance therapies, the drawbacks being the long list of side effects with penicillamine, some of which develop quite late after years of therapy, and the somewhat shorter list of side effects with trientine. The initial treatment of the liver presentation can also be carried out with one of these drugs. In fact, our current recommendation for treating the liver-failure presentation, assuming the failure is not so severe as to mandate liver transplantation, is a combination of trientine and zinc.

Both of these chelators are contraindicated for the treatment of the initial neurologic presentation of Wilson disease. Our survey data indicate a 50% rate of worsening of neurologic status in patients treated with penicillamine,[21] and our double-blind study indicates a 26% rate of worsening with trientine.[25] Many of the patients who worsen do not do well, never recover, and are left with severe lifelong disability and often an early death.

Because zinc and TM are the newer drugs, and are the major subject of this chapter, we will spend a little more time reviewing results of therapy with these drugs.

Zinc

The use of zinc in Wilson disease patients in recommended doses and away from food will block copper absorption, as shown by copper absorption studies, and this blockage correlates with the induction of intestinal cell MT.[39] The minimally effective dose of zinc in adults to cause a consistent negative copper balance is 25 milligrams three times per day, or 37.5 milligrams two times per day.[37,41] Giving 75 milligrams one time per day is not adequately affective. The standard recommended dose, to produce a safety factor, is 50 milligrams three times per day.

The use of 50 milligrams of zinc three times per day over many years of follow-up in patients previously treated with penicillamine has shown zinc to be a uniformly effective maintenance therapy.[43] It prevents the reaccumulation of copper and the reappearance or worsening of neurologic symptoms and LFT abnormalities. It is not uncommon for aspartate aminotransferase (AST) and/or alanine aminotransferase (ALT) levels to be at the upper limit of normal or a little higher than the upper limits of normal during chronic zinc therapy, but these values do not progressively increase and are not accompanied by abnormalities of other LFTs. An increase in AST or ALT is also seen in maintenance therapy with penicillamine, and it is probably due to the slow release of copper from liver stores, which remain high for many years.

As discussed earlier in this chapter, zinc therapy can be monitored by following 24-hour urine copper and zinc.[43] With effective zinc therapy, urine copper should level out at less than 125 μg/24 hours. It has been our experience that, when patients develop worsening of symptoms or worsening LFT values, the urine copper and zinc values always reveal a problem with compliance with the zinc regimen. Usually when confronted with the urine data, these patients admit poor compliance.

There are occasional isolated case reports of "failure" of zinc therapy.[60–62] When we have examined these reports, in no case have we found that there was evidence of good compliance. Generally these case reports have not included urine zinc data, which are necessary to be able to best check for noncompliance.

The other drugs available for maintenance therapy, penicillamine and trientine, are equally efficacious to zinc, given good compliance. Thus the choice of maintenance drug is based on differences in side effects. Here zinc is the clear winner because it appears to have no significant side effects, aside from a low frequency of gastric irritation, whereas penicillamine and trientine both have a significant number of side effects, some of them serious. Another factor in the choice of maintenance therapy, especially in developing counties, is cost. The approved pharmaceutical preparations of zinc sold in the United States, Europe, and Japan are relatively expensive, but salts of zinc (such as zinc gluconate and zinc sulfate) are inexpensive and sold over the counter in pharmacies and health food stores around the world. Use of this source of zinc allows therapy of Wilson disease in large numbers of patients around the world who could not otherwise afford it. If these preparations of zinc contain the labeled amount of zinc, they are as effective as the pharmaceutical preparations. Because they are not regulated, however, there is no verification that the label is correct and that they do not contain dangerous contaminants.

Zinc is also effective for the treatment of the presymptomatic patient from the beginning, and there is good follow-up in a fairly large number of presymptomatic patients to confirm efficacy.[13,43] Penicillamine or trientine is also efficacious in these patients. Again, choice depends on side effects.

The pregnant Wilson disease patient should continue maintenance anti-copper therapy to protect her own health. During the period when penicillamine was the only or primary maintenance therapy, many pregnant Wilson disease patients stopped their penicillamine because of the known teratogenic effects of penicillamine, and they suffered severe recurrence of their disease, including death.[6] Zinc is an excellent choice for therapy during pregnancy, protecting the health of the mother and generally allowing the birth of healthy babies.[45] In two cases of birth defects in babies from mothers on zinc therapy, copper control was quite tight.[45] Because copper deficiency is a known teratogen, it is suggested that control of copper levels be loosened during pregnancy, whether therapy is with zinc or another agent. According to scattered reports, trientine also seems to be a reasonable choice for therapy during pregnancy.[23] Penicillamine seems to be a poor choice because of its known teratogenicity.

Wilson disease should be treated as early as it is diagnosed, because there is evidence of liver damage occurring in children as young as three years.[3] Zinc is an excellent choice for the maintenance therapy of pediatric patients.[44,46] The doses that we have recommended are 25 milligrams two times per day until age six, 25 milligrams three times per day until age 15 or a body weight of 125 pounds has been reached, and then the adult dose. We have validated the efficacy of these doses in lengthy follow-up in a fairly large series of pediatric patients.[44] An Italian group, using our recommended doses, has done an excellent study in 20 pediatric patients followed for 10 years.[46] The group has confirmed the efficacy of these doses in pediatric Wilson disease. One of the good features of their study was a focus on younger children with 11 younger than six years and 20 younger than 10 years. An additional unique and exciting feature of their study was that they showed improvement in liver histology over the years of zinc therapy.

We do not believe that zinc alone is the optimum treatment for patients with the liver failure presentation of Wilson disease because it is too slow acting for these acutely ill patients. (We will hold off a discussion of zinc alone for treating the neurologically presenting patients until the next section on TM). Zinc in combination with trientine or penicillamine for the initial treatment of the liver-failure patient is the current treatment of choice, however.[24] The main reason for adding zinc to this initial therapy is that it will induce a high level of hepatic MT, which will safely sequester a significant amount of toxic hepatic copper while the faster-acting agent acts to deplete the body of copper.

We have chosen to use trientine as the fast acting chelator in combination with zinc, rather than penicillamine, because of trientine's more favorable safety profile. We have used the combination of trientine and zinc to treat nine

liver-failure patients with excellent results. To measure the severity of liver failure, we have used the Nazer prognostic index.[14] The Nazer index uses bilirubin
levels, AST levels, and prolongation of prothrombin time to develop a score that
ranges from 0 to 14, with 14 being severe disease. The Nazer group, doing their
work in the pretransplantation era, when only penicillamine therapy was available, found that patients with a score of 6 or less survived with penicillamine
therapy, whereas those with scores of 7 or more died on penicillamine therapy.
The score was developed on retrospective data, but a prospective study confirmed
its validity.[14]

In our study using trientine and zinc therapy, we were able to save the livers
(avoid hepatic transplantation) of patients with Nazer scores as high as 9.[24] We
believe that the improvement in the ability of medical therapy to save patients
from transplantation is the addition of zinc to the regimen, because we do not
believe that trientine is more efficacious than penicillamine, just less toxic. We
use the combination for four to six months, then transition to zinc maintenance
therapy.

Thus, we believe that the standard of care for treating liver-failure Wilson
disease patients with Nazer scores up to 9 is a combination of trientine and zinc.
For patients with higher Nazer scores, such as 10 or more, liver transplantation
should be immediately considered, to save the patient's life.

TM

The treatment of the neurologically presenting Wilson disease patient has been
problematic because the usual drug, penicillamine, causes a high frequency of
permanent neurologic worsening, trientine was an unknown but suspect because
it acts like penicillamine, and zinc was too slow acting for optimal therapy for
these acutely ill patients. It seemed that a new drug was needed, and we have
been developing TM to fill this therapeutic niche.

In an open-label study, 55 neurologically presenting patients were studied.[50]
Dose ranging was carried out. The study was an eight-week inpatient study in
which a semiquantitative neurologic examination (SQNE), in which the score
could range from 0 (normal) to 38, was carried out weekly. A replicable deterioration of 5 points in the score was set as indicating significant neurologic
deterioration. Of the 55 patients studied, only 2 (3.6%) reached criteria for neurologic worsening, a dramatic improvement over the estimated 50% rate for
penicillamine.[21] A dose of 120 mg/d – 20 milligrams three times per day with
meals and 20 milligrams three times per day between meals – was selected as the
dose of choice.

Subsequently, a double-blind study comparing this dose of TM to 1.0 g/d of
trientine was carried out.[25] Again, it was an eight-week inpatient study, with the
SQNE carried out weekly. The low rate of neurologic worsening with TM was
confirmed (1 in 25 patients, or 4%). Neurologic worsening in the trientine arm
occurred in 6 of 23 patients (26%), a significantly higher number than in the TM
arm ($p = 0.05$). Furthermore, five of the six patients who worsened in the trientine
arm did badly: Three patients died, and two never recovered functionally.

A problem with TM therapy is two side effects, a further increase in transaminase enzymes and anemia and/or leukopenia. For example, in the double-blind study, 4 of 25 (16%) patients had transaminase elevations, and 3 of 25 (12%) had anemia and/or leukopenia.[25] We think that the former is due to shifting copper pools in the liver, because it has not been seen in hundreds of non-Wilson patients taking TM.[55–58] The latter side effect appears to be due to bone-marrow depletion of copper, required for cellular proliferation, because the patients who develop this side effect have the lowest free copper levels in the study.[25]

Both side effects go away with a drug holiday and/or with halving the dose. Neither appear during the first weeks of therapy. Based on these facts, we designed a new double-blind study comparing the 120 mg/d, eight-week TM regimen to a new regimen.[63] The new regimen used a loading dose of 120 mg/d for 2 weeks, then a half dose of 60 mg/d for 14 weeks. A difference in this study from previous studies is that the between-meal doses were eliminated and the entire dose "away from food" was given as a single dose at bedtime. Thus during the 120 mg/d phase, patients took 20 milligrams three times per day with meals and 60 milligrams at bedtime. During the 60 mg/d phase, they took 10 milligrams three times per day with meals and 30 milligrams at bedtime.

We were able to accomplish our primary objective in this study in that 7 of 20 patients (35%) in the old (120 mg/d for eight weeks) regimen had one of the two side effects and only 1 of 20 (5%) in the new regimen had a side effect[63] – a statistically significant difference ($p < 0.02$). However, 3 of 20 patients in the new arm and 4 of 20 patients in the old arm reached criteria for neurologic worsening. These rates are higher than in our two previous studies (3.6 and 4%). We attribute these higher rates of neurologic worsening to the change in "away from food" dosing, from three between-meal doses to one single bedtime dose. Our current view is that the optimum regimen is the new regimen, but distributing the "away from food" doses as 20 milligrams three times per day between meals during the two weeks of 120 mg/d and 10 milligrams three times per day between meals during the 14 weeks of 60 mg/d.

Currently it appears that TM faces significant regulatory hurdles before FDA approval, which suggests that it may be some time before TM is available for the neurologically presenting patient. We believe that TM is by far the optimum therapy for these patients, but, until it is available, how should these patients be treated in the meantime? We believe that penicillamine and trientine are contraindicated in these patients because of the high risks and bad outcomes from neurologic worsening. Some have advocated a "baby-up" approach starting with low doses of these drugs, but, in our discussions with physicians who have used this approach, neurologic worsening still occurs with a high frequency.

In this situation, until TM is available, I recommend the use of zinc alone as initial therapy. Zinc is slow-acting, and there is risk of disease progression during the 6–12 months it takes zinc to control copper toxicity in this kind of patient. Indeed, in one of three patients with the neurologic presentation we treated with zinc alone, there was progression of a somewhat disabling tremor. Zinc does not cause drug-catalyzed worsening, as do both penicillamine and trientine, and I believe that the average outcome with zinc therapy alone will be considerably superior to that with penicillamine or trientine therapy.

FUTURE DEVELOPMENTS

I do not believe that there is a pressing need for new maintenance therapies because zinc is excellent for this purpose, with complete efficacy and no serious side effects. It is a nuisance, considering that it is lifelong therapy, to have to take it three times a day and avoid food with each dose. In the 10% or so of patients who can not take zinc because of gastric irritation, trientine seems to be a reasonable second choice.

I believe, however, that there is a need to improve zinc therapy. As with all lifelong therapies, particularly in young patients, there is a high rate of poor compliance. In our studies in patients who were followed closely and reminded if compliance became an issue, periodic poor compliance was approximately 25%, and serious noncompliance approximately 10%. Noncompliance can lead to serious relapse and even death. I believe that compliance could be substantially improved if zinc could be taken once daily instead of three times daily. In addition, occasionally poor compliance is due to the gastric irritation from the zinc salt taken on an empty stomach. Thus, a zinc preparation that could be taken once a day, and perhaps was developed so that it does not release a bolus of an irritating zinc salt in an empty stomach, would be a markedly better preparation.

There is obviously a pressing need for a therapy to initially treat the neurologically presenting Wilson disease patient. Based on our work to date, we believe that TM can fill this need well. We have shown excellent efficacy in terms of preventing neurologic deterioration while eliminating further copper toxicity. The drug is safe, with the two common side effects not being serious, and even these can be significantly reduced in frequency by using a 16-week, rather than an 8-week, drug regimen.

There are regulatory hurdles to be overcome, however, before TM can be approved. These are not insurmountable, but it appears likely that one more clinical trial will be required to achieve this goal.

Wilson disease is not a good candidate for newer techniques, such as gene therapy. The major problem is with disease recognition and diagnosis. After a patient is diagnosed, there are good drug therapies, but gene therapy would seem to add little. There is work going on in the liver-transplant area, such as partial transplants from living donors and the use of cultured normal liver cells for transplant. Of course, if stem cell technology begins to add effective treatment for more common movement disorders, such as Parkinson disease, it may become useful in Wilson disease patients with neurologic deficits.

REFERENCES

1. Brewer GJ. Recognition, diagnosis, and management of Wilson's disease. *Exp Biol Med.* 2000;223:39–46

2. Schilsky ML. Wilson disease: Genetic basis of copper toxicity and natural history. *Semin Liver Dis*. 1996;16:83–95

3. Scheinberg IH, Sternlieb I. Wilson's disease. L.H.J. Smith, ed. *Major Problems in Internal Medicine*, W.B. Saunders Company, Philadelphia, 1–171, 1984

4. Brewer GJ. *Wilson's Disease: A Clinician's Guide to Recognition, Diagnosis, and Management*, Kluwer Academic Publishers, Boston, 2001

5. Brewer GJ. Wilson's disease. AS Fauci, E Braunward, DL Kasper, Sl Hauser, DL Longo, JL Jameson, J Loscalzo, eds. *Harrison's Principles of Internal Medicine*, 17th edition, McGraw-Hill Companies, Inc., New York, 2449–2452, 2008

6. Brewer GJ, Yuzbasiyan-Gurkan V. Wilson disease. *Medicine*. 1992;71:139–164

7. Bhave SA, Pandit AN, Pradhan AM, Sidhaye DG, Kantarjian A, Williams A, Talbot IC, Tanner MS. Liver disease in India. *Arch Dis Child*. 1982;57:922–928

8. Starosta-Rubinstein S, Young AB, Kluin K, Hill G, Aisen AM, Gabrielsen T, Brewer GJ. Clinical assessment of 31 patients with Wilson's disease. Correlations with structural changes on magnetic resonance imaging. *Arch Neurol*. 1987;44:365–370

9. Fink JK, Hedera P, Brewer GJ. Hepatolenticular degeneration (Wilson's disease). *The Neurologist*. 1999;5:171–185

10. Brewer GJ, Fink JK, Hedera P. Diagnosis and treatment of Wilson's disease. *Semin Neurol*. 1999;19:261–270

11. Brewer GJ. Behavioral abnormalities in Wilson's disease. WJ Weiner, AE Lang, KE Anderson, eds. *Behavioral Neurology of Movement Disorders*, 2nd edition, Lippincott, Williams & Wilkins, Philadelphia, 262–274, 2005

12. Sternlieb I, Scheinberg IH. Prevention of Wilson's disease in asymptomatic patients. *N Engl J Med*. 1968;278:352–359

13. Brewer GJ, Dick RD, Yuzbasiyan-Gurkan V, Johnson V, Wang Y. Treatment of Wilson's disease with zinc. XIII: Therapy with zinc in presymptomatic patients from the time of diagnosis. *J Lab Clin Med*. 1994;123:849–858

14. Nazer H, Ede RJ, Mowat AP, Williams R. Wilson's disease: Clinical presentation and use of prognostic index. *Gut*. 1986;27:1377–1381

15. Bull PC, Thomas GR, Rommens JM, Forbes JR, Cox DW. The Wilson disease gene is a putative copper transporting P-type ATPase similar to the Menkes gene. *Nat Genet*. 1993;5:327–337

16. Tanzi RE, Petrukhin K, Chernov I, Pellequer JL, Wasco W, Ross B, Romano DM, Parano E, Pavone L, Brzustowicz LM Devoto M, Peppercorn J, Bush AI, Sternlieb I, Pirastu M, Gusella JF, Evgrafov O, Penchaszadeh GK, Honig B, Edelman IS, Soare MB, Scheinberg IH, Gilliam TC. The Wilson disease gene is a copper transporting ATPase with homology to the Menkes disease gene. *Nat Genet*. 1993;5:344–350

17. Yamaguchi Y, Heiny ME, Gitlin JD. Isolation and characterization of a human liver cDNA as a candidate gene for Wilson disease. *Biochem Biophys Res Commun*. 1993;197:271–277

18. Frommer DJ. Defective biliary excretion of copper in Wilson's disease. *Gut*. 1974;15:125–129

19. Cox DW, Roberts E. *Wilson Disease*, 2006 vol. Gene Clinics, University of Washington, Seattle, 1999

20. Walshe JM. Penicillamine, a new oral therapy for Wilson's disease. *Am J Med*. 1956;21:487–495

21. Brewer GJ, Terry CA, Aisen AM, Hill GM. Worsening of neurologic syndrome in patients with Wilson's disease with initial penicillamine therapy. *Arch Neurol*. 1987;44:490–493

22. Walshe JM. Treatment of Wilson's disease with trientine (triethylene tetramine) dihydrochloride. *Lancet*. 1982;1:643–647

23. Walshe JM. The management of pregnancy in Wilson's disease treated with trientine. *Q J Med*. 1986;58:81–87

24. Askari FK, Greenson J, Dick RD, Johnson VD, Brewer GJ. Treatment of Wilson's disease with zinc. XVIII. Initial treatment of the hepatic decompensation presentation with trientine and zinc. *J Lab Clin Med*. 2003;142:385–390

25. Brewer GJ, Askari F, Lorincz MT, Carlson M, Schilsky M, Kluin KJ, Hedera P, Moretti P, Fink JK, Tankanow R, Dick RB, Sitterly J. Treatment of Wilson disease with ammonium tetrathiomolybdate: IV. Comparison of tetrathiomolybdate and trientine in a double-blind study of treatment of the neurologic presentation of Wilson disease. *Arch Neurol.* 2006;63:521–527

26. Schouwink G. *De hepatocecerebrale degeneratie, met een onderzoek naar de zonkstrofwisseling.* MD thesis (with a summary in English, French, and German). University of Amsterdam, 1961

27. Hoogenraad TU, Van Den Hamer CJ, Van Hattum J. Effective treatment of Wilson's disease with oral zinc sulphate: Two case reports. *Br Med J (Clin Res Ed).* 1984;289:273–276

28. Hoogenraad TU, Van Hattum J, Van Den Hamer CJA. Management of Wilson's disease with zinc sulfate. Experience in a series of 27 patients. *J Neurol Sci.* 1987;77:137–146

29. Brewer GJ, Hill GM, Prasad AS, Cossack ZT, Rabbani P. Oral zinc therapy for Wilson's disease. *Ann Intern Med.* 1983;99:314–319

30. Hill GM, Brewer GJ, Prasad AS, Hydrick CR, Hartmann DE. Treatment of Wilson's disease with zinc. I. Oral zinc therapy regimens. *Hepatology.* 1987;7:522–528

31. Hill GM, Brewer GJ, Juni JE, Prasad AS, Dick RD. Treatment of Wilson's disease with zinc. II. Validation of oral 64copper with copper balance. *Am J Med Sci.* 1986;292:344–349

32. Brewer GJ, Hill GM, Dick RD, Nostrant TT, Sams JS, Wells JJ, Prasad AS. Treatment of Wilson's disease with zinc: III. Prevention of reaccumulation of hepatic copper. *J Lab Clin Med.* 1987;109:526–531

33. Brewer GJ, Hill G, Prasad A, Dick R. The treatment of Wilson's disease with zinc. IV. Efficacy monitoring using urine and plasma copper. *Proc Soc Exp Biol Med.* 1987;184:446–455

34. Yuzbasiyan-Gurkan V, Brewer GJ, Abrams GD, Main B, Giacherio D. Treatment of Wilson's disease with zinc. V. Changes in serum levels of lipase, amylase, and alkaline phosphatase in patients with Wilson's disease. *J Lab Clin Med.* 1989;114:520–526

35. Brewer GJ, Yuzbasiyan-Gurkan V, Lee DY, Appelman H. Treatment of Wilson's disease with zinc. VI. Initial treatment studies. *J Lab Clin Med.* 1989;114:633–638

36. Lee DY, Brewer GJ, Wang YX. Treatment of Wilson's disease with zinc. VII. Protection of the liver from copper toxicity by zinc-induced metallothionein in a rat model. *J Lab Clin Med.* 1989;114:639–645

37. Brewer GJ, Yuzbasiyan-Gurkan V, Dick R. Zinc therapy of Wilson's disease: VIII. Dose response studies. *J Trace Elem Exp Med.* 1990;3:227–234

38. Brewer GJ, Yuzbasiyan-Gurkan V, Johnson V. Treatment of Wilson's disease with zinc. IX: Response of serum lipids. *J Lab Clin Med.* 1991;118:466–470

39. Yuzbasiyan-Gurkan V, Grider A, Nostrant T, Cousins RJ, Brewer GJ. Treatment of Wilson's disease with zinc. X. Intestinal metallothionein induction. *J Lab Clin Med.* 1992;120:380–386

40. Brewer GJ, Yuzbasiyan-Gurkan V, Johnson V, Dick RD, Wang Y. Treatment of Wilson's disease with zinc: XI. Interaction with other anticopper agents. *J Am Coll Nutr.* 1993;12:26–30

41. Brewer GJ, Yuzbasiyan-Gurkan V, Johnson V, Dick RD, Wang Y. Treatment of Wilson's disease with zinc XII: Dose regimen requirements. *Am J Med Sci.* 1993;305:199–202

42. Brewer GJ, Johnson V, Kaplan J. Treatment of Wilson's disease with zinc: XIV. Studies of the effect of zinc on lymphocyte function. *J Lab Clin Med.* 1997;129:649–652

43. Brewer GJ, Dick RD, Johnson VD, Brunberg JA, Kluin KJ, Fink JK. Treatment of Wilson's disease with zinc: XV. Long-term follow-up studies. *J Lab Clin Med.* 1998;132:264–278

44. Brewer GJ, Dick RD, Johnson VD, Fink JK, Kluin KJ, Daniels S. Treatment of Wilson's disease with zinc XVI: Treatment during the pediatric years. *J Lab Clin Med.* 2001;137:191–198

45. Brewer GJ, Johnson VD, Dick RD, Fink JK, Kluin KJ, Hedera P. Treatment of Wilson's disease with zinc XVII: Treatment during pregnancy. *Hepatology.* 2000;31:364–370

46. Marcellini M, Di Ciommo V, Callea F, Devito R, Comparcola D, Sartorelli MR, Carelli G, Nobili B. Treatment of Wilson's disease with zinc from the time of diagnosis in pediatric patients: A single-hospital, 10-year follow-up study. *J Lab Clin Med*. 2005;145:139–143

47. Brewer GJ, Dick RD, Yuzbasiyan-Gurkan V, Tankanow R, Young AB, Kluin KJ. Initial therapy of patients with Wilson's disease with tetrathiomolybdate. *Arch Neurol*. 1991;48:42–47

48. Brewer GJ, Dick RD, Johnson V, Wang Y, Yuzbasiyan-Gurkan V, Kluin K, Fink JK, Aisen A. Treatment of Wilson's disease with ammonium tetrathiomolybdate. I. Initial therapy in 17 neurologically affected patients. *Arch Neurol*. 1994;51:545–554

49. Brewer GJ, Johnson V, Dick RD, Kluin KJ, Fink JK, Brunberg JA. Treatment of Wilson disease with ammonium tetrathiomolybdate. II. Initial therapy in 33 neurologically affected patients and follow-up with zinc therapy. *Arch Neurol*. 1996;53:1017–1025

50. Brewer GJ, Hedera P, Kluin KJ, Carlson M, Askari F, Dick RB, Sitterly J, Fink JK. Treatment of Wilson disease with ammonium tetrathiomolybdate: III. Initial therapy in a total of 55 neurologically affected patients and follow-up with zinc therapy. *Arch Neurol*. 2003;60:379–385

51. Bremner I, Mills CF, Young BW. Copper metabolism in rats given di- or trithiomolybdates. *J Inorg Biochem*. 1982;16:109–119

52. Gooneratne SR, Howell JM, Gawthorne JM. An investigation of the effects of intravenous administration of thiomolybdate on copper metabolism in chronic Cu-poisoned sheep. *Br J Nutr*. 1981;46:469–480

53. Mills CF, El-Gallad TT, Bremner I. Effects of molybdate, sulfide, and tetrathiomolybdate on copper metabolism in rats. *J Inorg Biochem*. 1981;14:189–207

54. Mills CF, El-Gallad TT, Bremner I, Weham G. Copper and molybdenum absorption by rats given ammonium tetrathiomolybdate. *J Inorg Biochem*. 1981;14:163–175

55. Gartner EM, Griffith KA, Pan Q, Brewer GJ, Henja GF, Merajver SD, Zalupski MM. A pilot trial of the anti-angiogenic copper lowering agent tetrathiomolybdate in combination with irinotecan, 5-flurouracil, and leucovorin for metastatic colorectal cancer. *Invest New Drugs*. 2009;27(2):159–165; epub 2008 Aug 20

56. Henry NL, Dunn R, Merjaver S, Pan Q, Pienta KJ, Brewer G, Smith DC. Phase II trial of copper depletion with tetrathiomolybdate as an antiangiogenesis strategy in patients with hormone refractory prostate cancer. *Oncology*. 2006;71:168–175

57. Redman BG, Esper P, Pan Q, Dunn RL, Hussain HK, Chenevert T, Brewer GJ, Merajver SD. Phase II trial of tetrathiomolybdate in patients with advanced kidney cancer. *Clin Cancer Res*. 2003;9:1666–1672

58. Pass HI, Brewer GJ, Dick R, Carbone M, Merajver S. A phase II trial of tetrathiomolybdate after surgery for malignant mesothelioma: Final results. *Ann Thorac Surg*. 2008;86:383–389

59. Brewer GJ, Yuzbasiyan-Gurkan V, Dick R, Wang Y, Johnson V. Does a vegetarian diet control Wilson's disease? *J Am Coll Nutr*. 1993;12:527–530

60. Mishra D, Kalra V, Seth R. Failure of prophylactic zinc in Wilson disease. *Indian Pediatr*. 2008;45:151–153

61. Walshe JM, Munro NA. Zinc-induced deterioration in Wilson's disease aborted by treatment with penicillamine, dimercaprol, and a novel zero copper diet. *Arch Neurol*. 1995;52:10–11

62. Lang CJ, Rabas-Kolominsky P, Engelhardt A, Kobras G, Konig HJ. Fatal deterioration of Wilson's disease after institution of oral zinc therapy. *Arch Neurol*. 1993;50:1007–1008

63. Brewer GJ, Askari F, Lorincz MT, Carlson M. Kluin KJ, Fink JK, Dick RB, Sitterly J. Treatment of Wilson's disease with ammonium tetrathiomolybdate V: New dosage regimen to reduce side effects. In preparation

14 Small copper complexes for treatment of acquired and inherited copper deficiency syndromes

Stephen G. Kaler

INTRODUCTION

Copper is a trace element present in nearly all tissues and is required for cellular respiration, connective tissue integrity, iron homeostasis, myelination of axons, neurotransmitter biosynthesis, peptide amidation, and pigment formation.[1] Human copper deficiency may be inherited or acquired, and both versions display a preferential impact on neurologic function, with effects ranging from major developmental brain abnormalities, as in classical Menkes disease, to myeloneuropathy and peripheral neuropathy, as in acquired copper deficiency. Other human neurological disorders also feature altered copper metabolism or aberrant copper–protein interactions.[2]

This chapter discusses the major copper deficiency conditions, delineates their varied neurological effects, and outlines the role of small molecule copper complexes as therapeutic interventions for these disorders.

ACQUIRED COPPER DEFICIENCY

It is known that adults with acquired copper deficiency due to excess zinc ingestion, malabsorption, gastric bypass surgery, or nephrotic syndrome may develop myeloneuropathy involving a profound sensory ataxia that improves or stabilizes in response to copper repletion.[3-7] Signs of lower motor neuron disease, including proximal and distal muscle weakness and bilateral foot drops, have also been reported in copper-deficient individuals.[8] Taken together, these reports indicate that (1) copper deficiency may cause disease via selective demyelination or other damage to the somatosensory pathways of the spinal cord, and (2) motor and sensory neurons of the peripheral nervous system in adults may be particularly sensitive to perturbations in copper homeostasis. Treatment with oral copper gluconate or copper sulfate, or parenteral cupric chloride or copper histidine, stabilizes or resolves the neurological symptoms.[3-8]

INHERITED COPPER DEFICIENCY SYNDROMES

Menkes disease

Menkes disease is an X-linked recessive disorder of copper transport caused by diverse mutations in a copper-transporting adenosine triphosphate (ATP)ase, ATP7A.[1] Newborns with this typically fatal neurodegenerative condition may respond well to early copper treatment if their mutation does not completely abrogate ATP7A function.[9,10]

As an X-linked disease, Menkes disease typically occurs in male infants who present at two to three months of age with loss of previously obtained developmental milestones and the onset of hypotonia, seizures, and failure to thrive. Characteristic physical changes of the hair and facies, in conjunction with typical neurological findings, often suggest the diagnosis. The presenting signs and symptoms of 127 patients reported in the medical literature up to 1985 were compiled.[11] The less distinctive appearance of young affected infants before the onset of neurodegeneration is discussed separately (see "Menkes disease in the neonatal period"). In the natural history of classical Menkes disease, death usually occurs by three years of age.[1,11]

The scalp hair of classically affected infants is short, sparse, coarse, and twisted. The hair is often less abundant and even shorter on the sides and the back of the head than on the top. The twisted strands may be reminiscent of those in steel wool cleaning pads. The eyebrows usually share the unusual appearance. Light microscopy of patient hair will illustrate pathognomonic pili torti (180-degree twisting of the hair shaft) and often other abnormalities, including trichoclasis (transverse fracture of the hair shaft) and trichoptilosis (longitudinal splitting of the shaft). The hair tends to be lightly pigmented and may show unusual colors, such as white, silver or gray, but in some cases is normally pigmented.

The face is jowly with sagging cheeks and ears that often appear large. The palate tends to be highly arched, and tooth eruption is delayed. Noisy, sonorous breathing is often evident. Pectus excavatum is a common thoracic finding. Umbilical and/or inguinal herniae may be present. The skin often appears loose and redundant, particularly at the nape of the neck and on the trunk.

Neurologically, profound truncal hypotonia with poor head control is invariably present. Appendicular tone may be increased with thumbs held in an adducted, cortical posture. Deep tendon reflexes are often hyperactive. The suck and cry are usually strong. Visual fixation and tracking are commonly impaired, whereas hearing is normal. Neurodevelopmental skills are invariably delayed. Growth failure commences shortly after the onset of neurodegeneration and is asymmetric, with linear growth relatively preserved in comparison to weight and head circumference.

Clinical diagnostic tests are often characteristic. White matter abnormalities reflecting impaired myelination, diffuse atrophy, ventriculomegaly, and tortuosity of cerebral blood vessels are typical findings on brain magnetic resonance imaging. Subdural hematomas are common in infants, and cerebrovascular accidents can occur in patients who survive longer. The "corkscrew" appearance of cerebral vessels is well-visualized by magnetic resonance angiography, a noninvasive method for study of the vasculature. Dysplastic coronary vessels may be detectable by echocardiography. Electroencephalograms are usually moderately to severely abnormal, although normal tracings have been recorded in some classically affected individuals. Pelvic ultrasonography reveals diverticula of the urinary bladder in nearly all patients. Radiographs often disclose abnormalities of bone formation in the skull (Wormian bones), long bones (metaphyseal spurring), and ribs (anterior flaring, multiple fractures).

The biochemical phenotype in Menkes disease involves (1) low levels of copper in plasma, liver, and brain due to impaired intestinal absorption; (2) reduced activities of numerous copper-dependent enzymes; and (3) paradoxical accumulation of copper in certain tissues (duodenum, kidney, spleen, pancreas, skeletal muscle, placenta). The copper-retention phenotype is also evident in cultured fibroblasts and lymphoblasts, in which reduced egress of radiolabeled copper is demonstrable in pulse-chase experiments. This constellation of biochemical findings denotes a primary defect of copper transport that begins with impaired absorption at the intestinal level and continues with failed utilization and handling of copper conveyed to other cells in the body.

Certain clinical features of Menkes disease are related to deficient activity of specific copper-requiring enzymes, and one can speculate on the effects that reduced activity of other copper enzymes would produce. Partial deficiency of dopamine beta-hydroxylase, a critical enzyme in the catecholamine biosynthetic pathway, is responsible for a distinctively abnormal plasma and cerebrospinal fluid (CSF) neurochemical pattern in Menkes patients.[9,12,13] The copper-dependent enzyme, peptidylglycine alpha-amidating monooxygenase (PAM), is required for removal of the carboxy-terminal glycine residue characteristic of numerous neuroendocrine peptide precursors (e.g., gastrin, cholecystokinin, vasoactive intestinal peptide, corticotropin-releasing hormone, thyrotropin-releasing hormone, calcitonin, vasopressin).[14] Failure to amidate these precursors can result in 100- to 1,000-fold diminution of bioactivity compared to the mature, amidated forms. Although deficiency of tyrosinase, a copper enzyme needed for melanin biosynthesis, is considered to be responsible for reduced hair and skin pigmentation in Menkes patients, PAM deficiency may also contribute to this feature through reduced bioactivity of melanocyte-stimulating hormone, an alpha-amidated compound. PAM deficiency may have more important and wide-ranging physiologic effects that contribute to the Menkes phenotype.

Deficient cytochrome *c* oxidase (CCO) activity may represent a major factor in the neuropathology of Menkes disease. Effects on the brain are quite similar to those in individuals with Leigh disease (subacute necrotizing encephalomyelopathy) in whom CCO deficiency is caused by complex IV respiratory chain defects. Deficiency of copper/zinc superoxide dismutase (Cu/Zn SOD) in Menkes disease could lower protection against oxygen free radicals and theoretically have cytotoxic effects. Localized brain damage due to such oxidant stress has been postulated as the pathogenetic basis of Parkinson disease. Mutations in the Cu/Zn SOD gene on chromosome 21 have been described in patients with amyotrophic lateral sclerosis, a motor neuron disease of adult onset.[15] The relative contribution of partial SOD deficiency to the neurodegenerative changes in patients with Menkes disease and its allelic variants is difficult to assign.

The pathology of the brain in Menkes disease includes marked neuronal cell loss in the cerebral cortex and cerebellum, severe demyelination, dystrophic Purkinje cells, mitochondrial proliferation, and vascular dilatation within the brain and spinal cord. Abnormal brain lipid composition, presumably reflecting impaired myelination, also has been documented.

Menkes disease in the neonatal period

Classical Menkes disease often escapes attention in the newborn period because of its subtle manifestations in neonates.[9,16] Several nonspecific physical and metabolic findings are commonly cited when birth histories of these babies are reviewed. These findings include premature labor and delivery, large cephalohematomas in cases where vaginal birth occurred, hypothermia that necessitated warming lights or an isolette, hypoglycemia for which early feeding or support with intravenous glucose was instituted, and jaundice that required several days of phototherapy. Pectus excavatum, and inguinal or umbilical herniae are found at birth in some affected patients. Occasionally, unusual hair pigmentation may suggest the diagnosis in newborns. Often, however, the appearance of the hair is unremarkable. As in healthy babies, Menkes newborns may show no hair, or have normally pigmented hair. The pili torti found on microscopic examination of hair from older Menkes patients is usually not evident in the hair of affected newborns. Neurologically, newborns with Menkes disease generally seem normal. Because the success of treatment with small copper complexes in this disorder depends heavily on early diagnosis and treatment, newborn screening based on neurochemical levels from dried blood spots or via high throughput molecular assays is urgently needed for Menkes disease.[9]

Occipital horn syndrome

Occipital horn syndrome (OHS) shares the connective tissue abnormalities of classical Menkes disease and also features the gradual development of distinctive calcifications within the tendons that attach the sternocleidomastoid and trapezius muscles to the occiput, from which the syndromic name was derived.[17] Because the neurological phenotype in OHS is mild (dysautonomia including syncope, orthostatic hypotension, and chronic diarrhea), affected individuals often escape detection until mid childhood or later.[18,19]

The molecular basis for typical OHS most often involves exon skipping with reduction of correct messenger ribonucleic acid (mRNA) processing.[18] Six of eight typical OHS mutations reported, as well as the molecular defect in a mouse-model OHS, involve such aberrant splicing. We reported on two brothers with typical OHS in whom we identified a novel missense mutation, N1304S, within the ATP-binding domain of ATP7A.[18] Characterization of this defect contributed to an understanding of the relationship between neurological phenotype and residual copper transport in OHS.

Copper-replacement treatment in OHS has been limited to date. Although patients with OHS have borderline low or low-normal serum copper levels, they may benefit from copper treatment, especially if provided prior to developing neurological symptoms. Based on experience with Menkes disease, copper treatment is not expected to improve the connective tissue manifestations, however.

ATP7A-related distal motor neuropathy

A third clinical phenotype was recently found to be associated with unique missense mutations (T994I and P1386S) in the ATP7A copper transporter gene.[20] This new allelic variant resembles Charcot-Marie-Tooth disease and involves progressive distal motor neuropathy with minimal or no sensory symptoms, and onset in the second or third decade of life, or older. Affected patients do not manifest the severe infantile central nervous system deficits observed in Menkes disease, the signs of autonomic dysfunction seen in OHS, or the hair and connective tissue abnormalities, or the typical biochemical findings found in both those phenotypes. Conversely, neither infants and children with Menkes disease nor adults with OHS (as old as 32 years) manifest distal motor neuropathy. These facts highlight the distinction between this isolated distal motor neuropathy and syndromes previously associated with ATP7A mutations. The phenomenon of late, often adult-onset, distal muscular atrophy implies that the described missense mutations, located in the carboxyl half of ATP7A, have attenuated effects and require years to provoke pathological consequences.

Although the subjects with ATP7A-related distal motor neuropathy evaluated to date have serum copper levels in the low-normal range (80–100 µg/dL, with levels between 75-150 µg/dL considered normal), they could potentially benefit from copper supplementation, based on the favorable treatment responses in sensory and motor neuropathy associated with acquired copper deficiency.[3,5,7,8]

Delineation of the precise mechanism(s) involved in this new form of ATP7A peripheral neuropathy will be helpful in clarifying rational treatment strategies.

Animal models of Menkes disease

The *mottled* mouse provides an excellent animal model for Menkes disease. The *mottled* (atp7a) and Menkes (ATP7A) loci are located in homologous regions of their respective X chromosomes, and numerous allelic variants have been recognized in the mouse, predicting the possibility of a similar situation in humans. One of the best-studied *mottled* mutants, the brindled (*Mo-br*) male hemizygote on a C57BL/6J background, shows decreased coat pigmentation, tremor, general inactivity, death at 13 days of age, increased intestinal copper levels with low levels in liver and brain, and decreased copper enzyme activities. In contrast to initial reports on the *Mo-br* mouse[21–23] (for which a precise genetic background was not reported), intraperitoneal copper treatment in the first week of life does not rescue C57BL/6J-Atp7a^{Mo-br} mice, recapitulating the principle that phenotypes associated with a specific mutation in mice can vary greatly depending on the genetic background on which the mutation is maintained.[24] The *mottled* blotchy mutant (*Mo-blo*) mouse, a model of OHS, shows normal viability and more pronounced connective tissue abnormalities.

The murine mutants serve as useful agents in the evaluation of potential new therapies for Menkes patients. Rescue of the *Mo-br* on a C57BL/6J background, a model of severe Menkes disease, was recently demonstrated using combination brain-directed therapies: 50 nanograms of copper chloride plus recombinant adeno-associated virus serotype 5 (AAV5) vector expressing a reduced-size human ATP7A.[25] Neither treatment alone was effective, but combination therapy dramatically shifted the Kaplan–Meier survival curve, with 5 of 16 (31%) combination-treated mutants surviving beyond 110 days of age ($p < 0.0002$). Identification of the mechanisms underlying this pronounced synergistic effect should help to illuminate the normal processes of copper transport in brain and the role of ATP7A in neuronal and neuroglial cells. In addition, this advance in gene transfer may have future clinical implications for Menkes disease caused by severe ATP7A mutations, and patients with ATP7A-related motor neuron disease.

SMALL COPPER COMPLEXES FOR TREATMENT

Various formulations of copper, including copper chloride, copper gluconate, copper histidine, and copper sulfate, have been used to treat individuals with acquired copper deficiency, Menkes disease, and OHS over the past 40 years. Figure 14–1 illustrates the coordination chemistry of these small molecules. Copper gluconate is available as an oral nutritional supplement, and copper chloride and copper sulfate are available commercially as injectable medications for prescription. In contrast, copper histidine is not yet commercially available, however, orphan drug designation by the U.S. Food and Drug Administration

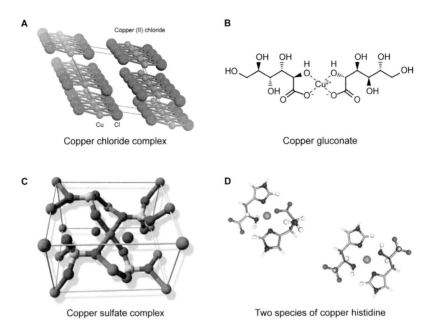

Figure 14–1: Models illustrate the fundamental coordination chemistry of four small copper complexes used for treatment of acquired and inherited copper deficiency syndromes. The abundance of albumin in human serum (500 micromolar concentration) and its high affinity for copper imply that this protein may compete for copper atoms introduced as small complexes. (A) Cupric (2+) Chloride. Copper atoms are pale red, chloride atoms are green, and coordination geometry is square planar. (B) In copper gluconate, four oxygen atoms coordinate a copper atom. (C) Copper sulfate complex. Sulfur atoms are yellow, oxygen atoms are red, and copper atoms are pale red. (D) Two species of copper histidine, based on density functional theory expected at physiological pH (7.3)[26] and modified to colorize nitrogen atoms (blue), oxygen atoms (red), and copper atoms (pale red). *See color plate.*

is currently pending, a status that often facilitates drug development for compounds useful in the treatment of rare disorders.

Copper chloride for human medical use is available from Hospira Inc. (Lake Forest, IL) in a concentration of 400 µg/mL. Therefore, subcutaneous injection of 500 microliters provides 200 micrograms of copper. Copper sulfate for human medical use is available from American Regent, Inc. (Shirley, NY) in a concentration 400 µg/mL. Copper histidine (U.S. Food and Drug Administration Investigational New Drug #34,166; holder, S. G. Kaler) is used in National Institutes of Health (NIH) clinical protocols #90-N-0149 and 09-CH-0059, and is a freeze-dried (for enhanced stability) preparation prepared by the NIH Pharmaceutical Development Service, using the following stepwise procedure:

1. Bubble nitrogen into water for injection for at least 20 minutes.
2. Weigh 1.345 grams of $CuCl_2$ dihydrate and 2.45 grams of L-histidine in separate beakers.
3. Dissolve $CuCl_2$ with water and do the same with L-histidine separately at room temperature; mix well.
4. Add both solutions together; blue color intensifies; mix well.

5. Adjust pH to 7.30–7.4 with 0.1 N NaOH or HCl.
6. Adjust volume to 1,000 milliliters.
7. Filter through a Silo filter U containing a 0.22-micrometer Durapore (Millipore, Billerica, MA) filter using sterile technique.
8. Aliquot, gravimetrically, two grams (two milliliters) into each five-milliliter sterile clear vial and place the vials on a tray for freeze-drying.
9. Freeze to –30° C and then freeze-dry until contents reach room temperature.
10. Stopper vials under vacuum, break off vacuum, and remove trays from freeze-dryer.
11. Seal vials with flip-off aluminum seals.
12. Refrigerate.

The product is stable for at least one month when stored as a freeze-dried product at room temperature. Patients' families typically store vials in their home freezers, however. For use in patients, contents of a vial are reconstituted with two milliliters of normal saline, providing a solution of 500 µg/mL for subcutaneous injection.

The dose of any copper preparation used for treatment should be calibrated based on serum copper and ceruloplasmin levels as well as response to treatment. In infants with Menkes disease, 200–500 µg/d administered by subcutaneous injection raises serum copper levels to the normal range (70–150 µg/dL).[9] Clinical neurodevelopmental outcomes in this population appear dependent on the age at which treatment begins, as well as the presence or absence of some residual function by the individual mutant ATP7A.[9] The major potential side effect in Menkes disease patients receiving exogenous copper is proximal renal tubular damage resulting in mild renal tubular acidosis. This process appears to be reversible, however, when the copper treatment is discontinued.[9] Treatment of acquired copper deficiency with 1-8 mg/day oral copper for several months typically stabilizes or resolves symptoms of myelopathy and/or peripheral neuropathy.[3,5–8]

Although there are well-defined systems mediating normal copper acquisition, distribution and regulation in mammalian species,[27] some fraction of exogenously administered copper complexes could have effects that do not rely on known copper transport mechanisms. The abundance of albumin in human serum (500 micromolar) and its high affinity for copper imply that this protein may compete for copper ions introduced as small complexes.[28]

COPPER ENTRY TO THE CENTRAL NERVOUS SYSTEM

The precise mechanisms of copper transport into the brain are not well understood. The blood–brain barrier is composed of brain capillary endothelial cells and astrocytes, and it is presumed that the endothelial cells localize ATP7A at their basolateral surfaces to accomplish copper delivery from the blood to the brain

A

Blood-brain barrier: Capillary endothelial cells

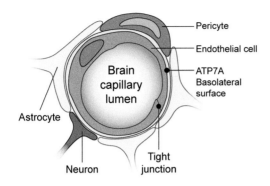

B

Blood-CSF barrier: Choroid plexus epithelium

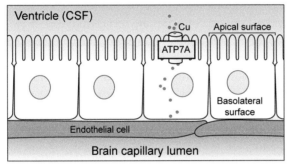

Figure 14–2: Paradigm of copper transport at the blood–brain barrier (A) and blood–CSF barrier (B). The usual basolateral membrane localization of ATP7A makes sense at the blood–brain barrier, however, apical localization in choroid plexus epithelial cells that comprise the blood–CSF barrier is proposed here. See text (Copper Entry to the Central Nervous System) for further explanation. *See color plate.*

(Figure 14–2, A). In cultured mammalian cells, ATP7A localizes to the trans-Golgi network in basal copper concentrations and relocates in small vesicles to the basolateral membrane in polarized epithelial cells exposed to elevated copper concentrations.[29] The epithelial cells of the choroid plexus (Figure 14–2, B) are polarized cells that mediate the rapid entrance of the trace metal manganese to rodent brain following intravenous infusion,[30] and we speculate that this process also occurs for copper. Rat choroid plexus epithelial cells express high levels of ATP7A, nearly threefold higher than the copper uptake gene, *Ctr1*.[31] However, the orientation of the choroid plexus epithelial cells is such that their apical, not basolateral, membranes protrude into cerebrospinal fluid. Based on this topology, we hypothesize that, for its copper exodus function, ATP7A in these cells probably localizes to the apical rather than its customary basolateral position (Figure 14–2, B). Precedent for this phenomenon exists from studies of the Na^+/K^+ ATPase, which is located on the basolateral surface in most polarized epithelia but which clearly resides at the apical membrane in choroid plexus epithelium.[32,33]

SUMMARY

Small molecule copper complexes are valuable for the treatment of nutritional copper deficiency and some inherited disorders of copper metabolism. Provision of copper to the developing brain is crucial for normal neurodevelopment, as exemplified by Menkes disease, in which mutation of the copper transporter ATP7A has devastating effects without early treatment. Some acquired and inherited forms of peripheral neuropathy may also respond to treatment with small copper complexes.

REFERENCES

1. Kaler SG. Menkes disease. L.A. Barness, ed. *Advances in Pediatrics*, Volume 41, C.V. Mosby, 263–304, 1994
2. Desai V, Kaler SG. The role of copper in human neurological disorders *Am J Clin Nutr.* 2008;88:855S–858S
3. Goodman BP, Bosch EP, Ross MA, Hoffman-Snyder C, Dodick DD, Smith BE. Clinical and electrodiagnostic findings in copper deficiency myeloneuropathy. *J Neurol Neurosurg Psychiatry* 2009;80:524–527.
4. Kumar N, Ahlskog JE, Klein CJ, Port JD. Imaging features of copper deficiency myelopathy: A study of 25 cases. *Neuroradiology.* 2006;48(2):78–83
5. Kelkar P, Chang S, Muley SA. Response to oral supplementation in copper deficiency myeloneuropathy. *J Clin Neuromuscul Dis.* 2008;10(1):1–3
6. Spain RI, Leist TP, De Sousa EA. When metals compete: A case of copper-deficiency myeloneuropathy and anemia. *Nat Clin Pract Neurol.* 2009;5(2):106–111
7. Zara G, Grassivaro F, Brocadello F, Manara R, Pesenti FF. Case of sensory ataxic ganglionopathy-myelopathy in copper deficiency. *J Neurol Sci.* 2009;277(1–2):184–186
8. Weihl CC, Lopate G. Motor neuron disease associated with copper deficiency. *Muscle Nerve.* 2006;34(6):789–793
9. Kaler SG, Holmes CS, Goldstein DS, Tang JR, Godwin SC, Donsante A, Liew CJ, Sato S, Patronas N. Neonatal diagnosis and treatment of Menkes disease. *N Engl J Med.* 2008;358:605–614
10. Kaler SG, Tang JR, Donsante A, Kaneski C. Translational read-through of a nonsense mutation in ATP7A. *Ann Neurol.* 2009;65:108–113
11. Baerlocher K, Nadal D. Das Menkes-syndrom. *Ergeb Inn Med Kinderheilkd.* 1988;57:77–144
12. Goldstein DS, Holmes CS, Kaler SG. Relative efficiencies of plasma catechol levels and ratios for neonatal diagnosis of Menkes disease. *Neurochem Res.* 2009;34:1464–1468
13. Kaler SG, Goldstein DS, Holmes C, Salerno JA, Gahl WA. Plasma and cerebrospinal fluid neurochemical pattern in Menkes disease. *Ann Neurol.* 1993;33:171–175
14. Eipper BA, Mains RE, Glembotski CC. Identification in pituitary tissue of a peptide α-amidation activity that acts on glycine-extended peptides and requires molecular oxygen, copper, and ascorbic acid. *Proc Natl Acad Sci USA.* 1983;80:5144–5148
15. Rosen DR, Siddique T, Patterson D, Figlewicz DA, Sapp P, Hentati A, Donaldson D, Goto J, O'Regan JP, Deng HX, et al. Mutations in Cu/Zn superoxide dismutase gene are associated with familial amyotrophic lateral sclerosis. *Nature.* 1993;362:59–62
16. Gunn TR, McFarlane S, Phillips LI. Difficulties in the neonatal diagnosis of Menkes' kinky hair syndrome-trichopoliodystrophy. *Clin Pediatr.* 1984;23:514–516
17. Sartoris DJ, Luzzatti L, Weaver DD, Macfarlane JD, Hollister DW, Parker BR. Type IX Ehlers-Danlos syndrome. A new variant with pathognomonic radiographic features. *Radiology.* 1984;152:665–670

18. Kaler SG, Gallo LK, Proud VK, Percy AK, Mark Y, Segal NA, Goldstein DS, Holmes CS, Gahl WA. Occipital horn syndrome and a mild Menkes phenotype associated with splice site mutations at the MNK locus. *Nat Genet.* 1994;8:195–202

19. Tang J, Robertson SP, Lem KE, Godwin SC, Kaler SG. Functional copper transport explains neurologic sparing in occipital horn syndrome. *Genet Med.* 2006;8(11):711–718

20. Kennerson ML, Nicholson GA, Kaler SG, Kowalski B, Mercer JF, Tang J, Llanos RM, Chu S, Takata RI, Speck-Martins CE, Baets J, Almeida-Souza L, Fischer D, Timmerman V, Taylor PE, Scherer SS, Ferguson TA, Bird TD, De Jonghe P, Feely SM, Shy ME, Garbern JY: Missense mutations in the copper transporter gene ATP7A cause X-linked distal hereditary motor neuropathy. *Am J Hum Genet.* 2010; 86:343–352

21. Fraser AS, Sobey S, Spicer CC. Mottled, a sex-modified lethal in the house mouse. *J Genet.* 1953;51:217–221

22. Hunt DM. Primary defect in copper transport underlies mottled mutants in the mouse. *Nature.* 1974;249:852–854

23. Hunt DM. A study of copper treatment and tissue copper levels in the murine congenital copper deficiency, mottled. *Life Sci.* 1976;19(12):1913–1919

24. Linder CC. Genetic variables that influence phenotype. *ILAR J.* 2006;47:132–140

25. Kaler SG, Donsante A, Tang J, Goldstein D, Holmes C, Sullivan P, Centeno J. Brain-directed AAV5 gene therapy, in combination with copper, rescues a murine model of severe Menkes disease. Session 42/Abstract 143, Annual Meeting of the American Society of Human Genetics. Available at: http://www.ashg.org/2009meeting/

26. Baute D, Arieli D, Neese F, Zimmermann H, Weckhuysen BM, Goldfarb D. Carboxylate binding in copper histidine complexes in solution and in zeolite. Y: X- and W-band pulsed EPR/ENDOR combined with DFT calculations. *J Am Chem Soc.* 2004; 126:11733–11745.

27. Kim BE, Nevitt T, Thiele DJ. Mechanisms for copper acquisition, distribution and regulation. *Nat Chem Biol.* 2008;4:176–185

28. McArdle HJ, Gross SM, Danks DM, Wedd AG. Role of albumin's copper binding site in copper uptake by mouse hepatocytes. *Am J Physiol.* 1990;258(6 Pt 1):G988–G991

29. Greenough M, Pase L, Voskoboinik I, Petris MJ, O'Brien AW, Camakaris J. Signals regulating trafficking of Menkes (MNK; ATP7A) copper-translocating P-type ATPase in polarized MDCK cells. *Am J Physiol Cell Physiol.* 2004;287:C1463–C1471

30. Aoki I, Wu YJ, Silva AC, Lynch RM, Koretsky AP. In vivo detection of neuroarchitecture in the rodent brain using manganese-enhanced MRI. *Neuroimage.* 2004;22:1046–1059

31. Choi BS, Zheng W. Copper transport to the brain by the blood-brain barrier and blood-CSF barrier. *Brain Res.* 2009;1248:14–21

32. Quinton PM, Wright EM, Tormey JM. Localization of sodium pumps in the choroid plexus epithelium. *J Cell Biol.* 1973;58:724–730

33. Alper SL, Stuart-Tilley A, Simmons CF, Brown D, Drenckhahn D. The fodrin-ankyrin cytoskeleton of choroid plexus preferentially colocalizes with apical Na+K+-ATPase rather than with basolateral anion exchanger AE2. *J Clin Invest.* 1994;93:1430–1438

Index

Abderhalden, Emil, 101
absolute oral bioavailability, 37
acquired copper deficiency, 202–203
active tubular secretion, 43
acute hereditary tyrosinemia, 115
adenosine triphosphate (ATP)
    ATP7A, 203
        distal hereditary motor neuropathy,
            206–207
        Menkes disease, 203
        OHS, 206
    nephropathic cystinosis, 103
agonists, 46
AKU. *See* alkaptonuria
AL deficiency. *See* argininosuccinate lyase
        deficiency
ALA. *See* aminolevulinic acid
alkaptonuria (AKU), 114, 118–121
    cardiac involvement, 119–120
    clinical presentation, 119
        arthritis as, 119
    diagnosis, 121
    dietary therapies, 120
    genetic factors, 121
    HGA, 118–119
    HPPD inhibition, 124
    incidence rates, 118–119
    nitisinone therapy, 125
        future developments, 130
        side effects, 127
        tyrosine levels, 129–130
    pathophysiology, 121
    renal transplants, 120
    vitamin therapy, 120
Alpha-1 Foundation, 21
ambrisentan, 11
amino acylation products, 142–144
aminolevulinic acid (ALA), 117–118
Ammonul, 144–145
    alternative therapy uses, 149
    dosage, 146
        overdosage, 147
    FDA status, 147
    HIP, 144–145

long-term therapy results, 147–149
    side effects, 147
antagonists, 46
apomorphine, 12
apoptosis, in cysteamine treatment, for
        nephropathic cystinosis, 103
apparent first-order kinetics, 40–41
apparent volume of distribution, 39
argininosuccinate lyase (AL) deficiency,
        135
argininosuccinate synthetase (AS)
        deficiency, 135
AS deficiency. *See* argininosuccinate
        synthetase deficiency
ATP. *See* adenosine triphosphate
ATP7A, 203
    distal hereditary motor neuropathy,
        206–207
    Menkes disease, 203
    OHS, 206

basal ganglion diseases, 60
    biotin therapy, 66
    inheritance factors, 63
Bench-To-Bedside Research Program,
        25
betaine, in homocystinuria treatment,
        176–179
    clinical evidence of, 176–177
    development, 176–177
    dosage, 177–178
    FDA status, 179
    future developments, 179
    for remethylation disorders, 177
        cblC disorder, 177
        MTHFR, 177
    side effects, 178–179
        case studies, 178–179
Bickel, Horst, 76
bioavailability, of drugs, 37–38
    absolute oral, 37
    bioequivalence and, 38
    relative, 37
    studies, 37

Printed in the United States
by Baker & Taylor Publisher Services